Electrical Stimulation and the Relief of Pain

Pain Research and Clinical Management

Editorial Board

G.F. Gebhart *(Iowa City, IA, USA)*	Chairman
A.I. Basbaum *(San Francisco, CA, USA)*	Neurobiology
J.N. Campbell *(Baltimore, MD, USA)*	Neurosurgery
M. Fitzgerald *(London, UK)*	Pediatric Pain
H. Flor *(Mannheim, Germany)*	Psychology
T. Jensen *(Aarhus, Denmark)*	Neurology
S.J. Linton *(Örebro, Sweden)*	Rehabilitation Medicine
P.J. McGrath *(Halifax, NS, Canada)*	Pediatrics
S. McMahon *(London, UK)*	Physiology
F. Porreca *(Tucson, AZ, USA)*	Pharmacology
R. Portenoy *(New York, NY, USA)*	Palliative Medicine
P. Reeh *(Erlangen, Germany)*	Neurophysiology
D. Turk *(Seattle, WA, USA)*	Psychology

Pain Research and Clinical Management

Volume 15

Electrical Stimulation and the Relief of Pain

Edited by

Brian A. Simpson

*Department of Neurosurgery, University Hospital of Wales, Heath Park,
Cardiff CF14 4XW, UK*

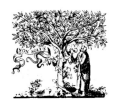

2003
ELSEVIER
AMSTERDAM • BOSTON • HEIDELBERG • LONDON • NEW YORK • OXFORD
PARIS • SAN DIEGO • SAN FRANCISCO • SINGAPORE • SYDNEY • TOKYO

MT

ELSEVIER B.V.
Sara Burgerhartstraat 25
P.O. Box 211, 1000 AE
Amsterdam, The Netherlands

First edition 2003
  Reprinted 2004

Library of Congress Cataloging in Publication Data
A catalog record from the Library of Congress has been applied for.

British Library Cataloguing in Publication Data
A catalogue record from the British Library has been applied for.

ISBN: 0-444-51258-6 (Hardbound)
ISBN: 0921-3287 (Series)

⊗ The paper used in this publication meets the requirements of ANSI/NISO X39.48-1992 (Permanence of Paper).
Printed in The Netherlands

3/1/06

Dedication

To Professor Patrick D. Wall

The father of modern therapeutic neurostimulation.

Foreword

This book deals with the subject of electrical stimulation of the nervous system for the relief of pain in a comprehensive way. As the editor of this book, Brian A. Simpson, notes in the Preface, due importance is given to clinical aspects. I strongly believe that indeed good clinical practice is not only good for the Patient, but also for Science and Technology. There is now overwhelming evidence that long-term relief (more than 30 years) of severe neuropathic pain can be observed, for example by peripheral nerve stimulation in a patient with a traumatic peripheral nerve lesion. Some of these very successful cases have to be stimulated frequently to be pain-free, some less so, and occasionally, the patient remains pain-free without further stimulation. Why?

It is also true that clinical outcome data vary widely between authors and that with the happier results there are the failures. Why the failures? Functional magnetic resonance imaging (fMRI) might be a tool to study, in these long-term patients, interesting aspects of the physiopathology of pain. It is the critical analysis of clinical data which offers the material to approach the scientific queries and I remember very well that Professor Wall, to whom this book is dedicated, listened with interest to detailed reports of patient stories and asked questions which were not so evident for the majority of clinicians, but must have been related to his thinking about neurophysiological mechanisms of some aspects of pain. Mentioning fMRI immediately raises the question of safety for the patient and for the implanted stimulator.

Pain clinicians are amongst the pioneers in neurostimulation and this book is a very timely one because the experience of these pioneers can now be found in one volume. This is good news for newcomers in the pain field but also useful for other applications of neurostimulation such as Parkinson's disease and other abnormal movement disorders, epilepsy and, who knows, even obsessive compulsive disorders (OCDs).

This last disorder should be approached very cautiously with a solid scientific know-how and integrity and ethical concern and poses a challenge to technology. Indeed, at the moment electrical energy consumption is high in this condition and a way should be found to recharge the battery of the implanted stimulator transcutaneously. The ability to do so would be good news for the patients treated with implant electro-stimulation technology, but also for the authorities responsible for health expenditure.

I think the future looks bright for neurostimulation and the authors of this book are to be congratulated for having produced a very fine state of the art account with a vision to the future of electrical stimulation of the nervous system for the relief of pain.

July 2003

Jan M. Gybels
Groenstraat 67
B-3050 Oud-Heverlee
Belgium

Preface

Since ancient times many cultures around the world have used electricity to combat pain. Until the late seventeenth century, when the first electrostatic generator was produced, only natural sources of electricity were available, predominantly species of fish. Once it became possible to store and control electricity, in the mid eighteenth century, it acquired enormous popularity as a nostrum and provided an excellent medium for quackery. Out of this undisciplined background there emerged a serious and prolific clinical use of electroanalgesia, particularly as an adjunct to dentistry and surgery, which was well established by the latter part of the nineteenth century. The present era of therapeutic electrical stimulation, characterised by transcutaneous (TENS) and implanted neurostimulators, was launched by the combination of the gate control theory of Ron Melzack and Pat Wall, published in 1965, and a new understanding of the way the nervous system responds to injury (including destructive surgery), to which Pat Wall also made a major, pioneering contribution.

Somewhere in the region of 50,000 neurostimulators are now implanted each year around the world, and the number is rising. The indications are diverse and increasing. There are wide geographical variations in practice; for example, ischaemic pain is a major indication for spinal cord stimulation in Europe but not in North America. The aim of this book is to present this broad field under one cover, to evolve an overall, comprehensive picture, to integrate the various strands and themes and not only to impart a good deal of useful factual knowledge and informed opinion but also to be thought-provoking and to allow some key conclusions to gestate and emerge.

There are three dimensions to this topic: the technological/scientific and the clinical are related symbiotically and the socio-economic determines the environment. The technology and the scientific knowledge are impressive but we must not lose sight of the art of medicine, particularly in this field. From the earliest planning stages of this book I felt it was important that the clinical perspective should be given due prominence and discussion, to provide the right context for authoritative scientific and technical chapters. I also felt that the right policy was to give the expert contributors a free reign in judging how to put their subject across rather than my being too prescriptive. I was delighted that every contribution came across contextually as I had hoped. It is only too easy for the hammer to see everything as a nail. Neurostimulation is only one class of weapon in the therapeutic armamentarium.

The authors have expressed their own views and opinions; the reader, and other contributors, may not agree with everything. Similarly, some authors have included an account of their own implantation technique(s); others might do it differently but there will still be useful tips to be gleaned from the accounts of these very experienced practitioners. Some parts of the book may be controversial and even provocative. This could include my own discussion of case selection and of assessment of outcome, which is in no way intended to ambush colleagues and co-contributors but rather to stimulate debate.

The book is arranged in what I hope is a logical sequence: after historical and scientific introductions we progress from the surface of the body via the peripheral nerves and the nerve roots to the spinal cord and then the brain, first its surface and, finally, the most invasive application: deep brain stimulation. The number of chapters on spinal cord stimulation reflects its present predominance as a target and their sequence is also intended to be logical. We end with a discussion, pragmatic rather than fanciful, of the issues that will influence and shape future practice. There is inevitably a degree of repetition and overlap for which I make no apology.

I am grateful to Pat Wall and to Elsevier for giving me the opportunity to put this book together; indeed I feel honoured. My only regret is that Pat did not live to see the finished product. It is also gratifying that so many extremely busy people agreed so willingly to contribute. This group of experts represents a broad church; 24 contributors from eight countries in three continents, representing several disciplines. It has been a pleasure to coordinate their considerable efforts. I gratefully acknowledge their hard work and the equanimity with which they dealt with all my emails. My secretary, Cath Gamble, has worked enormously hard, efficiently and uncomplainingly on this project and I am very grateful to her. Finally, I flatter myself by assuming that my work on this book must have had some impact on my family, Ann, Emma and Rachel, but I never heard them complain.

Brian A. Simpson
April 2003

List of Contributors

Giancarlo Barolat
Department of Neurosurgery, Thomas Jefferson University Hospital, 1015 Chestnut Street, Philadelphia, PA 19107, USA

Daniel S. Bennett
Integrative Treatment Centers, 8406 Clay Street, Denver, CO 80031-3810, USA

Daniel Brookoff
University of Tennessee College of Medicine, Comprehensive Pain Institute, 1265 Union Avenue, Memphis, TN 38104, USA

Eric Buchser
Anaesthesia and Pain Management Services, Hôpital de Morges, 1110 Morges, Switzerland

Tracy L. Cameron
Department of Biomedical Engineering, University of Texas Southwestern Medical School, Dallas, TX 75390, USA

Mike J.L. DeJongste
Department of Cardiology, Groningen University Hospital, Hanzeplein 1, P.O. Box 30 001, 9700 RB Groningen, The Netherlands

Tore Eliasson
Department of Internal Medicine, Multidisciplinary Pain Centre, Sahlgrenska University Hospital/Ostra, S-41685 Göteborg, Sweden

Jan Holsheimer
Institute for Biomedical Technology, Department of Electrical Engineering, Mathematics and Informatics, University of Twente, P.O. Box 217, 7500 AE Enschede, The Netherlands

Yves Keravel
Deparment of Neurosurgery, Hôpital Henri Mondor, 51 Avenue du Maréchal de Lattre de Tassigny, 94010 Créteil, France

Jean Pascal Lefaucheur
Department of Neurophysiology, Hôpital Henri Mondor, 51 Avenue du Maréchal de Lattre de Tassigny, 94010 Créteil, France

Bengt Linderoth
Department of Clinical Neuroscience, Section of Neurosurgery, Karolinska Institute/Karolinska Hospital, S-171 76 Stockholm, Sweden

Clas Mannheimer
Department of Internal Medicine, Multidisciplinary Pain Centre, Sahlgrenska University Hospital/Ostra, S-416 85 Göteborg, Sweden

Björn A. Meyerson

Department of Clinical Neuroscience, Section of Neurosurgery, Karolinska Institute/Karolinska Hospital, S-171 76 Stockholm, Sweden

Jean-Paul Nguyen

Department of Neurosurgery, Hôpital Henri Mondor, 51 Avenue du Maréchal de Lattre de Tassigny, 94010 Créteil, France

Richard B. North

Departments of Neurosurgery, Anesthesiology and Critical Care Medicine, Johns Hopkins University School of Medicine, 600 N. Wolfe Street, Meyer 8-181, Baltimore, MD 21287, USA

John C. Oakley

Yellowstone Neurosurgical Associates and Northern Rockies Pain and Palliative Rehabilitation Center, 2900 12th N, Billings, MT 59101, USA.

Joseph Ong

Department of Neurosurgery, Thomas Jefferson University Hospital, 1015 Chestnut Street, Philadelphia, PA 19107, USA

Umberto Rossi

Neurosurgeon, The Avenue Hospital, 40 The Avenue, Windsor, Victoria 3181, Australia

Ashwini Sharan

Department of Neurosurgery, Thomas Jefferson University Hospital, 1015 Chestnut Street, Philadelphia, PA 19107, USA

Brian A. Simpson

Department of Neurosurgery, University Hospital of Wales, Heath Park, Cardiff CF14 4XW, UK

Geert H. Spincemaille

Department of Neurosurgery, University Hospital Maastricht, P. Debyelaan 25, 6202 AZ Maastricht, The Netherlands

Michael Stanton-Hicks

Division of Anesthesiology, Department of Pain Management, Cleveland Clinic, 9500 Euclid Avenue, Cleveland, OH 44195, USA

Simon Thomson

Pain Management Services, Basildon and Thurrock University Hospital NHS Trust, Orsett Hospital, Rowley Road, Orsett, Essex RM16 3EU, UK

Volker M. Tronnier

Department of Neurological Surgery, University Hospital, Ruprecht-Karls-University Heidelberg, Im Neuenheimer Feld 400, D-69120 Heidelberg, Germany

Contents

Electrical Stimulation and the Relief of Pain
Pain Research and Clinical Management, Vol. 15
Edited by Brian A. Simpson

CHAPTER 1

Introduction

Brian A. Simpson*

Department of Neurosurgery, University Hospital of Wales, Heath Park, Cardiff CF14 4XW, UK

Therapeutic electrical stimulation of the nervous system has developed enormously over the last 30 or so years to the point where tens of thousands of units are implanted every year and yet one of the biggest criticisms is that there is a lack of high quality evidence of its efficacy. This theme emerges throughout this book. It is somewhat ironic that the same criticism nearly killed the modality in the 1970s. Indeed, deep brain stimulation (DBS) for pain is only now beginning to re-emerge on the back of the considerable recent developments in DBS for movement disorders; spinal cord stimulation has been more successful in securing acceptance and has been the mainstay of the invasive applications. Peripheral nerve stimulation is also beginning to enjoy a renaissance, facilitated by improvements in hardware and technique. Motor cortex stimulation was introduced relatively recently. Non-invasive neurostimulation (TENS) has been massively successful.

No matter how or where it is applied, with the exception of some acute conditions amenable to TENS, neurostimulation is used for *chronic* conditions. This has important implications. The outcome of treatments for acute conditions is very much easier to evaluate: the episode was controlled or aborted, the patient recovered, the episode did not recur, a cure was effected. Chronic conditions on the other hand exhibit spontaneous variation with time, may be influenced by many factors apart from the treatment, and are very likely themselves to have a variety of effects on the patient over time that either would not occur with acute conditions or would resolve after the event. Add to this the influence of adaptive mechanisms and the plasticity of memory and it can be seen that the whole field is very complex, particularly with regard to some of the neuropathic syndromes.

Since our relatively recent enlightenment regarding the neurophysiology of pain, we have discovered that electrical stimulation of almost any part of the nervous system can have a useful, sometimes dramatically beneficial, modulatory effect on a wide range of conditions, *but not always*. This in turn has tended to highlight the gaps in our knowledge of the pathophysiology of some conditions, e.g. the complex regional pain syndromes, but at the same time it has also added to our understanding. There is increasing awareness of a major neuropathic component in conditions such as interstitial cystitis. It seems that therapeutic stimulation has the potential to continue to add to our knowledge of neurological function; for example what does the relief of central pain afforded by motor cortex stimulation tell us about the integration of 'motor' and

*Correspondence to: Dr. B.A. Simpson, Department of Neurosurgery, University Hospital of Wales, Heath Park, Cardiff CF14 4XW, UK. Phone: +44 (29) 207 42708; Fax: +44 (29) 207 42560; E-mail: brian.simpson@cardiffandvale.wales.nhs.uk

'sensory' in the brain? It appears that, at least to some extent, spinal cord stimulation influences intrinsic, already available, modulatory systems whose function may or may not have been disturbed, to bring about 'normalisation'. This principle may apply both to neuropathic pain and to the 'maladaptive' changes occurring in ischaemia. What is astonishing is that something as crude as passing a simple electric current through a segment of the incredibly complex spinal cord can work at all.

Therapeutic neurostimulation crosses traditional boundaries at a professional level: neuroscience, anaesthetics, cardiology, vascular surgery, urology, orthopaedics, gastro-enterology etc. It also does so at a scientific level and provides a powerful reminder of the central role of the nervous system; it affects, and is affected by, every system in the body.

The selection of suitable candidates for this invasive (apart from TENS) and (initially) high cost treatment remains problematic. We still do not understand why patients with apparently the same diagnosis and with technically satisfactory stimulation respond differently. The difference can be dramatic, with enormous success in one and no relief at all in another. It may be that the diagnostic process is not sufficiently sophisticated; therapeutic electrical stimulation may help to improve it. Some of the conditions amenable to treatment with neurostimulation share the two characteristics of being both clinically florid and, until recently, poorly understood e.g. the complex regional pain syndromes and interstitial cystitis. The consequent accusations, or at least a suspicion, of a psychosomatic aetiology, malingering, embellishment etc. persist in some quarters and this does not help the cause of therapeutic neurostimulation.

At a basic clinical level there is a great deal to learn about the behaviour of patients, particularly their changing behaviour and responses over time. Why do some patients who seem suitable and who respond well to a trial of stimulation subsequently fail to obtain pain relief, sometimes months or years later? There is a strong tendency in a field like this to 'accentuate the positive' and ignore the negative. As a result, failures are not studied and a great deal of important information is simply not available, or, to put it more accurately, has not been collected and analysed. Failures, both of trials and of definitive stimulation, should be studied far more.

Complexity and chronicity have combined to make the measurement of, and the definition of, success very difficult in some parts of this field. It is essentially a clinical endeavour, the aim of which is to improve the quality of patients' lives, but success can be surprisingly difficult to determine. There are several simple examples of compounding factors. Reduction of neuropathic pain may permit a reduction or cessation of potent drug intake, making the patient feel better and more able to cope with any residual pain. What was the analgesic effect of the stimulator? Pain relief in peripheral ischaemia may permit more exercise and thereby improve the circulation, reducing the pain. Deciding on endpoints, on what is attributable, and so on can be difficult. In these respects the clinical aspects have not kept up with the scientific and technological developments.

Difficult though it may be to provide meaningful evidence, evidence is what is demanded, now more than ever. Those who use neurostimulation to treat patients with severe, chronic pain syndromes know that it can be extremely effective because they see the results. The two problems are: (1) how do you maximise the success *rate*; and (2) how do you produce the quality of evidence of efficacy demanded by the healthcare commissioner or reimbursement agency.

A plausible body of evidence of mechanisms of action is a very good start and several of the chapters in this book illustrate that we have come a long way in this respect. A considerable knowledge of physiology, anatomy, pharmacology, electronics and physics has been built up to show how neurostimulation *can* work, but not whether it *will* work, in a particular patient or group of patients.

Multidimensional, longitudinal studies are needed. Fully controlled randomised trials are not always possible because the sensations evoked by some stimulation prevent blinding but there are ways round this that do allow much better studies than have generally been published, such as the cluster randomised controlled trial. In this paradigm it is the treating centre that is randomised; different centres give different treatments.

The reader might reasonably have expected to find a chapter on cost effectiveness but the simple truth is that, at present, there is insufficient information. Cost effectiveness studies have started to appear relatively recently and the initial evidence is very supportive. Using cost effectiveness data in healthcare systems which generally rely on short term budgeting and in which "Yes, but that's a different budget" is heard all too often, is not straightforward. Economically, the biggest single driver is return to work but many patients who need stimulators are disabled, at least to a degree, and have been off work for a long time. Both these factors greatly impair the person's position in an employment market which is increasingly competitive. The biggest single cause of lost working days in the West is back pain and, not surprisingly, a good deal of effort has been invested in the application of SCS to this heterogeneous condition, which is why it has its own chapter in this book. Some progress has been made towards this 'holy grail'. A single treatment modality can only *contribute* to the management of a multifactorial condition; it cannot provide a comprehensive solution.

At present, invasive neurostimulation is regarded as a last resort but it is quite likely that better, possibly much better, results would be obtained in some conditions if it were used earlier. Better evidence of its efficacy is needed first, however, for society (and the payers) to accept this, which is something of a 'catch-22'. Many Western societies are drug-orientated and slow to relinquish the use of ever 'stronger' medication or complex cocktails of drugs in favour of considering a physical treatment such as neurostimulation, even when the former are relatively ineffective and having undesirable side effects. Perhaps this relative position will change, particularly as the hardware for neurostimulation continues to become more and more reliable and user friendly. As a generic treatment, neurostimulation is likely to be around for a long time, although the relative proportions of different modalities (peripheral nerve, nerve root, spinal cord, brain stimulation) will undoubtedly change. It may find an integrated role in combination with drug infusion systems and cell transplantation techniques. The hardware will become more sophisticated, perhaps incorporating feedback control systems. New indications will certainly be found and are already beginning to emerge, notably visceral and vascular conditions. It remains the case, however, that whatever developments occur in this valuable and exciting field, their implementation for the benefit of patients will be governed by socio-economic factors and the quality of the evidence of their effectiveness.

Hopefully this book, by presenting a synthesis of the present state of play, will raise awareness of the subject; bringing together all the diverse strands in one volume might have a potentiating effect and produce a critical mass.

Electrical Stimulation and the Relief of Pain
Pain Research and Clinical Management, Vol. 15
Edited by Brian A. Simpson

The history of electrical stimulation of the nervous system for the control of pain

Umberto Rossi*

Consulting Rooms, The Avenue Hospital, 40 The Avenue, Windsor, Victoria 3181, Australia

Abstract

The ancient peoples used the electromagnetic energy of some resins and stones as well as the numbing discharge of some electric fishes to treat pain. As they did not understand the physics involved, the treatment was founded on mystical beliefs or speculative philosophies. Mineral and piscean electricity remained the only source of electrotherapy until the first electrostatic friction machines were invented in the 17th century. In line with subsequent discoveries, electrical charges generated by friction, by chemical reaction or by induction were used for therapeutic purposes in the 18th and 19th centuries. The promulgation of the gate control theory of pain in 1965 produced a tsunami of research, which included an attempt to close the gate using electrical stimulation of the central and peripheral nervous system. Initial successes were dampened by too many failures due to uncritical use, inadequate equipment and surgical complications. A subsequent revival of interest brought on by improved technology and clinical discipline resulted in re-acceptance of the methodology, which is now an established adjunct to the armamentarium of interventional pain treatment.

Keywords: Electroanalgesia; Natural sources; Animal electricity; Man-made electricity; Quackery; Gate control theory; Implantable neurostimulators; Technology

"Indocti discant et ament meminisse periti"[1]
Hénault

1. Early days

Electrical stimulation for the treatment of pain has been used in one form or another by all manner of people in every culture for thousands of years. In antiquity, mystical and curative properties were attributed to 'animated minerals' and speculative philosophers considered that their prodigious effects emanated from 'fluid spirits'.

It is said that from circa 9000 BC, bracelets and necklaces of magnetite and amber were used to prevent headache and arthritis (Schechter, 1971a). The Roman writer, Pliny the Elder, mentioned in his *Historia Naturalis* that circa 1000 BC a Greek shepherd walking on Mt Ida noticed that the iron nails of his sandals were strongly drawn to some black rocks. That type of rock was then named *magnesian* from 'Magnes', the shepherd's name,

*Correspondence to: Dr. Umberto Rossi, 31 Olsen Road, Nar Nar Goon North, Victoria 3812, Australia. Phone: +61 3 5942 9157; Fax: +61 3 5942 9157; E-mail: urossi@netstra.com.au

[1] May those who do not know, learn – and may those who know, take pleasure in reminiscing.

and is now known as magnetite (Mourino, 1991; Basford, 2001). The Ancient Greeks called a fossilized resin today known as amber – from the old Arabic word *ambar* – 'electron'. As early as 600 BC, a Greek philosopher and mathematician, Thales of Miletus, noted the peculiar property of amber for attracting small pieces of material when rubbed with fur (Mourino, 1991). Thales believed that the amber became magnetic with friction because magnetite would attract iron without having to be rubbed. The observation remained a mystery for more than two millennia until the Italian mathematician and physician Girolamo Cardano realized, in 1551, that "the magnet stone and the amber do not attract in the same way" (Mourino, 1991). Half a century later the physician of Queen Elizabeth I, William Gilbert, widely regarded as 'the original electrician', pointed out that amber was not the only substance that, when rubbed, attracted light objects, and revealed the nature of electrostatic electricity and magnetism. He also introduced the term 'electric force' (Butterfield, 1991).

Much as ancient peoples were allured by the properties of the animated minerals, to a greater extent they stood in awe of the astounding forces discharged by certain fish. The ichthyological fauna comprises fish capable of discharging electrical current to stun or kill their prey. The freshwater, strongly electrogenic species include the electric catfish, which lives in the rivers of tropical Africa and the Nile valley, and the electric eel, which inhabits the rivers of South America. The saltwater, strongly electrogenic species include the electric rays, which are found in all tropical and temperate seas. The Ancient Egyptians acknowledged the power of the Nile catfish in tomb paintings and in hieroglyphs, describing it as the fish that 'releases the troupes', an implication that the fish's jolt of electricity forced fishermen to release the net so that the enmeshed fish could escape (Kellaway, 1946). The Greeks called the electric ray *narke* or 'numbness-producing', from which the word *narcosis* was coined (Schechter, 1971a). The Romans called it 'torpedo' from the word *torpor* as the name was synonymous with

the effect. The Ancient Egyptians apparently used the shocks from the Nile catfish for the treatment of neuralgia, headache and other painful disorders (Kane and Taub, 1975). However, the first written document on the medical application of electricity dates to AD 46 when the Roman physician, Scribonius Largus, mentioned in his work *Compositiones Medicae* the use of the torpedo's discharge to treat gout and headache (Kellaway, 1946; Fig. 1).

Electro-ichthyotherapy continued to be used in European medicine until the middle of the 19th century (Stillings, 1974a,b, 1983; Sheon, 1984; Kryzhanovsky, 1993). It is reported that South American Indians and primitive African tribes continued to employ it until modern times (Kellaway, 1946). In 1772 the effect of the torpedo fish was demonstrated to be 'absolutely electrical' by John Walsh (Walsh, 1773), an English surgeon, and the anatomy of their electric organs was described in detail by another English surgeon, John Hunter (Hunter, 1773). We now know that the electrogenic organs consist of stacks of vertically oriented cells (electroplaques) and that each cell acts like a miniature battery (Siegfried, 1978).

2. The advent of man-made electricity

The age of man-made electricity began in 1672 with the prototype of an electrostatic generator constructed by the German engineer, Otto von Guericke. This and subsequent friction machines were used to treat a variety of afflictions with limited success because the charge produced was relatively small. The Leyden jar (forerunner of the electrical capacitor), invented in 1745, extended the application of electricity for the treatment of pain by enabling energy to be stored and discharged for later use (Hoff, 1963). From then on the history of electrotherapy may be divided into definite periods demarcated by landmark discoveries of electromagnetism (Turrell, 1969).

The first stage of modern electrotherapy dates from the invention of the rotating-disc

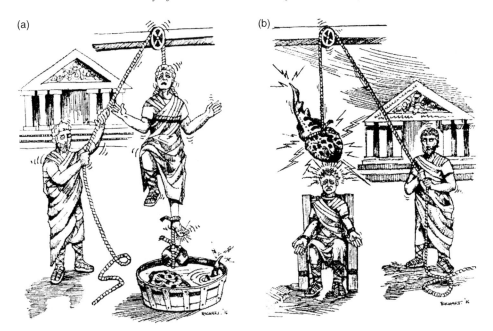

Fig. 1. Artist's impression of the treatment of gout (a) and headache (b) using torpedo fish. (Reproduced with permission: Perdikis, 1977.)

static-electricity machine invented by the English toolmaker, Jesse Ramsden, in 1766 (Geddes, 1984). The therapeutic application of static electricity was named 'Franklinism' after the American statesman and scientist, Benjamin Franklin, who, with his famous kite experiment in 1775, proved that lightning and electrostatic charge on a Leyden jar were identical. He also brought out the distinction between positive and negative electricity. By the middle of the 18th century electrostatic machines were used for electro-analgesia in English hospitals. John Wesley, the founder of Methodism, extolled the virtues of electricity in his book *The Desideratum* and advocated electrotherapy for angina pectoris, gout, headaches, pleuritic pain and sciatica (Gadsby, 1998). In 1782, John Birch, an English surgeon, gave case reports including treatment for low back pain and gout (Hymes, 1984). The most spectacular of the static electric therapies was the electric air-bath (Fig. 2), which was used, among other indications, for obstinate pain, particularly from rheumatism, and was recommended by Althaus for headache and neuralgia (Geddes, 1984).

The second stage of modern electrotherapy started with the Galvani–Volta controversy, which led to the discovery of the electrochemical battery in 1800. Interestingly, although Volta correctly refuted Galvani's theory of 'animal electricity' the energy produced by the Voltaic pile continued to be known as 'Galvanic' and the application of this current to the human body was termed 'Galvanism'. Although Volta has a secure place in the history of electricity an intriguing archeological discovery near Baghdad in 1936, dating back to the 2000-year-old Partian culture, raises doubt as to the originality of the concept of the electrochemical reaction of metals. The discovered device was composed of two dissimilar metals in an electrolyte resembling a 'Galvanic cell'. The similarity of the device with the Galvanic element led to its denomination as 'battery of Baghdad' and to the speculation that it may have been used for electro-analgesia (Keyser, 1993).

Therapeutic applications of 'contact electricity' improved pain treatments by delivering a current that was better tolerated than the static current because it did not produce painful sparks.

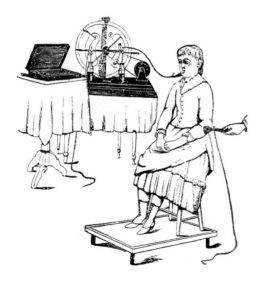

Fig. 2. The electric air-bath in a drawing from the book *Electrotherapeutics* by C.M. Haynes, published in 1896. One electrode from the electrostatic machine was connected to the ground and held in the hand of the therapist, who applied it to the painful parts. The other electrode was connected to the patient's clothing. Sparks were obtained with different types of electrodes: a ball, a point, a brush or a roller. (Reproduced with permission: Geddes, 1984.)

A popular form of generalized Galvanism was the electric bath, with the patient placed in a tub filled with water and a current passed via plate electrodes. However, localized Galvanism applied directly over the nerve supplying the ailing part became more popular (Geddes, 1984). Virtually all nerves were targeted, sometimes with tragic consequences such as loss of sight in the treatment of a case of ocular paralysis (Duchenne, 1855). In 1823, a French physician, Chevalier Sarlandière, considered that acupuncture, which had been brought back to France from the Far East by missionaries, could be enhanced with Galvanic current through needles, and introduced 'electro-acupuncture'. He was convinced that he could help those with gout and arthritis (Sarlandière, 1825). Others reported the beneficial effect of electro-acupuncture in sciatic and lumbo-sacral neuralgias (Hermel, 1844). In 1843, Golding Bird, assistant physician at Guy's Hospital in London, introduced electrical moxa obtained by local application of Galvanic current as a form of counter irritation.

The third stage of modern electrotherapy was reached with the discovery of electromagnetic induction. In 1819 the Danish scientist Hans Christian Oersted demonstrated that a magnetic field exists around an electric current. Michael Faraday, an English chemist and physicist, wondered: Given that an electric current produces a magnetic field, could magnetism produce electricity? In 1831 he showed that a changing current in one coil induced a voltage in a second coil. This paved the way for the introduction of the electric generator, the Inductorium, in 1848 by Du Bois-Raymond, which became the essential tool for stimulating excitable tissue (Geddes, 1984). The indirect current was termed 'Faradic' and the application of Faradic current to the human body was designated 'Faradization'. It came as a surprise to physiologists that the interrupted Faradic current could inhibit nerve conduction, and that observation increased interest for its use in the control of pain.

The French physician, Guillaume Duchenne de Boulogne, often called 'the father of electrotherapy', was the most distinguished promoter of Faradization (Devinski, 1993). He introduced the method of 'localized electrization' using cloth-covered surface electrodes. His book *De l'electrisation localisée et de son application à la pathologie et à la therapeutique* was the major electrotherapy event of the century (Gadsby, 1998). On the other side of the Rhine the German physician Robert Remak continued to defend Galvanization and introduced the concept of 'a catalytic action' of the Galvanic current on the inflammatory products that were the cause of neuralgia (Gadsby, 1998). Julius Althaus, a graduate of Berlin, introduced the work of Duchenne at King's College Hospital in London. He was the first to apply 'interrupted' current transcutaneously to peripheral nerves for the relief of pain (Kane and Taub, 1975). His book, *Treatise on Medical Electricity* (Althaus, 1859) contributed a great deal to the dissemination of electrical anaesthesia in Britain (Gadsby, 1998).

The history of electrotherapy in the New World followed the trail of that in Europe. By the mid-19th century this treatment modality was a major component of American medicine. In 1858, J.B. Francis, a physician in Philadelphia, described successful tooth extractions using a 'vibrating magnetic instrument'. The technique immediately spread through America. Subsequently 'electroanaesthesia' in dentistry was introduced to France, then to Germany and Italy in 1865 (Kane and Taub, 1975). In 1871 two physicians in New York, George Beard and Alphonse Rockwell (the latter is better known as the inventor of the electric chair) published the most influential American treatise on electrotherapy (Beard and Rockwell, 1891), with a specific chapter on neuralgia and low back pain (Hymes, 1984). Among the description of the applications, they reported the popular method of applying Faradic current with the electric-hand technique (Roth, 1977) (Fig. 3).

The 19th century became known as 'the golden age of medical electricity' (McNeal, 1977) but was also referred to as 'the electromagnetic era of medical quackery' (Macklis, 1993). A celebrated case was the 'Perkins Tractoration'. In 1796, Elisha Perkins, an American physician with a medical degree from Yale, secured the first patent to be issued for a medical device under the Constitution of the United States (Young, 1961). The device consisted of two pieces of metal that resembled horseshoe nails and were called 'tractors' (Schechter, 1971b) (Fig. 4). Perkins claimed that by sweeping the skin of the affected parts of the body with the tractors, a mysterious force would relieve the pain. Although Perkins was expelled from the Connecticut Medical Society for quackery, after his death the tractors were patented in England by his son with a profit of £10,000.

By the turn of the 19th century most doctors in America were using electrical machines in their offices without the blessing of science. This came to an end in 1910 when electrotherapy was legally excluded from clinical practice following the publication of the Flexner report, which triggered reforms in the standard of medical education. Electrical machines were removed from doctors' offices and were relegated to 'museums of quackery'

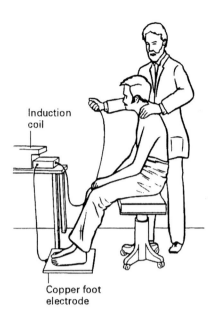

Fig. 3. The 'electric hand' method of Faradization, widely used in the late 1800s. One electrode from the induction coil generator was connected to the patient, the other to the therapist, who would use hand contact to massage the painful parts. (Reproduced with permission: Oschman, 2000).

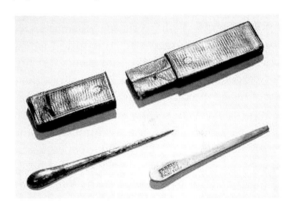

Fig. 4. The metallic tractors marketed in 1795. The inventor, Dr Elisha Perkins, affirmed that one tractor was an alloy of copper, zinc and gold; the other of iron, silver and platinum. They were sold at the retail price of 25 dollars a pair in America and 5 pounds a pair in England. (Young, 1961). (Photo: Courtesy of Clendening History of Medicine Library, University of Kansas Medical Center.)

(Oschman, 2000). The Golden Age of electroanalgesia also ended in Europe in the early 20th century. The association with quackery, the establishment of the drug industry and the appearance of X-ray treatments were probable reasons for the loss of interest (Gadsby, 1998).

Electrophysiological experiments in the early 1930s led to the development of induction coil techniques for 'remote' transfer of electrical energy through the intact body (Chaffee and Light, 1934; Eisenberg et al., 1965). An efficient variation employing radio-frequency as an induction method (Newman and Fender, 1937) was adopted by clinicians for cardiac pacing (Glenn et al., 1959). Subsequently produced neural stimulators were a spin-off of this technology.

3. The gate theory and the development of implantable neurostimulators

No single event had more impact on electro-analgesia than the Gate Theory of Pain (Melzack and Wall, 1965). The theory postulated central inhibition of pain by non-painful stimuli, a concept that had been predicted half a century earlier by the English neurologist Sir Henry Head. In 1965 Patrick Wall recruited William Sweet, Head of Neurosurgery at Harvard Medical School, to clinically test the gate theory. At first they experimented on their own infra-orbital nerves using needle-stimulating electrodes, and on superficial nerves, such as the ulnar nerve, using surface electrodes. They then used transcutaneous or percutaneous stimulation in three patients, who experienced partial or total relief of pain during stimulation (Wall and Sweet, 1967; Wall, 1985). Shortly thereafter the first peripheral nerve stimulator was implanted around the median nerve using a pair of split-ring platinum electrodes (Sweet and Wepsic, 1968).

Norman Shealy, a neurosurgeon in La Crosse, Wisconsin, thought that the 'gate' could be best closed by stimulating the dorsal columns, and confirmed this assumption experimentally in cats (Shealy et al., 1967a). When he presented the results of the study in April 1966 at a meeting of the American Association of Neurological Surgeons, the paper was considered so controversial that it was turned down for publication in the *Journal of Neurosurgery* (Shealy, personal communication).

In March 1967 Shealy implanted the first dorsal column stimulation device by laminectomy at D2-3 in a 70-year-old man (L.K.) suffering from inoperable bronchogenic carcinoma (Shealy et al., 1967b). The device was handmade by Tom Mortimer, a doctoral medical engineering student at Case Western Reserve University, Cleveland, Ohio. A vitallium electrode (cathode) was placed subdurally and maintained close to the cord by suturing it to the dura. The anode was placed in the intramuscular space. Connection between the electrodes and the external stimulator was made with subcutaneous jacks through hypodermic needles. Stimulation gave the patient good relief of pain until he died of complications related to his cancer, a few days after the implant (Mortimer, 1968). A second implant was done by Shealy in October 1967 in a 50-year-old lady (R.W.) suffering from intractable carcinomatous pelvic pain, using a radio-frequency-coupled stimulator (Fig. 5). The circuit design was based on a modified Medtronic device for stimulation of the carotid sinus to control angina and hypertension. This patient experienced approximately 50% relief of her pain, at times almost total control of pain, and was extensively evaluated until Mortimer successfully defended his Ph.D. thesis, 'Pain suppression in man by dorsal column electro-analgesia' in May 1968.

Subsequent implants were done by Shealy using similar devices manufactured by Medtronic. When he reported the results of his first six patients to the Harvey Cushing Society in 1969, many neurosurgeons became interested in the technique. A Dorsal Column Stimulation Group was formed with the intent of following 500 patients for 5 years before deciding if it was a valid procedure (Burton, 1973).

In late 1972 Avery Laboratories began marketing dorsal column stimulators to all neurosurgeons. Medtronic followed suit and changed the design of the electrodes from three solid plates of platinum to platinum twisted tinsel wire. This resulted in a major technical problem because

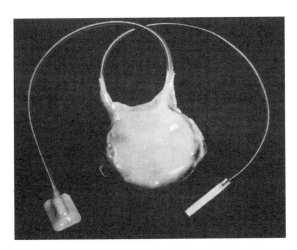

Fig. 5. Bottom view of assembled radio-frequency receiver and electrodes as implanted in Shealy's second patient (R.W.) on October 8, 1967. The coiled platinum–iridium wires connecting the electrodes to the receiver and the epoxy and glass portions of the receiver were covered with medical-grade silastic. The system was activated by a variable frequency transmitter-stimulator with a fixed pulse width. Frequency and amplitude were controlled by the patient. (Reproduced with permission: Mortimer, 1968.)

the tinsel wire oxidized and became ineffective after 6–12 months (Shealy, personal communication). Technical problems, surgical complications such as CSF leak, cord compression and adhesive fibrosis, as well as widespread use by inexpert implanters and uncritical selection of patients resulted in an initial high rate of failure of dorsal-column stimulation. Shealy was disappointed that the technology had been inadequately researched prior to clinical application, and progressively abandoned the modality. He performed his last implant in May 1973. For a few years the procedure fell into disfavour. Only a few dedicated neurosurgeons persevered.

Improved methods of implantation and screening contributed to a later resurgence of interest among neurosurgeons in Europe and America. Advances of the technique included the sequential 'endo-dural' method of placing the plate-type leads between dissected layers of the dura (Burton, 1973), percutaneous insertion of wire-like leads in the epidural space (Shimoji et al., 1971; Dooley, 1975; Cook, 1976; Zumpano and Saunders, 1976)

and pre-operative use of skin surface stimulation to 'demonstrate the sensation to be expected after implantation'. For this purpose Shealy resurrected the Electreat, a cumbersome battery-operated stimulator that used skin pads, which had been patented in 1918 by an osteopath. Although the FDA had forced the manufacturer to stop claiming that the device relieved pain, Shealy found that this claim was 'quite proper' (Shealy and Maurer, 1974). Donlin Long and others also noted that stimulation of the skin alone was often sufficient to provide pain control (Burton, 1973; Long, 1991).

On this basis Shealy, working in collaboration with Long, and each working independently, prompted the development of solid-state cutaneous electrical stimulators. The first commercial units were made by Medtronic and Stimulation Technology, Inc. Burton coined the term 'Transcutaneous Electrical Nerve Stimulation' (TENS). This has since become the most widely used form of electrotherapy.

The contribution of private industry was determinant to the success of electrical stimulation for pain control. The stimulators were gradually modified in synchrony with the demands of implanters and with the basic science research on the mechanisms of pain (Fig. 6). Technical improvements included the selective choice of material for electrodes, lead wires and coatings, and the development of integrated analogue and digital circuitry and high-density, long-life implantable batteries. Technological advances included progressive adjustment of the design of electrode arrays and to the programming capacity of the stimulating devices. The initially radio-frequency activated passive systems, with hard-wired contact combinations, gave way to multipolar, multi-channel, multiprogrammable neural stimulators (Waltz and Andreesen, 1981).

Advanced cardiac pacemaker technology provided the basis for the development of non-invasively programmable, totally implantable pulse generators (IPGs) (Lazorthes et al., 1985). Cordis introduced the first totally implantable

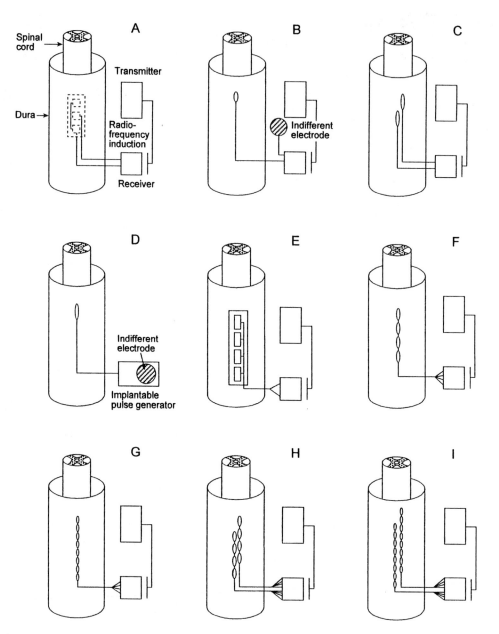

Fig. 6. Evolution of commercially available stimulation systems for SCS (Adapted from Augustinsson, 1985). (A) Radiofrequency (R/F)-coupled tripolar stimulation with plate-like lead implanted endo-durally by laminectomy; (B) R/F-coupled monopolar stimulation with wire-like lead implanted percutaneously in the epidural space and indifferent electrode placed subcutaneously; (C) R/F-coupled bipolar stimulation with percutaneously inserted epidural monopolar leads. Bipolar plate-like lead also available for the same system; (D) Monopolar stimulation with percutaneously inserted epidural lead. Indifferent electrode built into the receiver; (E) R/F-coupled quadripolar stimulation with plate-like lead implanted epidurally by laminectomy. Hardwired contact combinations; (F) R/F-coupled quadripolar multiprogrammable stimulation with wire-like or plate-like leads including dual bipolar configuration. Version with totally IPG available for the same system; (G) R/F-coupled octapolar multiprogrammable stimulation with wire-like or plate-like leads; (H) R/F-coupled dual quadripolar multiprogrammable stimulation with wire-like or plate-like leads. Version with totally IPG available for the same system; (I) R/F-coupled dual octapolar multiprogrammable stimulation with wire-like or plate-like leads.

neurostimulator (model 199A) in 1976. It was epoxy encapsulated, 'mercury battery' powered and had limited longevity. The programmability was restricted to four output current levels and four rates to a maximum of 30 pps. This IPG was initially used for stimulation of the spinal cord in movement disorders (primarily multiple sclerosis) and cerebellar stimulation for epilepsy by Ross Davis, a neurosurgeon in Miami (Marvin Sussman, personal communication). By 1980, the third generation Cordis IPG (model 900X – MK1) was powered by lithium–cupric sulfide batteries in a hermetically sealed titanium case and offered more choices of programmable parameters with a fixed pulse width. This unit was approved by the FDA for pain relief in 1981. The next model (904A; Fig. 7) featured a programmable pulse width and a thinner case that offered a more cosmetically acceptable implant (Peter Tarjan, personal communication).

Based on the pioneering work of Jay Law, a neurosurgeon in Denver, Colorado, who used complex array configuration for targeting the low back with stimulation (Law, 1987), dual multipolar lead systems were introduced (Fig. 8). This approach has been increasingly adopted but at the same time simpler electrode systems have continued to be developed. A transverse tripolar plate-like lead for spinal cord stimulation (SCS) is currently under evaluation (Struijk et al., 1998).

Over time the electrode arrays for peripheral nerve stimulation also evolved from 'split-cylinder' or 'wrap-around' designs to 'self-sizing spiral cuffs'. But they were all found to cause neural damage by compression, surgical trauma, lead tension and movement (Naples et al., 1990). Eventually a surgical implantation technique was developed that prevents direct contact with the nerve by using a quadripolar plate-like lead and putting a thin flap of fascia between the electrodes and the nerve (Racz et al., 1988). This has become an established routine implantation for peripheral nerve stimulation.

In 1977, McNeal wrote that "interest in the clinical application of electrical stimulation may be higher today than at any other time in its history."

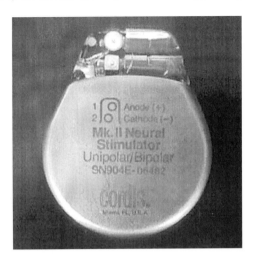

Fig. 7. The Cordis IPG (Model 904A – MKII) for pain relief. It included the features of programmable rates (10–100 pps), programmable currents (0.8–8.5 mA), programmable pulse width (75–315 µs), telemetry of lead resistance information and patient-adjustable amplitude using a magnet. (Courtesy Dr Peter Tarjan.)

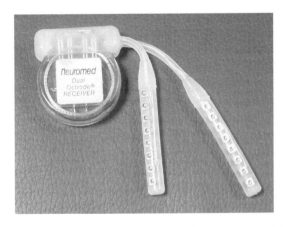

Fig. 8. Prototype of the receiver of the radio-frequency-coupled dual octapolar system for SCS manufactured by Neuromed (now Advanced Neuromodulation Systems) in 1991. The initial clinical evaluation in failed back surgery syndrome conducted in Australia (Rossi and Rabar, 1994) confirmed enhanced feasibility of stimulating the low back area with this configuration of electrodes, as predicted by Jay Law. The bulky connectors were eliminated in subsequent models.

At the same time Burton reported that "there were operating room personnel who would not assist in the implantation of neurostimulators because they perceived them to be against God." A major turning point for the acceptability of dorsal column stimulation came with the availability of percutaneous leads. The relative ease with which the leads could be inserted in the epidural space made the technique available to non-surgical disciplines. Anaesthesiologists became the most numerous implanters.

New terminology was introduced. The term 'dorsal column stimulation' was replaced by the term 'spinal cord stimulation' (SCS) because it appeared that structures other than the dorsal columns are involved in the analgesic effect (Barolat, 1999). Burton coined the term 'neuroaugmentive surgery' to denote that the implanted electronic devices 'augment' the function of the nervous system.

As the methods of neurostimulation became more complex, computer modelling of SCS was used (Coburn and Sin, 1985; Holsheimer, 1998; Wesselink, 1998) and patient-interactive computerized programming of stimulation was developed (North et al., 1992). The areas of stimulation expanded from the spinal cord and peripheral nerves to the sensory nuclei of the thalamus (Hosobuchi et al., 1973; Mazars et al., 1973), to the peri-aqueductal and peri-ventricular gray matter (Richardson and Akil, 1977), and of late to the motor cortex (Tsubokawa et al., 1993). The field of application of this modality also extended beyond the initial indication of failed back surgery to a wide range of conditions including ischaemic peripheral vascular disease (Cook et al., 1976; Dooley and Kasprak, 1976), atypical trigeminal neuralgia (Meyerson and Håkansson, 1980; Steude, 1984), refractory angina pectoris (Murphy and Giles, 1987), reflex sympathetic dystrophy (Barolat et al., 1989), interstitial cystitis (Feler, 1999), occipital neuralgia (Weiner and Reed, 1999), and ilioinguinal neuralgia (Alò et al., 1999).

The status of contemporary technology and applications of electroanalgesia are reviewed in recent publications (Stanton-Hicks and Salamon, 1997; Simpson, 1999; Lou, 2000; Alò, 2001) and are dealt with in subsequent chapters of this book. At the time of writing, therapeutic electrical neural stimulation is an established, systematic,

interdisciplinary field of science, with a continuing search for 'optimization' under the auspices of the International Neuromodulation Society.

The future is promising, as denoted by a quotation from the not-too-distant past: "There are many cells in the nervous system and many loci to stimulate. As technology advances, they will undoubtedly be stimulated" (Taub, 1975).

Acknowledgments

The author is grateful to Drs Norman Shealy, John Mortimer, Charles Ray, Ross Davis, Björn Meyerson, Peter Tarjan, Marvin Sussman and Mr Bill Borkan, who all kindly provided unedited information. I also wish to thank my daughter, Sandra, for her assistance with editing of the manuscript, and Ms Lindy Nelson of Mayne Health Library for pertinent searches and provision of literature. Thank you also to Mr Yang Qui Lin for preparing the artwork.

References

Alò, K. (2001) Recent advances in neurostimulation analgesia. Tech. Reg. Anesth. Pain Manage., 5(4): 142–151.

Alò, K., Yland, M., and Redko, V. (1999) Lumbar and sacral nerve stimulation (SNS) in the treatment of chronic pain: a novel anatomic approach and neurostimulation technique. Neuromodulation, 1: 23–31.

Althaus, J. (1859) Treatise on medical electricity, theoretical and practical and its use in the treatment of paralysis neuralgia and other diseases. Trubner, London.

Augustinsson, L.E. (1985) Epidural spinal cord electrical stimulation (ESCS) in chronic pain syndromes. Thesis. University of Göteborg, Göteborg, Sweden.

Barolat, G. (1999) History of neuromodulation. Neuoromod. News, 2: 3–9.

Barolat, G., Schwartzmann, R., and Woo, R. (1989) Epidural spinal cord stimulation in the management of reflex sympathetic dystrophy. Stereotact. Funct. Neurosurg., 53: 29–39.

Basford, J.R. (2001) A historical perspective of the popular use of electric and magnetic therapy. Arch. Phys. Med. Rehabil., 82: 1261–1269.

Beard, G., and Rockwell, A. (Eds.) (1891) *Medical and Surgical Uses of Electricity.* W. Wood Co, New York.

Burton, C. (1973) Seminar on dorsal column stimulation: summary of proceedings. Surg. Neurol., 1: 285–289.

Butterfield, J. (1991) Dr Gilbert's magnetism. Lancet, 338: 1576–1579.

Chaffee, E.L. and Light, R.E. (1934) A method for remote control of electrical stimulation of the nervous system. Yale J. Biol. Med., 7: 83.

Coburn, B. and Sin, W.K. (1985) A theoretical study of epidural electrical stimulation of the spinal cord. Part I: Finite element analysis of stimulus fields. I.E.E. Trans. Biomed. Eng., BME-32: 971–977.

Cook, A.W. (1976) Percutaneous trial for implantable stimulating devices. J. Neurosurg., 44: 650–651.

Cook, A.W., Oygar, A., Baggenstos, P., Pacheco, S., and Kleriga, E. (1976) Vascular disease of extremities. Electric stimulation of spinal cord and posterior roots. N.Y. State J. Med., 76: 366–368.

Devinski, O. (1993) Electrical and magnetic stimulation of the central nervous system: historical overview. Adv. Neurol., 63: 1–16.

Dooley, D.M. (1975) Percutaneous electrical stimulation of the spinal cord. Assoc. Neurol. Surg., Bal Harbour, Florida.

Dooley, D. and Kasprak, M. (1976) Modification of blood flow to the extremities by electrical stimulation of the nervous system. South. Med. J., 69: 1309–1311.

Duchenne (De Boulogne), G. (1855) De l'electrisation localisée et de son application à la pathologie et à la therapeutique. Baillière, Paris.

Eisenberg, L., Mauro, A., Glenn, W.W.L., and Hageman, J.H. (1965) Radio-frequency stimulation: a research and clinical tool. Science, 147: 578–582.

Feler, C.A., Whitworth, L.A., Brookoff, D., and Powell, R. (1999) Recent advances: sacral nerve root stimulation using a retrograde method of lead insertion for the treatment of pelvic pain due to interstitial cystitis. Neuromodulation, 2(3): 211–216.

Gadsby, J.G. (1998) Electroanalgesia: historical and contemporary development. Ph.D. Thesis. De Montfort University, Leicester, UK.

Geddes, L.A. (1984) A short history of the electrical stimulation of excitable tissue including electrotherapeutic applications. Physiologist, 27(1): S1–S47.

Glenn, W.W.L., Mauro, A., Longo, P., Lavietes, P.H., and Mackay, F.J. (1959) Remote stimulation of the heart by radiofrequency transmission. N. Engl. J. Med., 261: 948.

Hermel, E. (1844) Reserches sur les nevralgies et leur trestement. Am. Med. Psychol., 3: 209–230.

Hoff, H.E. (1963) An account of stimulation of tissue by electricity before Galvani. Arm. Sci., 1: 157.

Holsheimer, J. (1998) Computer modeling of spinal cord stimulation and its contribution to therapeutic efficacy (Review). Spinal Cord, 36: 531–540.

Hosobuchi, Y., Adams, J.E., and Rutkin, E. (1973) Chronic thalamic stimulation for the control of facial anesthesia dolorosa. Arch. Neurol., 29: 158–161.

Hunter, J. (1773) Anatomical observations on the torpedo. Phil. Trans. R. Soc., 63: 481–485.

Hymes, A. (1984) Introduction: a review of the historical uses of electricity. In J.S. Mannheimer, and G.N. Lampe (Eds.), *Clinical Transcutaneous Electrical Nerve Stimulation*. F.A. Davis Company, Philadelphia.

Kane, K. and Taub, A. (1975) A history of local electrical analgesia. Pain, 1(2): 125–138.

Kellaway, D. (1946) The William Osler Medal Essay. The part played by electric fish in the early history of bioelectricity and electrotherapy. Bull. Hist. Med., 20: 112–137.

Keyser, P.T. (1993) The purpose of the Parthian galvanic cells: a first-century A.D. electric battery used for analgesia. J. Near Eastern Studies, 52(2): 81–98.

Kryzhanovsky, L.N. (1993) The fishy tale of early electricity. Electronics World, February 1993, 119–121.

Law, J.D. (1987) Targeting a spinal stimulator to treat the "failed back surgery syndrome". Appl. Neurophysiol., 50: 437–438.

Lazorthes, Y., Siegfried, J., and Upton, A.R.M. (1985) A brief historical review of biostimulation. In Y. Lazorthes, and A.R.M. Upton (Eds.), *Neurostimulation: An Overview* (pp. 5–10). Futura Publishing Company, Mt. Krisco, New York.

Long, D.M. (1991) Fifteen years of transcutaneous electrical stimulation for pain control. Stereostact. Funct. Neurosurg., 56: 2–19.

Lou, L. (2000) Uncommon areas of electrical stimulation for pain relief. Curr. Rev. Pain, 4: 407–412.

Macklis, R.M. (1993) Magnetic healing, quackery, and the debate about the health effects of electromagnetic fields. Ann. Intern. Med., 118(5): 376–383.

Mazars, G., Merienne, L., and Ciolocca, C. (1973) Stimulations thalamique intermittentes antalgiques. Rev. Neurol., 128: 273–279.

McNeal, D.R. (1977) 2000 years of electrical stimulation. In F.T. Hambrecht, and J.B. Reswick (Eds.), *Functional Electrical Stimulation: Applications in Neural Prostheses* (pp. 3–35). Marcel Dekker, New York.

Melzack, R. and Wall, P.D. (1965) Pain mechanisms: a new theory. Science, 150: 971–979.

Meyerson, B.A. and Håkansson, S. (1980) Alleviation of atypical trigeminal pain by stimulation of the gasserian ganglion via an implanted electrode. Acta Neurochir. Suppl., 30: 303–330.

Mortimer, J.T. (1968) Pain suppression in man by dorsal column electroanalgesia. Ph.D. Thesis. Case Western Reserve University, Cleveland, Ohio, USA.

Mourino, M.R. (1991) From Thales to Lauterbur, or from the lodestone to MRI imaging: magnetism and medicine. Radiology, 180: 593–612.

Murphy, D.F. and Giles, K.E. (1987) Intractable angina pectoris: managements with dorsal column stimulation. Med. J. Aust., 146: 260.

Naples, G.G., Mortimer, J.T., and Yuen, T.G.H. (1990) Overview of peripheral nerve electrode design and implantation. In W.F. Agnew, and D.B. McCreery (Eds.), *Neural Prostheses. Fundamental Studies* (pp. 107–145). Prentice-Hall, M.C.

Newman, H. and Fender, F. (1937) cited by Eisenberg, 1965.

North, R.B., Fowler, K., Nigrin, D.J., and Szymanski, R. (1992) Patient-interactive, computer controlled neurological stimulation system: clinical efficacy in spinal cord stimulator adjustment. J. Neurosurg., 76: 967–972.

Oschman, J.L. (2000) Historical background. In: *Energy Medicine. The Scientific Basis.* Churchill Livingstone, Edinburgh, pp. 5–25.

Perdikis, P. (1977) Transcutaneous nerve stimulation in the treatment of protracted ileus. South African J. Surg. 17(2): 81–86.

Racz, G.B., Browne, T., and Lewis, R. (1988) Peripheral nerve stimulation implant for treatment of causalgia caused by electrical burns. Tex. Med., 84: 45–50.

Richardson, D.E. and Akil, H. (1977) Pain reduction by electrical brain stimulation in man. J. Neurosurg., 47: 178–194.

Rossi, U. and Rabar, J. (1994) Spinal cord stimulation in failed back surgery: A reappraisal – Presented at XIII Annual Scientific Meeting of the American Pain Society, Miami, FL.

Roth, N. (1977) The nineteenth-century revival of electrotherapy. Med. Instrum., 11(4): 236–237.

Sarlandière, J.B. (Ed.) (1825) *Memoires sur l'électro-puncture.* Delaunay, Paris.

Schechter, D.C. (1971a) Origins of electrotherapy. Part I. N.Y. State J. Med., May 1, 997–1008.

Schechter, D.C. (1971b) Origins of electrotherapy. Part II. N.Y. State J. Med., May 15, 1114–1124.

Shealy, C.N. and Maurer, D. (1974) Transcutaneous nerve stimulation for control of pain. Surg. Neurol., 2: 45–47.

Shealy, C.N., Taslitz, N., Mortimer, J.T., and Becker, D.P. (1967a) Electrical inhibition of pain: experimental evaluation. Anesth. Analg., 46(3): 299–305.

Shealy, C.N., Mortimer, J.T., and Reswick, J.B. (1967b) Electrical inhibition of pain by stimulation of the dorsal columns: preliminary clinical report. Anaesth. Analg., 46(4): 489–491.

Sheon, R.P. (1984) Transcutaneous electrical nerve stimulation: from electric eels to electrodes. Postgrad. Med., 75.5: 71–74.

Shimoji, K., Higashi, H., and Kano, T. (1971) Electrical management of intractable pain. Jpn. J. Anesthesiol., 20: 444–447.

Siegfried, J. (1978) I. – Introduction – Historique. In: Sedan, R., Lazorthes, Y. and Verdie, J.C: La neurostimulation electrique therapeutique. Neurochirurgue 24 (Suppl. 1): 5–10.

Simpson, B.A. (1999) Spinal cord and brain stimulation. In Wall, P.D., and Melzack, R. (Eds.), *Textbook of Pain.* 4th ed. (pp. 1353–1381). Churchill Livingstone, New York, NY.

Stanton-Hicks, M. and Salamon, J. (1997) Stimulation of the central and peripheral nervous system for the control of pain. J. Clin. Neurophysiol., 14(1): 46–62.

Steude, V. (1984) Radiofrequency electrical stimulation of the gasserian ganglion in patients with atypical trigeminal pain. Methods of percutaneous temporary test-stimulation and permanent implantation. Acta Neurochir., Suppl. 33: 481–486.

Stillings, D. (1974a) The Piscean origin of medical electricity. Med. Instrum., 8.5: 313. March–April.

Stillings, D. (1974b) The first observation of electrical stimulation. Med. Instrum., 815: 313. Sept.–Oct.

Stillings, D. (1983) Mediterranean origin of electrotherapy. J. Bioelectricity, 2(2–3): 181–186.

Struijk, J.J., Holsheimer, J., Spincemaille, G.H., Gielen, F.L.H., and Hoekema, R. (1998) Theoretical performance and clinical evaluation of transverse tripolar spinal cord stimulation. IEEE Trans. Rehabil. Eng., 6: 277–285.

Sweet, W.H. and Wepsic, J.G. (1968) Treatment of chronic pain by stimulation of fibers of primary afferent neurons. Tran. Am. Neurol. Ass., 93: 103–107.

Taub, A. (1975) Electrical stimulation for the relief of pain. Two lessons in technological zealotry. Perspect. Biol. Med., 19.1: 125–135.

Tsubokawa, T., Katamaya, Y., Yamamoto, T., Hirayama, T., and Koyama, S. (1993) Chronic motor cortex stimulation in patients with thalamic pain. J. Neurosurg., 78: 393–401.

Turrell, W.J. (1969) The landmarks of electrotherapy. Arch. Phys. Med. Rehabil., 50(3): 157–160.

Wall, P.D. and Sweet, W.H. (1967) Temporary abolition of pain in man. Science, 155: 108–109.

Wall, P.D. (1985) The discovery of transcutaneous electrical nerve stimulation. Physiotherapy, 71(8): 348–350.

Walsh, J. (1773) Of the electrical property of the torpedo. Phil. Trans. R. Soc., 63: 461.

Waltz, J.M. and Andreesen, W.H. (1981) Multiple-lead spinal cord stimulation: technique. Appl. Neurophysiol., 44(1-3): 30–36.

Weiner, R.L. and Reed, K.L. (1999) Peripheral neurostimulation for control of intractable occipital neuralgia. Neuromodulation, 2(3): 217–221.

Wesselink, W.A. (1998) Computer aided analysis of spinal cord stimulation. Ph.D. Thesis, University of Twente, Enschede, The Netherlands 108.

Young, J.H. (Ed.) (1961) *The Toadstool Millionaires: A Social History of Patent Medicines in America before Federal Regulation.* Princeton University Press, Princeton, New Jersey.

Zumpano, B.J. and Saunders, R.L. (1976) Percutaneous epidural dorsal column stimulation. Technical note. J. Neurosurg., 45: 459–460.

Electrical Stimulation and the Relief of Pain
Pain Research and Clinical Management, Vol. 15
Edited by Brian A. Simpson
© 2003 Elsevier Science B.V. All rights reserved

CHAPTER 3

Principles of neurostimulation

Jan Holsheimer*

Institute for Biomedical Technology, University of Twente, 7500 AE Enschede, The Netherlands

Abstract

Principles of neurostimulation and their impact on clinical applications are discussed in this chapter. The *activating function* as the driving force for the stimulation of (myelinated) nerve fibres is introduced. With this concept the various excitation and blocking effects of cathodic and anodic stimulation are described. The concept is also used to explain the differences between mono-, bi- and tripolar stimulation. Moreover, the activating function is used to describe the effects of fibre diameter and distance from the stimulating electrode to the target fibres on the threshold current of excitation, and the resulting order of fibre recruitment in a nerve trunk. A second basic concept introduced is the *strength–duration time constant*, or chronaxie, of neuronal elements. The relationship between threshold current and pulse width is described and it is explained why axons are the neuronal target elements when stimulating gray matter. Consequences of these principles in neurostimulation for clinical applications, such as spinal cord stimulation (SCS) for the management of chronic pain, deep brain stimulation (DBS) for the treatment of motor disorders, and motor cortex stimulation (MCS) for the management of central pain are described. Finally, the effects of pulse rate, the use of voltage-controlled and current-controlled pulse generators and safety aspects in neurostimulation are discussed. A list of symbols is included at the end of the chapter.

Keywords: Neurostimulation; Activating function; Strength–duration time constant; Chronaxie; Anodic excitation; Anodic block; Cathodic block; Electrical safety; Current-controlled stimulation; Voltage-controlled stimulation

1. Introduction

Electrical stimulation of the nervous system can be applied both at a cellular level by injecting current intracellularly by means of a microelectrode, and at a multicellular level by injecting current in the extracellular space surrounding the neuronal elements. In clinical applications relatively large electrodes, potentially stimulating a multitude of neurons, are generally used. Most pulse generators are voltage-controlled and create a preset potential difference between its two outputs (see Section 7), the electrode(s) connected to the positive output being the anode(s) and the one(s) connected to the negative output being the cathode(s). The injected current I depends on both the applied voltage V of the stimulation pulse and the impedance Z between the two stimulator outputs, according to Ohm's Law ($V = I \cdot Z$). This current is distributed in a 3-dimensional space made up of electrically conducting anatomical structures and obeys another law of physics: Poisson's law, which is derived from the basic Maxwell equations of electromagnetism (Malmivuo and Plonsey, 1995;

*Correspondence to: Dr. Jan Holsheimer, Faculty of Electrical Engineering, Mathematics and Informatics, University of Twente, P.O. Box 217, 7500 AE Enschede, The Netherlands. Phone: +31-53-489-2762; Fax: +31-53-489-2287; E-mail: j.holsheimer@utwente.nl

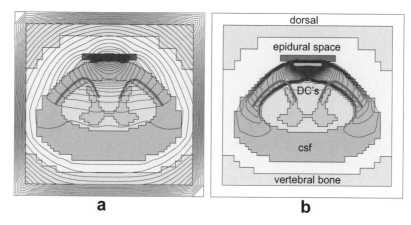

Fig. 1. Isopotential lines (a) and isocurrent density lines (b) in a transverse section of the 3-dimensional cervical SCS model including the mid-dorsal, epidural cathode; stimulation is applied monopolarly.

Guljarani, 1998). The resulting 3-dimensional electric field can be represented by its potential distribution and by its current density distribution. These distributions can be visualized by isopotential lines and isocurrent density lines, respectively, as shown in a transverse section of a spinal cord stimulation (SCS) model (Fig. 1).

The primary effect of an electrical stimulation pulse on a neuron is a change of its transmembrane voltage, being either a depolarisation or a hyperpolarisation. Due to a large difference between axonal and somadendritic electrical membrane properties the magnitude of the axonal membrane (de)polarisation resulting from a given stimulus exceeds the somadendritic membrane (de)polarisation by far (see Section 5.2). Therefore, the primary effect of stimulation is generally a (de)polarisation of nerve fibres. As long as these fibres are either depolarised by less than about 15 mV (subthreshold) or hyperpolarised, no further events will take place and at the end of the stimulus the transmembrane voltage will return to its resting state. When, however, the axon membrane is at least depolarised up to its threshold voltage, an action potential will be generated by the excitation mechanism first described by Hodgkin and Huxley (1952). In contrast to an action potential generated under normal physiological conditions (at the axon hillock of the cell body) and propagated orthodromically, a stimulation-induced action potential

propagates both orthodromically and antidromically along the fibre. As shown in Section 4 the nerve fibres most probably stimulated are large, myelinated nerve fibres. Therefore, this chapter is focused on stimulation of these fibres.

2. Stimulation of myelinated nerve fibres

2.1. Mechanism of nerve fibre stimulation

In Fig. 2a a schematic longitudinal section of part of a myelinated nerve fibre is shown. It consists of a cylindrical axon covered by a myelin sheath which is interrupted by a node of Ranvier at regular intervals. The electrical behaviour of a myelinated nerve fibre can be represented by a simple cable network as shown in Fig. 2b. This electrical equivalent includes the intra-axonal resistances R_a of each internodal section, the nodal membrane resistances R_m and the nodal membrane capacities C_m. The arrow in R_m indicates that this resistance is variable. It reflects the variation of Na^+ and K^+ channel conductivities during the generation of an action potential (Hodgkin and Huxley, 1952). Each node (n−1, n, n+1) has an intra-axonal potential V_a and an extracellular potential V_e. Accordingly, the membrane voltage at node n is $(V_{a,n}-V_{e,n})$ and the membrane current is $I_{m,n}$. It is assumed

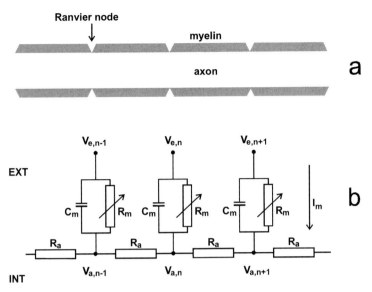

Fig. 2. Schematic longitudinal section (a) and electrical cable model (b) of a myelinated nerve fibre; for explanation see text and list of symbols.

that the internodal myelin sheath is a perfect insulator.

McNeal (1976) used the cable network shown in Fig. 2b to calculate how nodal transmembrane voltages are affected by a stimulation-induced extracellular field, represented by the field potentials V_e. Instead of the Hodgkin–Huxley equations based on measurements on unmyelinated giant axons of the squid (Hodgkin and Huxley, 1952), McNeal implemented the Frankenhaeuser–Huxley equations (Frankenhaeuser and Huxley, 1964) which represent the excitation mechanism of frog myelinated nerve fibres. He calculated that the rate of change of the membrane voltage at node n is primarily determined by the second order difference of the nodal field potentials V_e. This function, which is the driving force of the change of nodal transmembrane voltages, has been named the *activating function* AF (Rattay, 1986). For node n, the value of AF_n is thus calculated as the difference of two potential differences:

$$AF_n = (V_{e,n-1} - V_{e,n}) - (V_{e,n} - V_{e,n+1}) \\ = (V_{e,n-1} - 2V_{e,n} + V_{e,n+1}) \tag{1}$$

According to the model calculations of McNeal (1976) a positive value of AF_n results in a membrane depolarisation at node n, whereas a negative value gives hyperpolarisation. According to Eq. (1) depolarisation of node n occurs when $V_{e,n}$ is more negative than the average value of $V_{e,n-1}$ and $V_{e,n+1}$. This happens when the nerve fibre is near a negative electrode (cathode). The node closest to the cathode will have the most negative V_e and the largest AF, and will thus be depolarised most, as shown in Fig. 3. Fig. 3a represents a myelinated nerve fibre near a cathodic current source (e) in a 3-dimensional, homogeneous conducting medium. The spheric electric field is represented by isopotential lines centered at the current source, which gives a subthreshold pulse (−0.20 mA) of 0.5 ms duration. The nerve fibre model (10 μm diameter) is represented by a straight line at 1 mm distance from the cathode. The dots on this line represent the nodes of Ranvier at 1 mm intervals. The curve in Fig. 3b represents the (negative) field potential distribution along the fibre. The peak (∼ −50 mV) is at the node closest to the cathode. In Fig. 3c the AF value calculated from the nodal field potentials in Fig. 3b by using Eq. (1), is shown for each node.

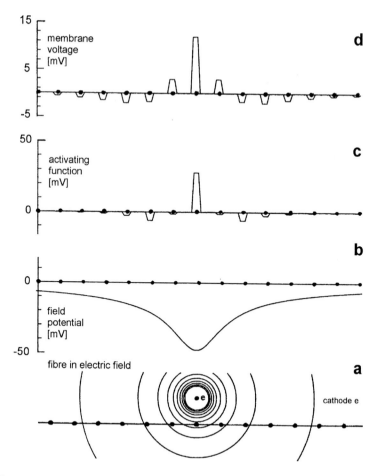

Fig. 3. Calculated distribution of quasi-static, subthreshold nodal membrane potentials elicited by stimulation; (a) myelinated nerve fibre (nodes indicated by dots) near a cathodic current source (e) in a 3D homogeneous conducting medium; (b) field potential distribution along the fibre; (c) distribution of nodal activating functions; (d) distribution of membrane voltage (depolarisation, hyperpolarisation).

The maximum AF corresponds to the minimum of the field potential curve in Fig. 3b, whereas the AFs at several nodes on both sides have smaller, negative values. In Fig. 3d the calculated changes of nodal membrane voltage at the end of the subthreshold pulse are shown. Although the maximum depolarisation corresponds to the maximum AF, the spatial distributions of membrane voltage and AF are somewhat different because the latter is just a first-order approximation of the calculated nodal membrane voltage.

The node closest to the cathode will be excited first when the stimulation current is sufficiently high. As the field potential gradients on both sides of this node get steeper, which occurs when the nerve fibre gets closer to the cathode, AF will rise and the stimulus needed for excitation will be reduced. The results of this theoretical approach are in accordance with the general observation that the threshold stimulus of nerve fibre excitation is smallest in the vicinity of a cathode and rises with increasing distance (Ranck, 1975). See also Section 4. The opposite response (membrane hyperpolarisation) applies to a nerve fibre in the vicinity of an anode.

The stimulation induced distribution of nodal membrane voltages (Fig. 3d) can also be explained as follows. The different nodal field potentials V_e

along a fibre give rise to simultaneous membrane currents I_m of opposite directions. Outward current leaving the axon at some nodes near the cathode and inducing membrane depolarisation enters the axon via other nodes on either side on its way from a distant anode, thereby inducing membrane hyperpolarisation. Although the total inward and outward currents are identical, the inward current is generally distributed over more nodes than the outward current. As a result cathodic stimulation gives rise to a depolarisation of one or few nodes, whereas a larger number of nodes on both sides are hyperpolarised to a lesser extent, as shown in Fig. 3d. In anodic stimulation the opposite occurs. These side effects of cathodic and anodic stimulation are named anodic and cathodic surround, or *virtual anode* and *virtual cathode* effects, respectively, and underly phenomena such as cathodic block and anodic excitation.

2.2. Cathodic and anodic stimulation

Apart from cathodic excitation other responses to electrical stimulation such as anodic excitation, cathodic block and anodic block are well known from experimental research (Ranck, 1975) and can simply be explained. When the *cathodic* current is increased the depolarisation and hyperpolarisation of nodal membranes, as shown in Fig. 3d are raised proportionally. At some cathodic current level the 'virtual anodic' hyperpolarisations are sufficient to compensate for the depolarisation induced by the action potential generated at the nodes in between. No action potential will be generated at these 'virtual anodic' nodes and propagation in either direction is blocked (*cathodic block*). When *anodic* current is applied to a fibre propagating an action potential, a few nodes closest to the anode are hyperpolarised and will block the propagation when the anodic current is large enough (*anodic block*). *Anodic excitation* of a fibre is feasible when the anodic current is so large that the 'virtual cathodic' depolarisation on either side of the hyperpolarisation will generate an action potential. These action potentials will propagate in opposite directions, as in cathodic stimulation.

The conditions for the various responses can be predicted with the model introduced by McNeal (1976). The calculated responses of a 10 μm diameter nerve fibre are shown in Fig. 4a–d as quasi 3-dimensional plots. The time scale (1.0 ms) is on the X-axis, while the Y-axis represents a nerve fibre with 60 nodes of Ranvier at 1.0 mm intervals. The intra-axonal potential at each node following (suprathreshold) stimulation is calculated as a function of time and the resulting 2-dimensional potential distribution is visualized by connecting points in the time–space domain having the same potential. These isopotential lines are drawn as solid lines at 10 mV intervals from 10 to 90 mV depolarisation. Similarly, membrane hyperpolarisation is indicated by dotted lines. In this way a propagating action potential is visualised. The duration of the action potential is ~0.35 ms.

In Fig. 4a the mechanism of *cathodic excitation* is illustrated. A suprathreshold cathodic pulse (−1.1 mA, 0.1 ms) is applied by a point source at 1.0 mm distance from the fibre next to node 31. Initially nodes 30–32 are depolarised, whereas several nodes on both sides are somewhat hyperpolarised (virtual anode effect). Subsequently, an action potential is generated at node 31 and as a result the initially hyperpolarised nodes are depolarised as well. Nodes 30 and 32 are excited next and the action potential propagates in either direction at a velocity of 57 m/s.

The mechanism of *cathodic block* is shown in Fig. 4b. Now a longer and somewhat larger cathodic pulse (−1.2 mA, 0.4 ms) is applied by the same point source. The initial response is a depolarisation and a subsequent excitation of nodes 30–32, similar to the response in Fig. 4a. Due to the increased 'virtual anodic' hyperpolarisation at the adjacent nodes, however, the propagation of the action potential is blocked in either direction. This block occurs only when the duration of the cathodic pulse is sufficiently long, i.e. similar to the duration of the action potential.

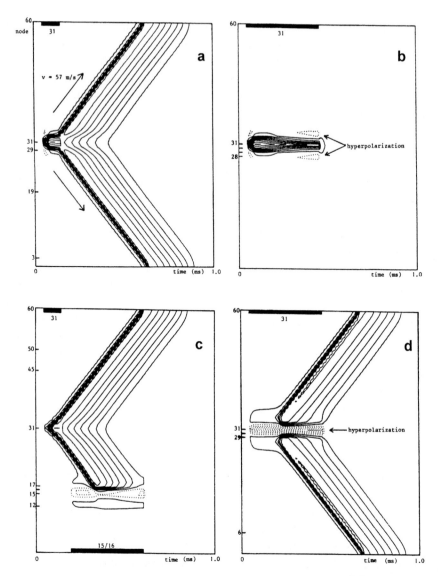

Fig. 4. Simulated generation and propagation of an action potential; X-axis: time scale (1 ms), Y-axis: length of the modelled fibre (60 nodes at 1 mm intervals), nodal membrane potentials represented by isopotential lines: depolarisation indicated by solid lines, hyperpolarisation by dotted lines; (a) cathodic excitation, (b) cathodic block; (c) anodic block, (d) anodic excitation; for details see text.

Otherwise the depolarisation resulting from the action potential present at nodes 30 and 32 may still exceed the excitation threshold of the previously hyperpolarised nodes 29 and 33.

In Fig. 4c the mechanism of *anodic block* is illustrated. As in Fig. 4a an action potential is generated by a cathodic current source near node 31 and is propagated in either direction.

An anodic pulse is applied by two point sources (0.55 mA and 0.4 ms each) at 1.0 mm distance from the fibre next to nodes 15 and 16, respectively, resulting in a hyperpolarisation of nodes 14–17. Due to a sufficient current and pulse width and despite some 'virtual cathodic' depolarisation at node 12 the propagation is blocked. When the anodic current is increased, the 'virtual cathodic' depolarisation of node 12 is increased as well and will, if sufficiently high, result in the excitation of this node and thus in a restored action potential propagation. In this situation the action potential 'jumps' over a couple of hyperpolarised nodes. To elicit a propagation block the anodic current has to be within a small amplitude window with a maximum current not exceeding twice the minimum block current.

Finally, the mechanism of *anodic excitation* is shown in Fig. 4d. An anodic pulse (1.2 mA, 0.4 ms) is applied by a point source at 1.0 mm distance from the fibre next to node 31. Nodes 30–32 are hyperpolarised and some nodes on both sides are depolarised (virtual cathode effect). The nodes depolarised most are 28 and 34 and these nodes are also excited first, as shown by the isopotential lines. Due to the large pulse width (0.4 ms) nodes 30–32 are not excited because they stay hyperpolarised until the propagating action potentials are vanished from the adjacent nodes.

According to the mechanisms described above, the threshold ratio of anodic and cathodic excitation will be equal to the ratio of the negative and positive peak values of the nodal membrane potentials as shown in Fig. 3d. In this case the ratio is ~ 6. This ratio may, however, vary due to variable stimulation conditions, such as the distance between the electrode and the nerve fibre, the diameter of the fibre, the size of the electrode and the pulse width. From their animal studies BeMent and Ranck (1969) reported that the anodic excitation threshold of central myelinated axons is 3–7 times their cathodic excitation threshold. Similar empirical ratios have been observed by Rijkhoff et al. (1994) for the anodic block threshold and the cathodic excitation threshold (5 to 8-fold). Ranck (1975) reported that the cathodic block threshold is more than 8 times the cathodic excitation threshold. High thresholds for both anodic excitation and anodic block as compared to cathodic excitation have been reported from studies on human peripheral nerve as well (Wee et al., 2000; Wee, 2001). Because in clinical neurostimulation currents

exceeding 3 times the value eliciting the initial response to cathodic stimulation are unlikely (except in electroconvulsive therapy), the occurrence of excitation and propagation block near an anode, as well as cathodic block, is very unlikely. In SCS, for example, the maximum therapeutic stimulation level (just below the discomfort threshold) does generally not exceed the perception threshold of paraesthesia by more than 40–70% (He et al., 1994; North et al., 2002).

3. Mono-, bi- and tripolar stimulation

Since the cathodic threshold current for nerve fibre excitation is 3–7 times lower than the anodic threshold current, cathodic stimulation is by far the more efficient way. In monopolar stimulation the active electrode (in or near the neuronal target) is therefore a cathode and the distant, indifferent electrode is an anode. Stimulation can be considered monopolar when the distance from the anode to the target is at least several times larger than the distance from the cathode to the target. In that situation the current injected by the cathode is distributed more or less evenly (depending on the electrical conductivities of the various tissues surrounding the cathode) in all directions. When the anode gets closer to the cathode, this uniform cathodic current distribution is gradually changing into a distribution with a preferential direction corresponding to the cathode–anode axis. Near the cathode the axial current density vector and thus the axial potential gradient and AF of nerve fibres parallel to this axis are increased (Section 2.1). As a result the threshold current to stimulate nerve fibres parallel to the cathode–anode axis is smaller in bipolar than in monopolar stimulation. If the cathode is flanked by an anode on either side ('guarded cathode') the threshold current is reduced even more. Accordingly, the threshold current will be larger when the nerve fibre axis is oblique or perpendicular to the bipole or tripole axis, as has been shown empirically (Ranck, 1975).

The effect of the (centre-to-centre) distance between the cathode and the anode(s) on the threshold current for stimulation of a nerve fibre parallel to the cathode–anode axis can be quantified by means of the corresponding AFs, due to the fact that these spatial functions can simply be superimposed. This is shown in Fig. 5a–c for the 'guarded cathode' configuration. The three electrodes (poles) are on a line (z-axis) parallel to a nerve fibre bundle. The triphasic AFs of the central cathode (C) and the two anodes (A1 and A2) are shown by solid lines. The central (highest) peak of the cathodic AF is positive and reflects depolarisation, whereas the corresponding peaks of the anodic AFs are negative and reflect hyperpolarisation. The position of each pole on the z-axis is represented by the position of the central peak of the corresponding AF. The peak values of the anodic AFs are only 50% of the cathodic peak value, because the anodic current is divided equally over the two anodes. The net AF ('sum'), obtained by superposition of the three AFs is indicated by the dotted line. In the situation shown in Fig. 5a the poles are so far apart that the anodic AFs do not influence the peak value of the cathodic AF. The three electrodes can thus be considered as independent monopoles. In Fig. 5b the poles are closer and one positive phase of each anodic AF ('virtual cathode') overlaps the central, positive phase of the cathodic AF, thus resulting in a larger positive AF peak at the cathode (dotted line). As a result, the threshold current for excitation of a fibre parallel to the axis of the tripole is reduced. In Fig. 5c the poles are so close that the central, negative phases of the anodic AFs partly overlap the central, positive phase of the cathodic AF, thus resulting in a smaller positive peak of the superimposed AFs and an increased threshold current. When in bi- and tripolar 'guarded cathode' stimulation the distance between the poles gets smaller, the threshold current to excite nerve fibres parallel to the electrode array is first gradually reduced and then steeply raised. This is shown by the curve in Fig. 6, based on data from SCS modelling

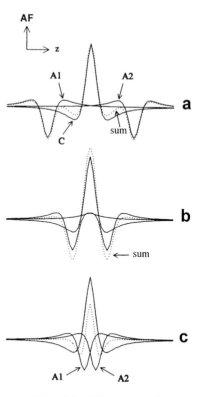

Fig. 5. Superposition of the AFs corresponding to the cathode (C) and the two anodes (A1, A2) of a tripole ('guarded cathode'), dotted line (sum) is the superimposed AF; (a) large anode–cathode distance, cathodic peak value is not affected by the anodic AFs; (b) smaller electrode distance, summed cathodic peak value is larger; (c) small electrode distance, summed cathodic peak value is smaller.

(Holsheimer and Wesselink, 1997). Under these model conditions the minimum threshold is 23% less than the value at a large electrode distance. It was calculated that the threshold for dorsal column fibre stimulation will be lowest when the (centre-to-centre) distance of the electrodes is ~1.7 times the distance between the target (dorsal columns) and the electrode array (Holsheimer and Wesselink, 1997). Obviously, any superposition effect of AFs is absent when the electrode array is very close to, or in direct contact with the neuronal target tissue, as in deep brain stimulation.

The current needed to stimulate a nerve fibre bundle can thus be minimized by stimulating tripolarly ('guarded cathode') with an electrode

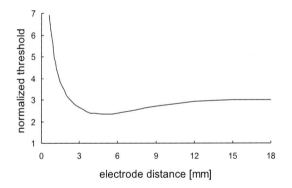

Fig. 6. Effect of cathode–anode distance on the threshold stimulus in tripolar 'guarded cathode' stimulation.

array in parallel to this bundle, e.g. in SCS where the electrode array is in parallel to the dorsal column fibres. Assuming that the mean distance between the epidural electrode array and the dorsal columns is ∼ 3.5 mm, the inter-electrode distance providing maximum battery life would be ∼ 3.5 × 1.7 = ∼ 6 mm. Currently available SCS systems have electrode distances ranging from 7 to 18 mm.

If nerve fibres with various orientations are present near an electrode array, bipolar and 'guarded cathode' stimulation can also be used to stimulate preferentially nerve fibres in parallel to the electrode array. This effect is due to the selective reduction of their stimulation threshold and plays a role in SCS. The longitudinal orientation of the electrode array may favour dorsal column stimulation over dorsal root stimulation, the latter being most likely responsible for the undesirable sensations at discomfort threshold. The number of dorsal column fibres stimulated below the discomfort threshold can be maximized by 'guarded cathode' stimulation, although in many cases this selective threshold reduction is not sufficient to compensate for the relatively low stimulation threshold of dorsal root fibres (Holsheimer, 1997). The preference of chronic pain patients for stimulation with a 'guarded cathode' over all other combinations of a quadripolar SCS array has been shown empirically by North et al. (1991). Despite the rather large

electrode distance they used (10 mm), the preference was statistically significant. A more apparent preference for 'guarded cathode' stimulation would have been observed if an array with an electrode distance of 7 mm or less had been used in this study.

4. Recruitment order of nerve fibres

The order in which fibres in a peripheral nerve, a spinal root or a central pathway (e.g. the dorsal columns) are excited by a stimulus pulse is predominantly related to both the fibre diameter and the distance between the fibre and the cathode. In Fig. 7a the calculated threshold stimulus of a 12 μm fibre as a function of its depth in the dorsal columns is presented (Holsheimer, 2002). From the dorsal border up to 0.7 mm deep the threshold is increased by ∼ 220%. In the conductive media around an electrode the current density is inversely proportional to the 2nd–3rd power of the distance. Accordingly, the threshold current to excite a nerve fibre is increased at the same rate, as shown empirically (Ranck, 1975). In Fig. 7b the calculated threshold stimulus of a fibre at the dorsal border of the dorsal columns as a function of its diameter is presented (Holsheimer, 2002). It is shown that the threshold stimulus of a fibre is inversely related to its diameter and that the threshold current to excite a 5 μm fibre is 4.4 times the value of a 15 μm fibre at the same position. This relationship of fibre size and threshold stimulus can simply be understood from the effect of fibre size on AF. As the internodal distance of a nerve fibre is proportional to its diameter (100 times as a rule of thumb), the potential differences between nodes and thus the peak value of AF will be less for a smaller fibre than for a larger one (see Fig. 2 and Eq. (1)).

From the two relationships shown in Fig. 7a–b the recruitment order of fibres in a bundle can be predicted. The first fibres to respond will generally be the largest ones closest to the cathode. At an increased amplitude the largest fibres will be

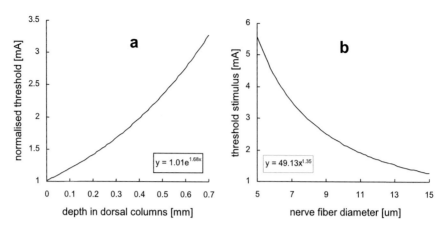

Fig. 7. (a) Relationship between median depth in dorsal columns and normalized threshold stimulus of a 12 μm fibre, calculated with SCS model; (b) inverse relationship of nerve fibre diameter and threshold stimulus of a fibre at the median dorsal column border, calculated with SCS model.

recruited at an increased distance from the cathode, and in addition somewhat smaller fibres close to the cathode will be excited. With increasing stimulus amplitude this process continues. A fibre bundle with a small cathode (c) on one side is drawn schematically in Fig. 8a–b. The increase of fibre recruitment is shown by a number of contour lines indicating the outer border of the activated fibres of each diameter (in μm) separately, with the line of the largest fibres ahead and followed by the contour lines of subsequently smaller fibres. All these contours move away from the cathode when the stimulus amplitude is increased.

Due to the generally limited amplitude range in clinical applications of neurostimulation only the larger fibres will be recruited. For example, the maximum therapeutic amplitude in SCS does generally not exceed 170% of the perception threshold of paraesthesia (cf. Section 2.2). Since the largest dorsal column fibres are ∼12 μm (Feirabend et al., 2002) it was calculated that the maximum depth in the dorsal columns at which these fibres can be recruited is less than 0.3 mm when stimulating bipolarly with electrodes having a center-to-center distance of 9 mm (Holsheimer, 2002). It was also calculated that fibres smaller than ∼9 μm will not be recruited at all.

Another relevant aspect of these recruitable large fibres is their density. It has been established

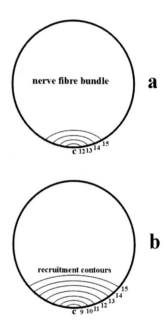

Fig. 8. Recruitment of nerve fibres of different diameters (in μm) in a fibre bundle by a cathode, **c**, at a low current (a) and a high current (b).

that only 0.5% of the fibre population in the superficial part of the T10–T11 human dorsal columns has a diameter ≥ 10.7 μm (Feirabend et al., 2002). This corresponds to a density of only ∼1 fibre per 10,000 μm² and a mean of ∼67 fibres larger than 10.7 μm in the outer 0.3 mm layer of a single low thoracic dorsal column. Taking into account that several smaller fibres will be recruited as well, only ~1% of the population of dorsal column fibres may be activated by SCS and may – apart from large cutaneous dorsal root fibres – elicit paraesthesia and pain relief. This low density of recruitable dorsal column fibres will limit the probability of targeting all dermatomes represented by some of these afferents.

5. Sensitivity of neuronal elements to stimulation

5.1. Relationship between pulse amplitude and duration

When the duration of a stimulus pulse PW is varied the *threshold current* I_{th} to elicit a response changes as well. The relationship between PW and I_{th} is known as the strength–duration relationship. An example of this inverse, non-linear relationship is presented in Fig. 9. By this *strength–duration curve* it is shown that I_{th} is large when PW is small and falls with increasing PW towards a minimum, the *rheobase current* I_{rh}. The shape of a strength–duration curve is generally characterized by two parameters, I_{rh} (mA) and the *strength–duration time constant* τ_{sd} (ms), and is described by the following equation

$$I_{th} = I_{rh}(1 + \tau_{sd}/PW) \qquad (2)$$

According to this equation $\tau_{sd} = PW$ when $I_{th} = 2I_{rh}$, which means that τ_{sd} is identical to the *chronaxie*, defined as the pulse width at twice the rheobase current (see Fig. 9).

When both sides of Eq. (2) are multiplied by PW the following equation, known as Weiss's law (1901), is obtained

$$I_{th} \cdot PW = I_{rh}(PW + \tau_{sd}) \qquad (3)$$

with $I_{th} \cdot PW$ being the charge (µC) of the threshold pulse. It has been demonstrated that empirical strength–duration data fit well to this equation

(Nowak and Bullier, 1998a; Mogyoros et al., 1999). Apart from the non-linear strength–duration curve, calculated according to Eq. (2) with $I_{rh} = 1.0$ mA and $\tau_{sd} = 0.07$ ms, the corresponding linear *charge–duration curve* is also presented in Fig. 9. This curve shows that the charge needed for a threshold pulse rises considerably when PW is enlarged. An increase of PW from 0.1 to 0.4 ms is accompanied by a 2.7-fold increase of the threshold charge of a pulse. Battery life is thus favoured by short stimulation pulses (although higher voltages may also require additional current), which is of particular interest when an implanted, battery powered pulse generator is used in clinical neurostimulation.

The value of τ_{sd} is primarily determined by the value of the *membrane time constant* τ_m (Bostock, 1983), which is defined as

$$\tau_m = R_m \cdot C_m \qquad (4)$$

with R_m being the membrane resistance and C_m the membrane capacity (Fig. 2) of the neuronal target. However, τ_{sd} is also influenced by various other factors including the distance from the stimulating electrode(s) to the target cells (West and Wolstencroft, 1983) and the conductivities of the tissues in between, the geometry of the electrode(s) (Bostock, 1983), the electrode

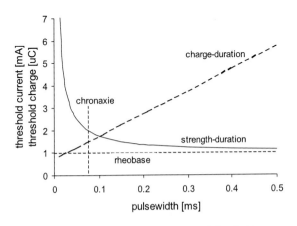

Fig. 9. Relationship between pulse width and threshold current (strength–duration curve), and between pulse width and threshold charge (charge–duration curve); see text for details.

configuration (e.g. mono- or bipolar), the size of the neuronal target elements, and the level of membrane polarisation at the moment of stimulation (Mogyoros et al., 1999). Due to these variables τ_{sd} may vary considerably as demonstrated by e.g. Mogyoros et al. (2000), but has generally a larger value than the corresponding τ_m.

The τ_m values of a somadendritic membrane and the nodal membrane of a myelinated axon are about 1–15 and 0.04–0.06 ms, respectively, thus differing roughly 100-fold. This difference is due to their different membrane resistivities, whereas the capacitances of the axonal and somadendritic membranes have most likely similar values ($C_m = \sim 1\ \mu\text{F} \cdot \text{cm}^{-2}$). Despite the large variability of the corresponding τ_{sd} values, being ~ 0.05–0.4 ms for Aα and Aβ fibres, ~ 0.4–0.8 ms for Aδ and C fibres, and ~ 1–20 ms for cell bodies and dendrites, these ranges do not overlap. Therefore, the potential targets of stimulation (cell bodies and dendrites, large and small axons) can generally be identified on the basis of their τ_{sd} values calculated from strength–duration measurements (Ranck, 1975; Nowak and Bullier, 1998a).

Among nerve fibres an inverse relationship between propagation velocity v and τ_{sd} has been demonstrated. West and Wolstencroft (1983) reported that the mean τ_{sd} of small bulbospinal fibres ($v = 5$–15 m/s) is 2.2-fold the mean value related to large ones ($v = 16$–63 m/s). Swadlow (1992) has shown an inverse relationship between v and τ_{sd} for a wide diameter range of neocortical efferent fibres ($v = 0.2$–23 m/s). Wesselink et al. (1999), who modelled human myelinated sensory nerve fibres with a τ_m value of 47 μs, calculated a τ_{sd} value of 202 and 126 μs for a 5 and a 15 μm fibre, respectively.

Because both τ_{sd} and I_{rh} are related to R_m, smaller fibres have a larger τ_{sd} value and a higher I_{rh} value than larger fibres. Differences in I_{th} value among fibres with different diameters can be reduced by increasing PW, as shown by the two strength–duration curves in Fig. 10, having τ_{sd} values of 0.06 and 0.145 ms, respectively. The dissimilarity of strength–duration curves of nerve

fibres with different diameters may underly the observation that in SCS the body area covered with paraesthesia gets generally larger when PW is increased (Krainick et al., 1975). An explanation of this phenomenon could be that smaller A$\alpha\beta$ fibres in the dorsal columns are not stimulated when PW is small, but that they are activated in addition to the largest A$\alpha\beta$ fibres when PW has a larger value.

5.2. The neuronal elements targeted by stimulation

During electrical stimulation ionic current passes neuronal membranes, thereby polarizing or depolarizing these membranes. Because membranes are complex impedances represented by a membrane resistance R_m in parallel to a membrane capacity C_m (Fig. 2), the rate of (de)polarisation is directly related to R_m and C_m, constituting τ_m (Eq. (4)). When τ_m has a small value, as in large axons, the membrane will (de)polarise considerably faster than e.g. a somadendritic membrane, as shown by the curves in Fig. 11, representing the calculated responses to a long pulse ($PW > 1$ ms). It is shown that after ~ 0.3 ms the depolarisation of an axon membrane ($\tau_m = 0.1$ ms) is at 95% of its maximum (14.25 mV), whereas at that moment a somadendritic membrane ($\tau_m = 5$ ms) is depolarised by only

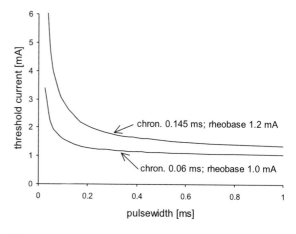

Fig. 10. Calculated strength–duration curves of a large nerve fibre (chronaxie 0.06 ms, rheobase 1 mA) and a smaller fibre (chronaxie 0.145 ms, rheobase 1.2 mA).

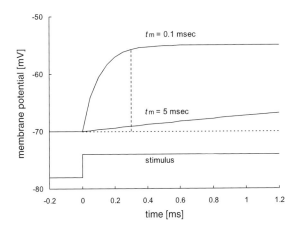

Fig. 11. Depolarisation of nodal membrane ($\tau_m = 0.1$ ms) and somadendritic membrane ($\tau_m = 5$ ms) with the same stimulus.

0.87 mV ($\sim 6\%$). Assuming that the axonal excitation threshold is reached, an action potential will be generated by an axon, whereas a somadendritic membrane is hardly depolarised by the same stimulus.

When a stimulation electrode is placed in the grey matter of the brain which includes both somadendritic elements, afferent and efferent axons, it is thus highly probable that axons are the neuronal elements responding to the stimulation. This hypothesis has been confirmed empirically. Nowak and Bullier (1998a) stimulated cortex preparations of the rat and determined the I_{th} values to evoke responses at different pulse widths. The resulting τ_{sd} values (mean 0.38 ms) suggest that axons are the targets. In the accompanying paper Nowak and Bullier (1998b) demonstrated that afferent fibres were predominantly responding. In a study on human subjects with a DBS electrode array in the thalamic ventral intermediate (Vim) nucleus or the internal globus pallidus (GPi) for the treatment of Parkinson's disease and essential tremor, Holsheimer and colleagues (2000b) determined the threshold voltage to stop the tremor at different PW values. The resulting τ_{sd} values (mean ~ 0.14 ms) suggest that large axons are responding to the stimulation. Because in this study only threshold voltages could be determined (instead of threshold currents), the

resulting τ_{sd} values were adapted according to Holsheimer et al. (2000a) to account for the PW-dependent electrode impedance.

5.3. Mechanisms in deep brain stimulation and cortex stimulation

Under the assumption that nerve fibres are predominantly activated when grey matter is stimulated, several mechanisms underlying the neurophysiological effect of high frequency (> 100 pps) stimulation of deep brain nuclei (DBS) have been proposed. Due to the dominating GABA-mediated input of GPi (striatal and external pallidal efferents) it is likely that the stimulation of afferents in GPi results in an increased inhibitory synaptic input of GPi neurons, thus reducing the GPi efferent activity. This hypothesis has been validated by e.g. Boraud and colleagues (1996) in an animal model of Parkinson's disease. They applied high frequency stimulation (120 pps) to the GPi of MPTP-treated rhesus monkeys and recorded the activity of its neurons. It was observed that stimulation induces a mean reduction of the spontaneous firing rate of about 19%. A similar mechanism is likely to occur in high frequency stimulation of the subthalamic nucleus (STN), receiving its major (GABA-mediated) input from the pallidum. Benazzouz and colleagues (1995) observed a powerful inhibition of STN cells in normal rats following high frequency stimulation of this nucleus.

Because action potentials elicited by stimulation are not only propagated by the afferents towards their synaptic endings (orthodromically), but also antidromically towards their cell bodies in other nuclei, other mechanisms have also been hypothesized (Benabid, 2002; Dostrovsky and Lozano, 2002). When afferent axons in STN are stimulated, action potentials will also be propagated antidromically to the external globus pallidus (GPe) and will activate this nucleus, as has been observed by Benazzouz in rat (1995). The hyperexcited GPe may then inhibit STN and GPi via its strong GABAergic projections to these nuclei.

The implicit assumption of the hypotheses regarding DBS is that the simultaneous stimulation of efferent fibres is of little concern. Afferents have many branches innervating a multitude of cells in a nucleus, whereas each cell has just a single efferent fibre. Due to this difference in fibre density and because it is unlikely that all parts of a nucleus will be stimulated, only part of the efferent fibres may be stimulated, whereas most neurons may be inhibited by the afferent fibres.

In motor cortex stimulation (MCS) the situation is different. PET-scan imaging during MCS in chronic pain patients revealed that during stimulation the regional cerebral blood flow (rCBF) in the cortex below the epidural electrode was not increased (García-Larrea et al., 1999). Since a higher rCBF results predominantly from an increase in synaptic activity, it was concluded that cortical afferents near the electrode are not activated. In contrast, other brain structures innervated by motor cortex efferents showed increased metabolism during MCS. Because in MCS the stimulus amplitude is kept low to avoid muscular activity, it is likely that in the precentral cortex only efferent fibres to the medial thalamus are activated.

In SCS, stimulation of nerve fibres is limited by the narrow amplitude window of the stimuli between the perception threshold of paraesthesiae and the discomfort threshold. It was calculated that only $A\alpha\beta$ fibres in dorsal rootlets near the cathode, and less than 140 $A\alpha\beta$ fibres in the outer layer of the dorsal columns (< 0.3 mm) can be stimulated. (See Section 4).

6. Effects of pulse amplitude, pulse width and pulse rate

Generally, electrical stimuli have a rectangular shape and are referred to as pulses. The common way to raise the stimulus intensity is by increasing its amplitude (current, voltage). According to the relationship between the threshold amplitude of a pulse and its duration (see Section 5.1), the stimulus intensity can also be raised by increasing the pulse duration while keeping the amplitude constant. According to the shape of the strength–duration curve (Fig. 9) the stimulus intensity is most sensitive to variations in pulse duration in a range up to the chronaxie (τ_{sd}). When the pulse duration exceeds τ_{sd} the stimulus intensity is changed more efficiently by varying the pulse amplitude.

When a nerve fibre is stimulated by a train of identical pulses it will generate an action potential following each single pulse as long as the pulse rate is not too high. According to the channel kinetics of the neural membrane (Hodgkin and Huxley, 1952) each action potential is followed by a temporary inactivation of the sodium channels. The corresponding time interval of a few milliseconds, the *refractory period*, is inversely related to the nerve fibre diameter.

When a nerve fibre bundle is stimulated at a low rate, all recruited fibres will respond simultaneously to each single pulse. When the pulse interval becomes smaller than the refractory period of some of the fibres, the activation pattern of the fibre bundle will become desynchronised. The largest fibres may still follow the stimulus pulse rate, whereas smaller ones will only be excited by each second pulse, etc. Only an unphysiologically high pulse rate (300–500 pps or more) may block neural transmission of the applied stimuli and thereby prevent a (therapeutic) effect, either by inactivation of sodium channels in the nerve fibre membranes (*depolarisation block*), or by depletion of neurotransmitter substance in their presynaptic endings.

When stimulus pulses are given at a 'physiological' rate (below ~ 300 pps), as in most clinical applications of neuromodulation, an increasing rate will induce an increasing postsynaptic effect, being either a larger depolarisation or hyperpolarisation, mediated by excitatory and inhibitory synapses, respectively. Because these postsynaptic neurons are generally part of a *non-linear* network, an increase of the (therapeutic) effect will only occur over a limited range of pulse rates.

Beyond a particular rate the effect may deteriorate. Such a non-linear effect has been shown in the treatment of Parkinsonian and essential tremor with DBS (Benabid et al., 1991). Whereas no effect on tremor can be obtained at pulse rates below ~ 60 pps, the pulse amplitude needed to suppress tremor is initially reduced and subsequently increased at a progressive increase of the pulse rate. The threshold amplitude is lowest when the pulse rate is about 150 pps, implying that this optimal rate corresponds to a minimum number of neurons that need to be stimulated.

7. Voltage-controlled and current-controlled stimulation

Historically, clinical implantable neurostimulation systems have generally been voltage-controlled as are cardiac pacemakers. In contrast, current-controlled stimulation is common in experimental studies. Voltage-control means that during a stimulation pulse the output voltage V of the pulse generator is regulated. Generally V is kept constant, thus creating a rectangular voltage pulse. The related current I is automatically adapted to obey Ohm's law: $I = V/Z$, where Z is the actual load impedance. Z consists of the complex, time varying impedances of the electrode–tissue interfaces in series with the resistances of the tissue and the cable connections to the pulse generator (Holsheimer et al., 2000a). In contrast, a current-controlled pulse generator keeps I constant, whereas V is automatically adapted according to the actual value of Z. This value may vary over time due to initial oedema after implantation, growth of a fibrous tissue layer encapsulating the electrodes, and scar tissue growth near the electrodes. These morphological changes generally occur within 6–12 weeks after implantation.

Because AF and thus the excitation of nerve fibres is directly related to the injected current I (Section 2.1), the pulse amplitude needed to activate fibres with current-controlled pulses is not influenced by the value of Z. In chronic stimulation the initial current setting (mA) generally requires no correction over time, except when a change in excitability of the target nerve fibres occurs. In voltage-controlled stimulation, however, the voltage needed is influenced by the value of Z and may thus vary over time. In chronic, voltage-controlled stimulation the amplitude setting (V) has to be adapted regularly, particularly in the first few months after implantation.

The relationship between V and I is more complex when multiple cathodes and/or anodes are active in voltage- or current-controlled stimulation with a single pulse generator. The current ratio of e.g. two anodes in tripolar 'guarded cathode' stimulation will change when the Z-ratio of the two anodes varies over time. This change in current distribution among electrodes results in a change of the electric field and may alter paraesthesia coverage and pain relief, particularly when cathodes are concerned. The only way to control the electric field and thus paraesthesiae in multiple electrode stimulation is by controlling the current of each cathode and anode independently, i.e. by providing each cathode and anode with its own current source.

Since current consumption determines battery life of an implanted pulse generator, it is important that stimulation current can be determined in the first place. This is, however, impossible when a voltage-controlled pulse generator is used, because I is determined by both the selected V and the unknown Z. Nevertheless, it is often erroneously assumed that a reduction of V implies a reduction of I, and vice versa. When, e.g. in SCS monopolar stimulation is replaced by bipolar stimulation, the perception threshold voltage V_p is increased because Z is raised, although the perception threshold current I_p is reduced. When bipolar stimulation is changed into tripolar 'guarded cathode' stimulation, V_p is reduced because both Z and I_p got less. When, however, a second cathode instead of an anode has been added, V_p would not change, whereas I_p would be increased.

By these examples it is shown that V is an unreliable indicator of I and thus an unreliable predictor of battery life.

The foregoing demonstrates that current-controlled pulse generators have advantages over voltage-controlled stimulators. Recently, the first current-controlled SCS system found its way to the neurostimulation market.

8. Safety aspects of neurostimulation

Stimulation related tissue damage may have various origins. The insertion of an electrode causes some tissue disruption and oedema, usually resulting in a temporary inactivation ('shock') of the neuronal tissue surrounding the electrode. The insertion of a DBS electrode in e.g. the Vim nucleus of a patient with Parkinson's disease may result in a temporary block of the tremor before any stimulation is given.

Any implant is recognized as a foreign body and provokes the generation of a fibrous tissue layer encapsulating all parts of the implant. If any mechanical stress imposed by the implant on the surrounding tissue is absent, as would be expected with an electrode in the brain, this encapsulation layer will be small (~ 70 μm). If, however, mechanical stress is exerted by the implant on the surrounding tissue, possibly accompanied by movement of the implant with respect to this tissue, excessive connective tissue growth may occur locally, giving rise to additional pressure and eventually electrode dislocation. This process may happen in SCS, where the electrode is in a small volume of epidural fat with both flexible and firm structures dorsally: the vertebral arches and ligaments. In SCS mechanical stress is frequently present, as shown by the dislocation of SCS electrodes. An excessive connective tissue layer covering cathode(s) and anode(s) will reduce the efficacy of the stimulation, because stimulation voltages are increased.

Another mechanism potentially damaging the nervous tissue to be stimulated is caused by electrochemical reactions at the electrode–tissue interface. Because a noble metal is generally used as the electrode material (platinum), this material will not be oxidized and dissolved at the anode surface. There will thus be no toxic effect of metal ions in the tissue surrounding the anode. At the cathode, however, oxygen molecules present in the interstitial fluid are electrochemically reduced and this process is accompanied by the irreversible formation of free radicals. These highly reactive and toxic species are known to damage cell membranes, protein molecules and DNA molecules. In their study Morton and colleagues (1994) demonstrated that a substantial quantity of oxygen molecules is reduced to cations during a typical neurostimulation pulse. It is, therefore, important to minimize the amount of free radicals diffusing from the cathode into the neighbouring tissue, particularly because neural stimulation takes place near the cathode (see Section 2.2). Different stimulation parameters should be considered to achieve this goal.

Part of the free radicals generated near a cathode can be neutralized by oxidation when the cathodic pulse is followed by an anodic one. Morton and colleagues (1994) concluded that the reduction of oxygen, and thus the generation of free radicals, is restricted most when the cathodic pulse has a small width and when this pulse is immediately followed by an anodic pulse which holds the same charge. This principle is known as biphasic, charge-balanced stimulation (Lilly et al., 1955). Most neurostimulation systems deliver pulses of this type.

The amount of reduced oxygen and free radicals produced by stimulation is most probably proportional to both the current density (or charge density) at the cathode–tissue interface and the transported charge/phase (current times cathodic phase duration). McCreery and colleagues (1990) investigated the neural damage in cortical grey matter resulting from stimulation with different combinations of charge density and charge/phase of biphasic, charge-balanced pulses. The authors proposed maximum safe values for the combination of these stimulation parameters to be used in the stimulation of grey matter. Haberler's group (2000) observed that no damage was present in the brain tissue near the DBS electrode in the thalamic Vim nucleus (6 cases) and STN (2 cases) of patients with Parkinson's disease after continuous stimulation for up to 70 months.

McCreery and colleagues (1992) compared the early axonal degeneration of the sciatic nerve of cats resulting from continuous stimulation during 8 h at 50 pps with two different waveforms. They demonstrated that biphasic, charge-balanced pulses of 50 µs/phase without any delay between the two phases results in less degeneration than biphasic pulses of 100 µs/phase and a 400 µs delay between the two phases. These results support the suggestions made by Morton and colleagues (1994). With both waveforms, the threshold current for early axonal degeneration exceeded the current required to excite all large axons in the sciatic nerve.

Because the transported charge is also related to the rate at which pulses are given, McCreery's group (1995) investigated the effect of pulse rate and pulse amplitude on the early axonal degeneration of the sciatic nerve in cats after 7 days of continuous stimulation, using biphasic, charge-balanced pulses. They concluded that continuous stimulation at 50 pps and an amplitude that recruits all large fibres in a peripheral nerve is not harmful.

It is highly unlikely that electrochemical damage to the spinal cord and the motor cortex will result from SCS and MCS, respectively, because in both cases the epidural electrode is separated from the neuronal tissue by the dura mater, the arachnoid, the pia mater and the cerebro-spinal fluid (CSF). Wesselink and colleagues (1998) calculated the charge/phase and the maximum charge density under various conditions similar to those in clinical SCS. They concluded that of all selectable stimulation parameters only *PW* affects the charge/pulse and the charge density in the nervous tissue, whereas both *PW* and the electrode surface area strongly affect these parameters in the non-neural tissue surrounding the epidural electrodes.

9. Conclusions

- In bi-, tri- and multipolar stimulation, activation of nerve fibres happens near a cathode because much lower currents are needed than in anodic stimulation. Monopolar stimulation is, therefore, always applied by a cathode.
- For optimal stimulation of the neuronal target, the position of the cathode(s) is more critical than the position of the anode(s).
- Stimulation-induced excitation of a nerve fibre is followed by bidirectional propagation of the action potential: orthodromic and antidromic.
- In clinical neurostimulation (PNS, SCS, DBS, MCS), phenomena such as cathodic block, anodic excitation and anodic block are unlikely to occur.
- Tripolar 'guarded cathode' stimulation and, to a lesser extent, bipolar stimulation selectively favour the activation of fibres in parallel to the bi/tripole axis. In SCS these electrode combinations most likely improve paraesthesia coverage in chronic pain patients.
- The threshold current to stimulate a nerve fibre increases with the distance between the fibre and the cathode, and is inversely related to the fibre diameter.
- The preferential stimulation of large nerve fibres is favoured most when short pulses (~60 µs) are applied. Smaller fibres can be activated more easily when pulses are wider. In SCS wide pulses (0.5–1 ms) may result in improved paraesthesia coverage.
- Therapeutic effects achieved through neuronal activation (including inhibitory effects) will occur only within a limited range of frequency; unphysiologically high rates (300–500 pps or above) may cause a depolarisation block or depletion of neurotransmitter.
- When a brain nucleus or cortical grey matter is stimulated, axons are the neuronal elements

responding to the stimulation. Whether afferent or efferent fibres are predominantly stimulated depends on the stimulation conditions.

- Due to changes in the tissue impedance around the electrodes, the amplitude setting of a voltage-controlled pulse generator needs regular corrections for an optimal clinical effect, particularly in the first 2–3 months after implantation. A current-controlled system does not need such corrections.
- Current consumption is minimized and battery life is maximized when stimulation is given with a 'guarded cathode' parallel to the fibre bundle to be stimulated in PNS (nerve trunk) and SCS (dorsal columns).
- Battery life is also favoured by a short pulse width, because the charge/pulse rises substantially when the pulse width is increased.
- The amplitude (V) of a voltage-controlled pulse generator is an unreliable predictor of battery life.
- Biphasic, charge-balanced pulses with a short initial phase and a minimum phase interval should be used to minimize electrochemically induced neuronal damage. Axonal damage is unlikely to occur under clinical stimulation conditions.

List of symbols

AF	activating function [V]
I	stimulation current [mA]
I_p	paraesthesia threshold current [mA]
I_{th}	threshold current for nerve fibre excitation [mA]
I_{rh}	rheobase current [mA]
τ_m	membrane time constant [ms]
τ_{sd}	strength–duration time constant [ms]
V	voltage between stimulator outputs [V]
V_p	paraesthesia threshold voltage [V]
v	propagation velocity of action potentials [m/s]
Z	impedance between stimulator outputs [Ohm]

Parameters of myelinated axon model

R_m	membrane resistance [Ohm]
R_a	intra-axonal resistance of an internodal section [Ohm]
C_m	membrane capacity [µF]
$I_{m,n}$	transmembrane current at node n [mA]
$V_{e,n}$	extracellular potential at node n [V]
$V_{a,n}$	intracellular potential at node n [V]

Stimulation modalities and anatomical structures

DBS	deep brain stimulation
MCS	motor cortex stimulation
PNS	peripheral nerve stimulation
SCS	spinal cord stimulation
GPe	external pallidum
GPi	internal pallidum
STN	subthalamic nucleus
Vim	ventral intermediate nucleus

References

BeMent, S.L. and Ranck, J.B. (1969) A quantitative study of electrical stimulation of central myelinated fibers with monopolar electrodes. Exp. Neurol., 24: 147–170.

Benabid, A.L. (2002) Mechanisms of deep brain stimulation (Commentary). Mov. Disord., 17(Suppl. 3): S73–S74.

Benabid, A.L., Pollak, P., Gervason, C., Hoffmann, D., Gao, D.M., Hommel, M., Perret, J.E., and De Rougemont, J. (1991) Long-term suppression of tremor by chronic stimulation of the ventral intermediate thalamic nucleus. Lancet, 337: 403–406.

Benazzouz, A., Piallat, B., Pollak, P., and Benabid, A.L. (1995) Responses of substantia nigra pars reticulata and globus pallidus complex to high frequency stimulation of the subthalamic nucleus in rats: electrophysiological data. Neurosci. Lett., 189: 77–80.

Boraud, T., Bezard, E., Bioulac, B., and Gross, C. (1996) High frequency stimulation of the internal globus pallidus (GPi) simultaneously improves parkinsonian symptoms and reduces the firing frequency of GPi neurons in MPTP-treated monkey. Neurosci. Lett., 215: 17–20.

Bostock, H. (1983) The strength–duration relationship for excitation of myelinated nerve: computed dependence on membrane parameters. J. Physiol. (Lond.), 341: 59–74.

Dostrovsky, J.O. and Lozano, A.M. (2002) Mechanisms of deep brain stimulation. Mov. Disord., 17(Suppl. 3): S63–S68.

Feirabend, H.K.P., Choufoer, H., Ploeger, S., Holsheimer, J., and Van Gool, J.D. (2002) Morphometry of human superficial dorsal and dorsolateral column fibres: significance to spinal cord stimulation. Brain, 125: 1137–1149.

Frankenhaeuser, B. and Huxley, A.F. (1964) The action potential in the myelinated nerve fibre of Xenopus Laevis as computed on the basis of voltage clamp data. J. Physiol. (Lond.), 171: 302–315.

García-Larrea, L., Peyron, R., Mertens, P., Gregoire, M.C., Lavenne, F., Le Bars, D., Convers, P., Mauguière, F., Sindou, M., Laurent, B. (1999) Electrical stimulation of motor cortex for pain control: a combined PET-scan and electrophysiological study. Pain, 83: 259–273.

Guljarani, R.M. (1998) *Bioelectricity and Biomagnetism*, Wiley, New York.

Haberler, C., Alesch, F., Mazal, P.R., Pilz, P., Jellinger, K., Pinter, M.M., Hainfellner, J.A., and Budka, H. (2000) No tissue damage by chronic deep brain stimulation in Parkinson's disease. Ann. Neurol., 48: 372–376.

He, J., Barolat, G., and Ketcik, B. (1994) Stimulation usage range for chronic pain management. Analgesia, 1: 75–80.

Hodgkin, A.L. and Huxley, A.F. (1952) A quantitative description of membrane currents and its application to conduction and excitation in nerve. J. Physiol. (Lond.), 117: 500–544.

Holsheimer, J. (1997) Effectiveness of spinal cord stimulation in the management of chronic pain: analysis of technical drawbacks and solutions. Neurosurgery, 40: 990–996.

Holsheimer, J. (2002) Which neuronal elements are activated directly by spinal cord stimulation. Neuromodulation, 5: 25–31.

Holsheimer, J. and Wesselink, W.A. (1997) Optimum electrode geometry for spinal cord stimulation: the narrow bipole and tripole. Med. Biol. Eng. Comput., 35: 493–497.

Holsheimer, J., Dijkstra, E.A., Demeulemeester, H., and Nuttin, B. (2000a) Chronaxie calculated from current-duration and voltage-duration data. J. Neurosci. Methods, 97: 45–50.

Holsheimer, J., Demeulemeester, H., Nuttin, B., and De Sutter, P. (2000b) Identification of the target neuronal elements in electrical deep brain stimulation. Eur. J. Neurosci., 12: 4573–4577.

Krainick, J.U., Thoden, U., and Riechert, T. (1975) Spinal cord stimulation in post-amputation pain. Surg. Neurol., 4: 167–170.

Lilly, J.C., Hughes, J.R., Alvord, E.C., and Galkin, T.W. (1955) Brief, noninjurious electric waveform for stimulation of the brain. Science, 121: 468–469.

Malmivuo, J. and Plonsey, R. (1995) Bioelectromagnetism, Principles and Applications of Bioelectric and Biomagnetic Fields. On website: www.tut.fi/~ malmivuo/bem/bembook.

McCreery, D.B., Agnew, W.F., Yuen, T.G.H., and Bullara, L.A. (1990) Charge density and charge per phase as cofactors in the induction of neural injury by electrical stimulation. IEEE Trans. Biomed. Eng., 37: 996–1001.

McCreery, D.B., Agnew, W.F., Yuen, T.G.H., and Bullara, L.A. (1992) Damage in peripheral nerve from continuous electrical stimulation: comparison of two stimulus waveforms. Med. Biol. Eng. Comput., 30: 109–114.

McCreery, D.B., Agnew, W.F., Yuen, T.G.H., and Bullara, L.A. (1995) Relationship between stimulus amplitude, stimulus frequency and neural damage during electrical stimulation of sciatic nerve of cat. Med. Biol. Eng. Comput., 33: 426–429.

McNeal, D.R. (1976) Analysis of a model for excitation of myelinated nerve. IEEE Trans. Biomed. Eng., 23: 329–337.

Mogyoros, I., Lin, C., Dowla, S., Grosskreutz, J., and Burke, D. (1999) Strength–duration properties and their voltage-dependence at different sites along the median nerve. Clin. Neurophysiol., 110: 1618–1624.

Mogyoros, I., Lin, C., Dowla, S., Grosskreutz, J., and Burke, D. (2000) Reproducibility of indices of axonal excitability in human subjects. Clin. Neurophysiol., 111: 23–28.

Morton, S.L., Daroux, M.L., and Mortimer, J.T. (1994) The role of oxygen reduction in electrical stimulation of neural tissue. J. Electrochem. Soc., 141: 122–130.

North, R.B., Ewend, M.G., Lawton, M.T., and Piantadosi, S. (1991) Spinal cord stimulation for chronic, intractable pain: superiority of "multichannel" devices. Pain, 44: 119–130.

North, R.B., Kidd, D.H., Olin, J.C., and Sieracki, J.M. (2002) Spinal cord stimulation electrode design: prospective, randomized, controlled trial comparing percutaneous and laminectomy electrodes. Part I: Technical outcomes. Neurosurgery, 51: 381–389.

Nowak, L.G. and Bullier, J. (1998a) Axons, but not cell bodies, are activated by electrical stimulation in cortical gray matter. I. Evidence from chronaxie measurements. Exp. Brain Res., 118: 477–488.

Nowak, L.G. and Bullier, J. (1998b) Axons, but not cell bodies, are activated by electrical stimulation in cortical gray matter. II. Evidence from selective inactivation of cell bodies and axon initial segments. Exp. Brain Res., 118: 489–500.

Ranck, J.B. (1975) Which elements are excited in electrical stimulation of mammalian central nervous system: a review. Brain Res., 98: 417–440.

Rattay, F. (1986) Analysis of models for external stimulation of axons. IEEE Trans. Biomed. Eng., 33: 974–977.

Rijkhoff, N.J.M., Koldewijn, E.L., Van Kerrebroeck, P.E.V., Debruyne, F.M.J., and Wijkstra, H. (1994) Acute animal studies on the use of an anodal block to reduce urethral resistance in sacral root stimulation. IEEE Trans. Rehabil. Eng., 2: 92–99.

Swadlow, H.A. (1992) Monitoring the excitability of neocortical efferent neurons to direct activation by extracellular current pulses. J. Neurophysiol., 68: 605–619.

Wee, A.S. (2001) Anodal excitation of intact peripheral nerves in humans. Electromyogr. Clin. Neurophysiol., 41: 71–77.

Wee, A.S., Leis, A.A., Kuhn, A.R., and Gilbert, R.W. (2000) Anodal block: can this occur during routine nerve conduction studies?. Electromyogr. Clin. Neurophysiol., 40: 387–391.

Weiss, G. (1901) Sur la possibilité de rendre comparables entre eux les appareils servant à l'excitation électrique. Arch. Ital. Biol., 35: 413–446.

Wesselink, W.A., Holsheimer, J., and Boom, H.B.K. (1998) Analysis of current density and related parameters in spinal cord stimulation. IEEE Trans. Rehabil. Eng., 6: 200–207.

Wesselink, W.A., Holsheimer, J., and Boom, H.B.K. (1999) A model of the electrical behavior of myelinated sensory nerve fibres based on human data. Med. Biol. Eng. Comput., 37: 228–235.

West, D.C. and Wolstencroft, J.H. (1983) Strength-duration characteristics of myelinated and non-myelinated bulbospinal axons in the cat spinal cord. J. Physiol (Lond.), 337: 37–50.

Electrical Stimulation and the Relief of Pain
Pain Research and Clinical Management, Vol. 15
Edited by Brian A. Simpson

CHAPTER 4

Transcutaneous and peripheral nerve stimulation

Michael Stanton-Hicks*

Department of Pain Management, Division of Anesthesiology, Cleveland Clinic, 9500 Euclid Avenue, Desk C-25,
Cleveland, OH 44195, USA

Abstract

From its origins in the 1960s, peripheral nerve stimulation showed promise in the management of neuropathic pain that is not amenable to other forms of neurostimulation or pharmacological treatment. The ability to achieve analgesia by the application of electrical energy to a nerve in the distribution of which a source of neuropathic pain resides is an attractive concept. As is described in this chapter, the main limitation to successful treatment is the availability of specific electrodes that conform to the size and shape of the target nerves and are highly reliable. Early experience with peripheral nerve stimulation was fraught with unreliable equipment and a failure to appreciate the micro-anatomy of nerve function which led to an unacceptable morbidity and to abandonment of the technique by many physicians. However, in the hands of a few dedicated individuals, the technique has developed to a point where it is now used not only for peripheral nerves in the extremities, but also for other segmental nerves, cranial nerves and nerve roots. These latter applications are limited only by the availability of specific electrodes.

Transcutaneous electrical nerve stimulation (TENS) was studied and underwent development in parallel with peripheral nerve stimulation. While its application is much less specific and it is frequently used for myofascial pain syndromes that are associated either with neuropathic pain or with other pathology, the principle of using electrical energy to achieve analgesia is similar to that of direct peripheral nerve stimulation.

Keywords: Peripheral nerve stimulation (PNS); Transcutaneous electrical nerve stimulation (TENS); Neurostimulation; Neuromodulation; Electrode; Pulse generator

1. Background

Work by Wall and Sweet (1967), which showed that electrical stimulation of a nerve could achieve hypaesthesia and analgesia distal to the point of stimulation, opened up the era of what has come to be known as stimulation produced analgesia (SPA) (MacKay, 1841; Reynolds, 1969; Mayer and Liebeskind, 1974; Long and Hagfors, 1975).

It is no accident that electrical stimulation has been used by man for the treatment of painful conditions for millennia. Various fishes related to the families torpedinidae and narkidae were used by the ancient Egyptians, Greeks and Romans for the treatment of gout, headache and other maladies. Even Althaus (1859) noted in a treatise of medical electricity that analgesia and anaesthesia developed with the onset of paraesthesiae

---
*Correspondence to: Dr. Michael Stanton-Hicks, Department of Pain Management, Division of Anesthesiology, Cleveland Clinic, 9500 Euclid Avenue, Desk C-25, Cleveland, OH 44195, USA. Phone: + 1-216-445-9559; Fax: + 1-216-444-9890; E-mail: stantom@ccf.org

during electrical stimulation of major nerve trunks. It was not until the publication by Melzack and Wall (1965) of the Gate Control Theory, however, that interest in its practical application was galvanized. During early clinical experimentation with spinal cord stimulation (SCS) it became clear that for many patients their pain remained unrelieved (Sweet and Wepsic, 1974). As a result, an interest in other methods of stimulation, including transcutaneous stimulation (TENS) and peripheral nerve stimulation (PNS) increased (Picaza et al., 1975; Nashold et al., 1979, 1982; Stanton-Hicks and Salamon, 1997).

Long and Hagfors (1975) found that a square wave pulse stimulator with controllable amplitude and frequency was effective in reducing or relieving some types of neuropathic pain. Although there is a large body of information containing clinical reports of TENS, the success rate, at least for early intervention, is quite consistent, being around 60–80% (Sweet, 1976; Cooperman et al., 1977; Long et al., 1979; Taylor et al., 1981; Bourke et al., 1984; Roche et al., 1985). However, the types of pain for which TENS is commonly used vary greatly and it is evident that a placebo effect is particularly important to its successful response. This will be discussed at greater length.

2. Anatomical considerations

2.1. Nerve fibres and fascicular anatomy

Nerve fibres consist of a cylindrical core – *the axon* – that is enclosed by a membrane, the axolemma, surrounded by a complex sheath. This latter structure varies in size depending on the presence or absence of myelin. A myelinated fibre consists of multiple laminae forming the *internodes*, which are interrupted by nodes at varying intervals, depending on the size of the fibre. The myelin sheath is invested in a membrane, the *endoneurium* or endoneural tube, which in non-myelinated fibres may contain several axons, whereas the myelinated fibre contains only a single axon. Of note is the fact

that a given axon may vary in diameter throughout its length from as little as 2 microns (μm) to 11.75 μm (Hubbard, 1976; Peters et al., 1976).

Nerve fibres undergo extensive branching, not only in the subserved tissue, but also in the trunk itself. This anatomical arrangement ensures that activity in a comparatively large mass of tissue can be influenced by a single neuron. The practical lesson from this is that referred pain may originate not only by multiple branching so that nociception mediated by an injured branch is referred to undisturbed tissue, but it may, by axon reflex via branching axons, cause the release of algesic substances in otherwise non-injured tissue. This has a bearing on the effects of neurostimulation, which will be discussed later.

The main physiological types of nerve fibres are motor, the diameter of which varies from 2 to 20 μm; sensory fibres, which vary in diameter from 1.5 to 20 μm and post-ganglionic sympathetic fibres, the diameter of which is less than 2 μm. As a reminder, Table I identifies the functions of the different fibre types.

2.2. Microstructure of nerve trunks

Nerve fibres are collected into fasciculi, each fasciculus being surrounded by a thin laminated sheath of perineural cells and fine collagen tissue.

TABLE I

Summary of characteristics of different nerve fibre types

Nerve fibre		Nerve fibre (diameter in μm)	Conduction velocity (m/s)	Function
A	Alpha	12–20	70–120	Motor, extrafusal muscle fibres, proprioceptors
	Beta	5–12	30–70	Touch, pressure
	Gamma	3–6	15–30	Motor, intrafusal muscle fibres
	Delta	2–5	10–30	Nociceptors, touch, temperature
B		1.5–3	3–15	Pre-ganglionic sympathetic fibres
C		< 2.0	0.5–2	Post-ganglionic sympathetic fibres

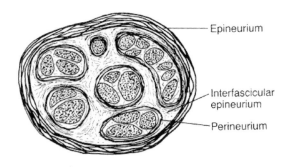

Fig. 1. Cross-section of a nerve trunk showing composition of the epineurium extending between the fasciculi invested by perineurium.

Within this framework are the endoneural tubes surrounding each nerve fibre. All of the fasiculi in a nerve trunk are invested by the loose areolar tissue – the *epineurium* (Fig. 1).

2.3. Fascicular anatomy

Of great importance to neurostimulation is the fact that fasciculi are not arranged in parallel strands, but they repeatedly divide and unite to form plexuses. These plexuses can be demonstrated throughout the entire length of a nerve and continue in this fashion even to the terminal branches – i.e., digital nerves. Most fasciculi vary in size from 0.04 to 2 mm, but occasionally may be as large as 4 mm. Fasciculi are more numerous where a nerve crosses a joint and, with regard to the median and ulnar nerves, there are fewer fasciculi above the elbow compared to the forearm. Of interest is that in certain nerves, nerve fibres may be collected into a single fasciculus for a short distance, i.e. the ulnar nerve behind the medial humeral epicondyle and the radial nerve in the spiral groove, the axillary nerve behind the shoulder and common peroneal nerve in the lower thigh. This fact may have a bearing on placement of neurostimulator electrodes (Sunderland, 1945, 1978; DiRosa et al., 1988).

As each individual nerve trunk passes distally to its regional distribution, the localization of any particular branch system, which in the proximal part of the nerve is random, becomes discrete as the fasciculi approach their terminal branches (Fig. 2a,b).

2.4. The epineurium and blood supply of nerves

The epineurium provides the supporting framework for nerve trunks and gives a normal nerve the distinctive cord-like structure that sets it aside from surrounding tissues. The proportion of epineurial tissue varies between 30 and 75% of a nerve trunk. The only exception to this is the sciatic nerve which may contain as much as 88% epineurial tissue. This too has a bearing on the application of electrical energy from neurostimulator electrodes.

Perineural tissue, as described earlier, is the thin dense sheath that invests each fasciculus. The perineurium is a diffusion barrier and as such does affect local anaesthetic nerve action. The thicker the perineurium and fewer the fasciculi, the more difficult it is to block the nerve.

The blood supply, or vasa nervorum, to a peripheral nerve is shown in Fig. 3. This is provided from neighbouring vessels in an irregular fashion. These nutrient vessels are tortuous to allow for considerable translational movement of the nerve and are most numerous near a joint. The main nutrient artery enters a nerve before branching into its main ascending and descending branches, either on the surface or some distance from and parallel to the nerve. Anastomoses from adjacent vessels occur at intervals along the course of the nerve in a manner similar to reinforcement of the spinal arteries. Because of the irregular anastomotic supply from nutrient arteries, it is imperative during dissection of the nerve that these nutrient vessels be preserved to prevent a comparatively long 'watershed', which under the circumstances of dissection or subsequent scarring, might render the nerve ischaemic. These superficial longitudinal vessels often maintain a constant position on the surface of a nerve. Unlike the blood supply to the spinal cord, the arteriae nervorum are not end-arteries, but have an extensive microvascular network that ensure the

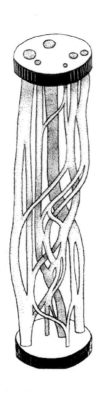

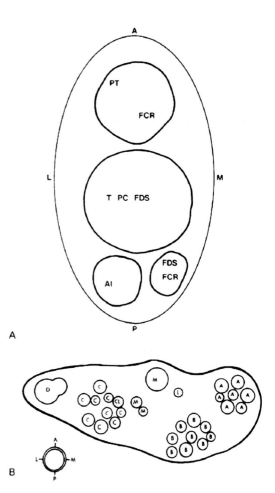

Fig. 2. (a) Reconstruction from transverse sections of musculocutaneous nerve of the arm. (Reproduced with permission from Sunderland: Nerve injuries and their repair. Edinburgh, Churchill Livingstone, 1991, p 32). (b) Transverse section of median nerve, (A) at elbow and (B) at wrist, showing separation of fasciculi as the nerve reaches its distal distribution. M = thenar motor; PT = pronator teres; PC = palmar cutaneous; AI = anterior interosseous; L = lumbrical; FCR = flexor carpi radialis; FDR = flexor digitorum sup.; ABC = 1st, 2nd and 3rd cutaneous to digital areas; D = cutaneous to radial aspect thumb (after Sunderland, 1991).

nutrition of all the elements of the nerve trunk. Having stated this however, it is clear, as in the case of mobilizing the ulnar nerve for example, that the nutrient vessels between the axilla and wrist can be sacrificed without impairing its blood supply. Nevertheless, care should be taken to ensure that these nutrient vessels are separated well away from the nerve in order to maintain satisfactory blood flow to the longitudinal arterial chains on which the nerve is so dependent for an effective collateral circulation.

Although the undisturbed blood supply is in excess of normal metabolic needs, mobilization

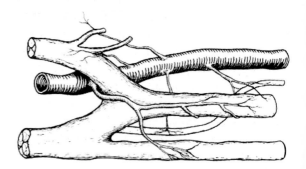

Fig. 3. Vascular supply to axillary nerves from the axillary artery. (Reproduced with permission from Sunderland. Nerve injuries and their repair. Edinburgh, Churchill Livingstone, 1991, p 53.)

and transposing a 2–3 cm segment of the ulnar nerve anterior to the medial humeral epicondyle has been shown to reduce the intraneural flow for 3 days (Ogata and Naito, 1986). Also, mobilization of proximal and distal segments of a nerve to facilitate end-to-end union should not extend beyond a critical limit of 8 cm (Smith, 1966a,b). Other indirect and direct evidence has implicated sclerosing pathology that narrows or occludes nutrient arteries, in reducing the development of collateral circulation and nutrition of nerve fibres. Much of the morbidity associated with early peripheral nerve stimulation electrodes can be attributed to interference with the nutritional supply by a stricture and intra-epineural sclerosis. In summary, it can be stated that the peripheral re-supply to nerve trunks by adjacent anastomotic vessels is important to the maintenance of structural and functional integrity of peripheral axons, and therefore every attempt should be made to preserve this during any surgical procedure on a nerve.

3. Transcutaneous electrical nerve stimulation (TENS)

One of the principal foundations of the Gate Control Theory applied to neurostimulation is that stimulation of primary afferent (A fibres) can inhibit C fibre evoked activity. This has been confirmed by electrophysiological, behavioural and chemical studies. An extensive literature attests to the prolonged relief of symptoms in about 60% of patients with acute pain and 30% with chronic pain by TENS. Wall and Sweet's description in 1967 was the first to demonstrate that prolonged stimulation of peripheral nerves by percutaneously placed needle electrodes can modify neuropathic pain or noxious stimuli. By using vibration (and stimulation of A-beta fibres), TENS or peripheral nerve stimulation, local inhibitory circuits within the dorsal horn of the spinal cord, and no doubt other sites rostral in the neuraxis, can be activated to modify or eliminate noxious input. Generally, low amplitude electrical stimulation is required.

3.1. Technical considerations

Electrical stimulation is provided by a pulse generator in which various configurations of pulse width – rectangular, triangular, sine wave, exponential, bi-phasic or a combination of these wave forms – are used in conjunction with varying rates (frequency) or 'bursts' of low or high frequencies. Because of varying impedance due to the interface between the delivering electrode and the skin, this can be achieved by use of a constant current generator that will provide constant stimulation in spite of changing impedance. Conversely, a constant voltage amplifier would be unpleasant and not therapeutic due to the consequences of sudden changes in impedance. The typical range of parameters that are therapeutically effective is a current varying between 1 and 50 milliamperes (mA), frequencies between 1 and 100 Hertz (Hz) and a pulse width that varies between 0.1 and 0.5 milliseconds (ms). Generally, rectangular pulse waves provide greatest utility although many theories and 'voodoo' would suggest bi-phasic pulses and combinations of different parameters may have more therapeutic effect.

Electrodes used for the delivery of TENS therapy are generally a dual electrolyte-impregnated sponge, silver/silver clad electrodes/tapes or a rubber-silicone material that is impregnated with carbon particles (Brennan, 1976). Depending on the atopic characteristics of the individual, it may be necessary to try different electrodes in order to find a compatible system. Maintaining the electrode–skin interface is probably the most difficult aspect in successful TENS therapy. The typical resistance of a silicone-rubber/carbon electrode is about 10 Ω/cm^2 and the current density falls off exponentially in a centrifugal fashion. Because the typical current density for TENS is 1–5 mA/cm^2, electrodes must be a minimum of 4 cm^2; otherwise skin irritation from high current density will preclude their use (Mason and MacKay, 1976). Furthermore, if there is an increase in impedance due to drying of electrolyte or distraction of the electrode surface, the otherwise pleasant feeling of vibration will be replaced by a disagreeable burning or prickling pain, and thermal damage to the outer layer of the skin can occur (Woolf and Thompson, 1994). Another factor determining satisfactory TENS therapy is varying skin thickness yielding changing impedance (Seligman, 1982). Also, electrochemical changes below the skin can result in the formation of an ionic bi-layer with an increase in impedance and reduction in current density which has been an argument for the use of bi-phasic electrical stimulation, although Seligman and others showed that cathodal rectangular pulses do not contribute to the ionic bi-layer as the interval is of sufficient duration between pulses to allow for anodal charge recovery (Bütikofer and Lawrence, 1979; Seligman, 1982).

3.2. Practical application

The aim of TENS is to activate sensory myelinated fibres without causing motor defects or dysaesthesia. The site of stimulation should be proximal to the source of pain and should be directed to afferent nerve endings in the vicinity rather than the nerve trunk itself. High frequencies, which would activate A-delta fibres, are not tolerated and, therefore, low frequency stimulation in the vicinity of 40–70 Hz and a pulse width of 0.1–0.5 ms are best tolerated. Therapeutic efficacy of TENS may be achieved as early as 20 min, but in some patients it may require several hours. In the case of chronic pain, it is evident that a cumulative effect of TENS will cause the relief of pain to occur with continuous stimulation requiring several weeks (Thompson, 1986; Thompson and Filshie, 1993). Interestingly, some patients receive relief from TENS therapy only after the stimulation has been removed.

3.3. TENS trial

As with most indications for neurostimulation, it is necessary to first trial the procedure to: (a) ensure that pain is not aggravated, (b) familiarize the patient with the system and (c) ensure that the relief of symptoms is realized. Obviously, in some cases, this may require several weeks. From earlier statements, it should be repeated that a trial of less than an hour is probably inadequate.

Transcutaneous electrical nerve stimulation management is determined during the trial. After directions have been given to the patient, a trial for 1 h, 3 times a day, should be undertaken with adjustments being made as needed. Patients should also be instructed on how to compare continuous with intermittent stimulation. After 1 month TENS use should be reviewed and this should be repeated at 3-month intervals for the first year. If adequate analgesia and/or significant improvement in function is realized, it may be appropriate for the patient to persist with the therapy for as long as it is needed.

3.4. Indications for TENS

The most effective indications for TENS therapy are angina pectoris, failed laminectomy syndrome, post-herpetic neuralgia, diabetic neuropathy and many mononeuropathies (Meyer and Fields, 1972; Nathan and Wall, 1974; Loeser et al., 1975; Mannheimer et al., 1986). Other applications are pain from radiculopathy, compression syndromes, chronic facial pain (atypical facial pain and trigeminal neuralgia; Cauthen and Renner, 1975); central pain states such as brachial plexus avulsion injuries, spinal injury pain and, in some cases, referred visceral pain. A particular indication that has proved salutary is uncontrollable itch.

Transcutaneous electrical nerve stimulation may also be very effective in certain acute pain conditions such as that arising from trauma, from fractured ribs, orofacial pain (Myers et al., 1977; Hansson and Ekblom, 1983; Eriksson et al., 1984) and periodontal infections, including pulpal inflammation, pain associated with acute arthritis, acute myalgia and particularly the myofascial syndrome associated with complex regional pain syndrome (CRPS). TENS has been used successfully for the treatment of labour pain in which case at least 2 sets of electrodes are generally required

(Augustinsson et al., 1977). Some forms of post-operative pain can be treated by TENS, particularly that after abdominal surgery and Caesarian section (Smith et al., 1986). Its use after thoracic surgery, hip replacement, hand operations and lumbar spinal surgery is also reported (Cooperman et al., 1977).

The efficacy of TENS therapy is described mostly in anecdotal reports because of the difficulty of blinded comparisons. Sham stimulation usually involves a device (TENS unit) without the capacity to deliver a current. However, it is difficult to accept the argument that sham stimulation represents a placebo effect when the patient is aware that stimulation paraesthesiae are absent. More recently, however, double blinded, randomized controlled trials would seem to have vindicated the earlier anecdotal reports that this form of electrical stimulation is, in fact, therapeutic (Pike, 1978; Solomon et al., 1980). Certainly, a placebo effect of approximately 33% is apparent, but the continuing efficacy of TENS stimulation underscores a therapeutic effect that is not placebo. In one study by Harrison and colleagues (1986) in which TENS was compared with sham stimulation for labour pain, the authors found that patients were thoroughly impressed by the use of TENS, in spite of the fact that there was no reduction in their peak pain. The authors suggested that the modality might reduce the 'disturbing nature' of pain without materially affecting its intensity. Many controlled studies (for example Thorsteinsson et al., 1977) found that TENS was 3 times more effective than placebo in the management of chronic neuropathies. Likewise, Long and colleagues (1979) noted that the placebo effect was highest on the first day, but was negligible by the end of the first month. A double blinded study of 1 year duration in which TENS was used to treat the pain of osteoarthritis found that the pain relief from stimulation was far greater than any placebo effect, even at the end of the 12-month period (Taylor et al., 1981).

An interesting study reported that the indirect changes in post-operative oxygen tension (pO_2),

lung capacity and functional residual capacity of patients treated by TENS after upper abdominal surgery were much less affected than in sham stimulated patients (Ali et al., 1981). The obvious conclusion was that TENS minimized the tendency towards decremental changes in respiratory mechanics due to pain-induced splinting of the diaphragm.

3.5. Stimulation parameters

It is difficult to make a specific recommendation for stimulation parameters when so many contradictory schemes are described in the literature (Linzer and Long, 1976; Mannheimer and Carlsson, 1979). Frequencies from 1–5 Hz to as much as 100–150 Hz are described. Most patients, however, when given a choice of frequency will select a range between 40 and 70 Hz. When low-frequency stimulation is used, a much higher intensity is necessary to evoke unpleasant symptoms equivalent to those obtained at high frequencies (Andersson et al., 1976). The disadvantage of high intensity/low frequency stimulation is the possibility of causing unpleasant muscle contraction.

Tolerance to TENS therapy is not as significant a phenomenon as that which is frequently seen with pharmacologic agents, although Loeser and colleagues (1975) noted that 68% of 198 patients obtained short-term relief with TENS but this number fell to 12% over a prolonged period. In a carefully supervised 3-year trial, Ericksson et al. (1979) reported that at 2 months, 55% of patients had effective pain relief but this number dropped to 41% relief at 12 months. In spite of this, patients were noted to have a significantly reduced analgesic drug requirement. Others have reported similar reductions in efficacy over time.

3.6. Conclusions (TENS)

From the published literature and this author's own experience, TENS therapy is an effective treatment for the management of pain that is of a neuropathic nature. It can be predictably used in patients suffering from chronic musculoskeletal pain of the trunk or limbs, and for pain after trauma or surgery. The outcome of TENS therapy is determined by three factors: (1) the patient, (2) the stimulator (electrodes and settings) and (3) how the outcome is measured; i.e. analgesia, its onset, any post-TENS analgesia and the nature of side effects. The results of two important studies by Johnson et al. are paraphrased in Table II (Johnson et al., 1991a,b).

The implications of these observations is that physicians should give TENS the benefit of the doubt. Furthermore, a minimum of 1 h pre-trial should determine whether the modality is likely to be effective, recognizing that it may take a more protracted use over a month to be more realistic in establishing its overall efficacy. The fact is that TENS can be useful in a variety of acute and chronic painful states and its placebo effect may be an equally important attribute. TENS therapy should be considered an adjunct to other treatments and, as stated, may be quite effective in reducing the dose or need for opiate analgesics.

TABLE II

Transcutaneous electrical nerve stimulation (TENS)

1. No correlation was found in any patient regarding: diagnosis, stimulator or outcome variable or anatomical region.
2. Stimulation was set to give strong, topographic paraesthesiae.
3. In 75% of patients analgesic onset occurred within 0.5 and in 95% of patients within 1 h.
4. TENS reduced the intensity of pain by >half in 47% of patients.
5. Post-TENS analgesia lasted >30 min in 51% of patients; for >1 h in 30% and for >2 h in 20% of patients.
6. TENS was used daily in 75% of patients and in 30% for ≥49 h/week (7 h daily).
7. Pulsed (burst) mode of stimulation was used by 44% of patients.
8. A strong individual preference for pulse frequency and patterns, with continual adjustment, was noted.
9. Skin irritation occurred in one-third of patients due in part to desiccation of the electrode jelly, and in part a result of atopic reaction to the adhesive or its constituents.

Modified from: Johnson et al. (1991a,b).

4. Peripheral nerve stimulation (PNS)

4.1. General and historical considerations

Initial enthusiasm for peripheral nerve stimulation was tempered by the morbidity associated with the electrode design and with the surgical techniques that were used for their implantation (Long et al., 1981). By the early 1980s there were but a mere handful of surgeons in different countries still performing the technique (Kirsch et al., 1975; Campbell and Long, 1976; Nashold et al., 1979, 1982; Law et al., 1981). As a modality for the treatment of neuropathic pain in one or two nerves, PNS is ideal, particularly when its influence is directed to the distribution of the affected nerves. The early investigations by Wall and Sweet (1967) and Sweet and Wepsic (1974) have determined the different approaches adopted. The use of large surface metal electrodes which were the prototype for TENS therapy has already been discussed. Temporary percutaneous electrodes were initially used by the same implanting physicians to test the feasibility of PNS. This method was used by Sweet and Wall for the stimulation of each other's infra-orbital nerves. A trial of PNS by 'open' surgery with the placement of electrodes either on or inside the epineurium, by microdissection, may be undertaken.

From the early experience, it is clear that PNS can be highly successful if: (1) electrophysiologic studies – electromyography (EMG) or somatosensory evoked potentials (SSEP) – can demonstrate abnormalities in the distribution of a peripheral nerve, (2) repeated nerve blocks are effective in relieving pain distal and in the region subserved, (3) a percutaneous trial stimulation proximal to the peripheral nerve lesion provides 50% relief of symptoms, (4) if pain relief in the nerve distribution is less than 50%, but there is a significant improvement in function, blood flow, control of allodynia/hyperalgesia and use of the extremity, (5) the patient understands the limitations and objectives of the therapy and is motivated for success, (6) the patient understands that the modality will reduce, but probably not eliminate, their pain and that it will not cure the condition.

It is worth reviewing some of the early reports, which, although anecdotal, clearly describe those medical conditions that are most likely to respond to this modality. Most of the early electrodes were of a button, bipolar or cuff design. Nashold advocated functional nerve mapping using circumferential electrical stimulation to localize sensory and motor fascicles (Nashold and Goldner, 1975; Nashold et al., 1982; Fig. 4). By paying attention to this detail the authors claimed that it is possible to position an electrode in such a manner that optimal stimulation of afferent fascicles is achieved. While the orientation of sensory and motor fibres in peripheral nerves constantly changes in the more proximal portion of a nerve trunk (*vide supra*; Sunderland, 1945, 1978), the regional motor and sensory components are much more localized in the distal segment (e.g. upper arm vs. forearm). However, unlike the orderly disposition of nerve tracts in the central nervous system, no common map of fibre orientation exists for peripheral nerves. Law and

colleagues (1981) reported a 60% success rate in 20 of 22 patients who had upper extremity post-herpetic/post-traumatic neuropathy. A number of investigators have reported that PNS surgery in the lower extremity is not as successful when it is compared with stimulation of nerves in the upper extremity (Kirsch et al., 1975; Picaza et al., 1975; Campbell and Long, 1976; Sweet, 1976). The difference in efficacy was felt to be a function of electrode placement in which the stress or traction affecting its proximity to the nerve was influenced by weight bearing and movements of the lower extremity (Waisbrod et al., 1985; Gybels and Kupers, 1987). The large diameter of the sciatic nerve was also considered to be a factor affecting efficacy because many afferent fibres deep in the centre of the nerve may not be influenced by surface stimulation (the stimulation amplitude being limited by the threshold of motor fibre stimulation; Goldner et al., 1982).

With the introduction of flat, paddle type electrodes, the success rate of peripheral nerve stimulation increased by an order of magnitude. Two reports by Racz (Racz et al., 1988, 1990) described the use of a 4-contact paddle electrode (Resume® Medtronic, Inc., Minneapolis MN, USA) that is physically separated from the nerve by a thin layer of tissue harvested from an adjacent fascia or tendon. These authors felt that separating the electrode from the epineurium would prevent some of the neurofibrosis from developing that was previously described by Picaza and colleagues (1975). This technique was adopted by other groups (Cooney 1991, 1997; Strege et al., 1994; Hassenbusch et al., 1996; Novak and MacKinnon, 1999) with consistently good results.

The scope of PNS has broadened during the past decade. While the commonest application has been neuropathic pain in the upper and lower extremities with radial, ulnar, median and sciatic nerves or their branches being the most frequent targets, stimulation of a number of other nerves, such as the cranial sensory nerves, occipital, sacral, genitofemoral, ilioinguinal and iliohypogastric nerves has recently been described.

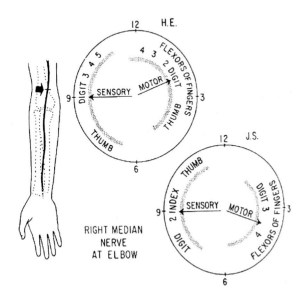

Fig. 4. Functional mapping of a median nerve at elbow. (Reproduced with permission from Nashold and Goldner (1975).)

4.2. Electrode design

While there has been a steady improvement in the technical aspects of PNS, electrode design has languished as a result of the early failures and relative abandonment of the technique for almost 15 years. Reliability of the electronic pulse generators in parallel with cardiac pacemakers is excellent; the two areas that now require close attention, if PNS is to replace central neuraxial stimulation for specific peripheral neuropathic pain conditions, are electrode (lead) design and reliability of the transmission system.

At the present time, the most common electrode used for peripheral nerve stimulation in the United States is the 'Resume®' or 'On-Point®' electrode (Medtronic Corporation). The On-Point® electrode, as can be seen in Fig. 5, has a thin mesh surrounding the paddle which facilitates its fixation to adjacent tissues. In the United States this procedure is approved by the Food and Drug Administration (FDA) for peripheral nerve stimulation in association with a radio frequency (RF) receiver–transmitter system. Many new concepts for electrode design have been proposed. One such example as an alternative to the On-Point®

electrode is shown in Fig. 6. Manifestly, use of a flat electrode with four button contacts of a standard size is ill-equipped to provide uniform stimulation to a 'cylinder' (nerve trunk) the diameter of which may vary in size from 3 to 24 mm. Furthermore, unreliability related to its longitudinal translation, lateral rotation or distraction that can result from fibrosis combined with continuous movements of the adjacent muscles, demands that an electrode placed on the surface of the nerve must conform to the shape of the nerve without inducing any constriction-related morbidity ('ring barking') of the nerve trunk. Another approach is to use a subperineural electrode that is introduced by microdissection. This is a tiny, flexible, platinum multiple contact electrode that has been described by Buschman and Oppel (1999). This type of electrode has undergone extensive research and development for functional (efferent motor) electrical stimulation (Brummer and Turner, 1977a,b,c). Clearly, improvements incorporated in electrode design will ultimately determine whether the full potential for peripheral afferent nerve stimulation is to be realized.

4.3. Surgical technique

Before surgery is contemplated, patients must satisfy the criteria that are outlined in Table III.

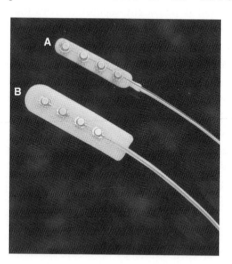

Fig. 5. Peripheral nerve electrodes currently approved by the Food and Drug Administration (FDA) for use in the United States. A. – 'Resume®' and B. – 'On-Point®' Medtronic Corporation.

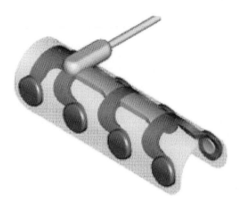

Fig. 6. Example of proposed peripheral nerve electrode. One of the many concepts that have been suggested for this purpose.

TABLE III

Criteria and indications for patient selection for peripheral nerve stimulation

1. Pain in an extremity or nerve distribution that is neuropathic.
2. Demonstration by 1–3 targeted nerve blocks that pain is relieved.
3. EMG demonstration of axonal impact, if appropriate.
4. Pain reduction with a trial of TENS.
5. Psychological testing to exclude psychiatric pathology or specific pain related behaviour.
6. Other factors outlined in Table II.

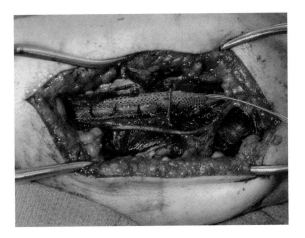

Fig. 7. 'On-Point®' (Medtronic) electrode shown attached to the ulnar nerve. N.B. 4.0 monofilament sutures through nylon gauze and epineurium.

Although any peripheral nerve may be amenable to electrode implantation, the most common nerves for which this procedure is currently used are: the median, ulnar and, radial nerves in the upper extremity, and, in the lower extremity, the sciatic, common peroneal, posterior tibial, femoral, saphenous and sural nerves. Particular nerves are exposed in the following areas: median and ulnar in the brachial groove at the level of the mid humerus; radial nerve in the spiral groove at the same level; common peroneal behind the biceps femoris muscle, superior to the popliteal space; the sciatic nerve is found by the same approach, slightly higher; and the posterior tibial nerve is accessed proximal to the medial malleolus. A length of nerve sufficient to accommodate the electrode is exposed in a manner that preserves the vasa nervorum and will minimize the amount of scar formation.

The procedure may be performed in two stages, the first requiring location of a stimulating electrode adjacent (in apposition) to the target nerve. Although there has been a movement at some centers to abandon the interposition of fascial tissue between electrode and nerve (Fig. 7), this procedure will be described as follows: A flap of fascial tissue is fashioned from an adjacent muscle or, if no convenient tissue is available, a free fascial graft is harvested from a distant muscle and interposed between the electrode and nerve. After ensuring that all four electrode contacts are in close proximity with the nerve, the mesh and fascia are secured using 4.0 or 5.0 monofilament nylon sutures that pass through the mesh, graft and epineurial tissue. If a trial of electrical stimulation is to be undertaken, the electrode lead is then connected to an externalized extension through a stab wound some 15 cm from the main incision. The extension is secured by a purse string suture to the skin. This is followed by a trial period of 1 or 2 days during which time any necessary adjustments to ensure adequate analgesic stimulation are made. The second stage involves fashioning a pocket for the implantable/intracorporeal pulse generator (IPG) and making a tunnel through which the extension cable is drawn. After connecting this to the electrode lead and IPG, it is important to perform intra-operative impedance testing before wound closure. For implants in the upper extremity it is most convenient and cosmetic to fashion a pocket for the RF receiver or IPG on or under the pectoralis fascia near to its tendon and below the clavicle. In a similar manner, a pocket for the RF receiver or IPG is made in the buttock for PNS in the lower extremity. In this latter case, an imaginary line between the posterior superior iliac spine and the greater trochanter at a point that is 45° to the sagittal plane determines the most comfortable site to center the pocket. This author has found that fixation of the larger IPGs (Versitrol®, Synergy®;

Medtronic Corporation) to the fascia or, in thin individuals, beneath the fascia overlying the gluteus medius muscle will avoid any complaints of discomfort without degrading telemetric programmability. It should also be noted, that in a similar manner, the smaller Itrel® (Medtronic Corporation) IPG can also be placed much deeper without any adverse effect on its programmability.

Although all of the early experience was gained with the RF system, the only system currently approved for use with PNS in the United States by the FDA, it has been replaced by most surgeons with the IPG. Because the functional outcome of PNS is so good, and the fact that surgical placement of the electrode accounts for the bulk of the surgical procedure, many surgeons now elect not to subject the patient to a trial, thereby avoiding the second surgical stage. This decision is obviously predicated on very strict criteria and surgical indications for peripheral nerve surgery. These outcomes can also be attributed to good psychological testing as a component of the indications above.

4.4. Stimulation parameters

The range of settings commonly employed for PNS is far narrower than those parameters used for spinal cord stimulation for the following reasons: While some nerves may be purely sensory, the majority of nerves that lend themselves to peripheral nerve stimulation are mixed nerves and the nature of their fascicular architecture makes for a comparatively narrow range between those settings that achieve analgesia through sensory stimulation and settings that reach the threshold for motor stimulation. Treatment parameters commonly used for peripheral nerves range from 0.5 to 2 V, a pulse width that varies between 120 and 180 ms and rates that vary between 50 and 90 Hz (Racz et al., 1990; Weiner, 2000). It is usual to use a continuous stimulation mode until the patient is completely familiar with their system and with the level and manner in which pain relief and function are realized. After 6 months it may be

possible for the patient to experiment with cycling modes. Battery usage with PNS is minimal in comparison with other applications of neurostimulation, 9–10 years' use commonly being reported before battery exhaustion requires replacement of the IPG.

4.5. Outcome of peripheral nerve stimulation

The results of clinical outcome studies most recently reported are in general agreement. Cooney's group recently summarized data on 60 patients that have been followed for over 2 years (Cooney, 1991; Strege et al., 1994). The success in terms of pain relief was over 80% with about 60% having almost complete pain relief and 20% reporting a level of tolerable pain relief. The authors emphasize the need to have complete pain relief following a peripheral nerve block in the affected nerve and appropriate psychiatric assessment before selection for peripheral nerve surgery. Most of their patients had had chronic pain for several years with significant adverse effect on their function. In the study by Hassenbusch and colleagues (1996), 30 patients were treated for complex regional pain syndrome type II of the upper or lower extremities. The authors reported an overall success of 63%. Only five patients experienced no relief and subsequently had their system removed. Of interest in this study is the gradual loss of efficacy between the first and second year of approximately 35%, after which most patients in this group went on to have fair, long term relief, now at 9 years. Twenty-three percent of the successful group either returned to work full-time or changed from no employment to part-time employment. A total of 148 patients have now received peripheral nerve stimulators for complex regional pain syndrome type II or other mononeuropathies.

Schetter's group (1997) have reported their results in 117 patients who have been followed for up to 53 months. In their series, all patients underwent a trial of stimulation, then progressed to surgical implantation of the IPG

(Shetter et al., 1997). The authors reported greater than 70% relief of pain in males and 80% in females; increased activities of daily living in more than 65%, an improvement in sleep and a greater than 75% approval of this form of therapy. A similar return to work experience to that in the Hassenbusch et al. (1996) study is reported by Novak and MacKinnon (1999). These investigators described their experience with PNS in 17 patients (7 men and 10 women) with a mean follow-up time after implantation of 21 months. Eleven patients had good to excellent pain relief, four had fair and two poor relief. In terms of function, the authors noted that of the 12 patients who were unable to work before their surgery, six returned to work afterwards.

In summary, peripheral nerve stimulation for neuropathic pain in an extremity has proven to be a very useful modality in a difficult patient population. Its ultimate success is limited only by the development of appropriate electrodes and perhaps a better understanding of applied physics.

4.6. Stimulation of specific nerves

4.6.1. Occipital nerve stimulation

Occipital neuralgia, a chronic paroxysmal pain in the distribution of the greater/lesser occipital nerves, is a particularly intractable ailment that has been described by Weiner (2000), Weiner and Reed (1999) and Weiner et al. (1999) as being amenable to PNS. To determine the efficacy of neurostimulation, a trial screening procedure can be undertaken by means of a subcutaneous electrode that is introduced at the level of the atlas vertebra. Patients may be placed either prone or in the lateral decubitus position to facilitate fluoroscopic imaging. Under local anaesthesia, a curved introducing needle is directed subcutaneously below the superior nuchal line. A percutaneous quadripolar electrode, Pisces Quad Plus® (Medtronic) or Quattrode® (Advanced Neuromodulation Systems Inc., Plano, TX 75024, USA) is then inserted (Fig. 8a,b). The full

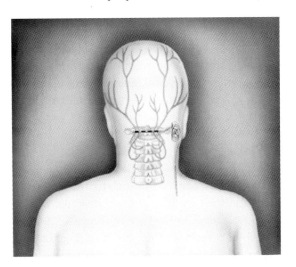

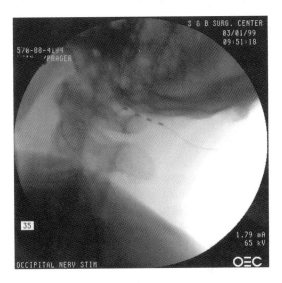

Fig. 8. (a) A sketch showing position of a percutaneous quadrapolar electrode for treatment of occipital neuralgia. (Courtesy of Richard L. Weiner, M.D., Dallas Neurological Associates, 8230 Walnut Hill Lane, Suite 220, Dallas, TX 75231, USA). (b) Radiograph showing an occipital nerve electrode from an oblique projection. (Courtesy of Joshua Prager, M.D., 100 UCLA Medical Plaza, Suite I 760 SP, Los Angeles CA 90095, USA).

length of the needle has to cross either the ipsilateral greater and lesser occipital nerves or, in case of bilateral pain, the contralateral occipital nerves. After removing the needle, test stimulation should be perceived as paraesthesiae in the occipital nerve distribution. After suturing the electrode to the skin, the patient should undergo a trial of neurostimulation for 5–7 days to ensure that sustained pain control is achievable.

If the trial is successful, and the pain unilateral, a single quadripolar plate electrode, or dual quadripolar plate electrodes if bilateral, are placed under local anaesthesia through a midline incision into one or two small lateral pockets that are large enough to accommodate the electrodes snugly. The electrodes can be sutured to the superficial fascia and their lead wires brought down midline through a tunnel to the base of the neck. A strain relief loop is fashioned as shown in Fig. 8a. This author has found it simpler to implant the pulse generator posterolateral in the buttock as described for PNS implantation in the lower extremity. The lead(s) are connected to the pulse generator via the tunnelled extension cable.

4.6.2. Trigeminal nerve trunk stimulation

Meyerson and Håkanson (1980) originally described the treatment of trigeminal neuropathy by electrical stimulation. The technique has since been used in various forms, mostly by a percutaneous approach with the electrode being directed through the foramen ovale (Meglio, 1984; Taub et al., 1997). Because the electrode is subject to dislodgment in some cases, many neurosurgeons prefer an intracranial to a percutaneous approach. However, if sufficient electrode is placed through the foramen ovale into Meckel's cave, its distraction will generally be prevented. Comparatively low voltage – 0.5–1.5 V – with a pulse width of 100–200 ms and rate 30–100 Hz is sufficient to induce analgesia. Analgesia will not be possible in the absence of afferent pathways, which may occur in some cases of post-herpetic neuralgia – a potentially good indication for trigeminal stimulation.

4.6.3. Supra-orbital and supra-trochlear neuralgia

Stimulation of the supra-orbital and supra-trochlear nerves can be achieved by percutaneous electrode placement (Dunteman, 2002). In a manner similar to that described for placement of an occipital nerve electrode, a small (Compact

Pisces®; Medtronic) electrode is passed under local anesthesia through a curved Tuohy-type needle that is introduced anterior to the auricle at the level of the superior orbital margin. Care should be taken not to disturb the auriculotemporal nerve and vessels. In a manner similar to that for occipital nerve stimulation, a trial of 5–7 days should be adequate to demonstrate whether it is effective in relieving the neuropathic pain (Alo and Holsheimer, 2001; Dunteman, 2002; Fig. 9).

4.6.4. Miscellaneous nerves

In their recent report, Buschman and Oppel (1999) described the use of a small flexible subepineurial platinum electrode for use in peripheral neuropathies in the following nerves: upper extremity – ulnar, median and radial; lower limb – peroneal, sciatic, saphenous, tibialis, femoralis and lateral femoral cutaneous; trunk, head and neck – genitofemoral, ilioinguinal, the 5th thoracic root, occipital and trigeminal. Their technique, which exposes a small (approximately 2 cm) length of nerve with the help of an operating microscope and electrophysiological monitoring, facilitates placement of the flexible platinum electrode. This is retained in position by epineurial sutures.

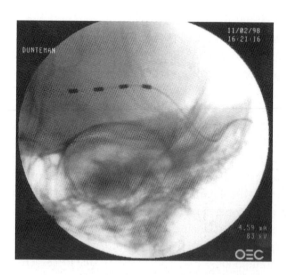

Fig. 9. Radiograph of supraorbital/supratrochlear nerve electrode for the management of pain in the trigeminal distribution. (Reproduced from Dunteman (2002), with permission.)

This group adopted a period of trial stimulation of several days during which time the patient participated in active physical therapy. The authors had performed this technique in 52 patients since 1991 with good to excellent results in 80% of their patients. Even more significant is the fact that of the 42 patients who had ceased to work as a result of their neuropathic pain, 13 returned to their full-time occupation, nine returned to part-time work and two changed their vocation.

4.6.5. Sacral root stimulation

Sacral stimulation for pelvic and rectal pain, interstitial cystitis and vulvodynia has shown considerable promise for the management of these very intractable conditions. Both transsacral and retrograde approaches to the sacral nerve roots are described (Alo et al., 1999; Chancellor and Chartier-Kastler, 2000; Wyndaele et al., 2000; Fig. 10). The reader is also referred to Chapter 5.

For midline pain, a transforaminal approach allows the introduction of electrodes through the posterior sacral foramina, to exit through the anterior sacral foramina adjacent to the S2, S3 and S4 anterior roots. Bilateral stimulation of the anterior roots of S4 is used for rectal pain. A period

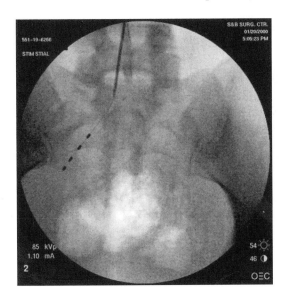

Fig. 10. Radiograph showing retrograde placement of electrodes on the S3 and S4 roots for the management of pelvic pain.

of 3–5 days' trial stimulation is generally sufficient to determine if this modality will be effective. Permanent electrodes are placed through the posterior and anterior sacral foramina. An electrode system that has been designed and approved for this purpose is Interstim® (Medtronic). After their introduction, the electrodes are secured to the periosteum and are then connected to the extension lead, which is tunnelled to a pocket in the buttock for the IPG; previously described.

4.7. Conclusions and future predictions

In the more than 30 years since Wall and Sweet first described the analgesic action of peripheral nerve stimulation, the 'dark ages' which eclipsed the period of early advances have now passed and are succeeded by a new era of clinical curiosity, entrepreneurial development and technical innovation. In spite of all the pharmacological advances and use of membrane stabilizing agents with the promise of receptor specificity and targeted molecules, our contemporary management of neuropathic pain is still far from adequate. We can train some of our patients to live with their symptoms, but in the final analysis the disability, loss of function and social ostracism takes its toll on family, work place, society and the individual affected.

Peripheral nerve stimulation as a treatment modality has shown great promise. The cumulative evidence, both anecdotal and scientific, would suggest that early rather than later implantation is much more successful in the management of pain that is neuropathic and distal in the affected nerve. Considerable experimental experience with nerve injury models has demonstrated that the plastic changes which occur in the central neuraxis in response to chronic neuropathic pain may degrade the efficacy of PNS and cause the development of tolerance, or worse, disinhibition when the modality is applied late.

Although there are, to this date, no randomized, prospective controlled studies to scientifically validate the therapeutic efficacy of peripheral nerve stimulation similar to Kemler's study of the treatment of complex regional pain syndrome by spinal cord stimulation (Kemler et al., 2000), reports during the last 5 years using more acceptable outcome measures of function, return to work data and reduction or cessation of narcotic use support the success of PNS. In comparison to other forms of neurostimulation, in particular spinal cord stimulation, the volume of peripheral nerve surgical implants is quite small, but growing. The principal limitations of growth in the United States are: (1) the lack of appropriate electrode designs and (2) the failure to acknowledge this form of treatment at the time surgical procedural coding was introduced, resulting in anomalous and poor reimbursement. This latter anomaly occurred at a time of increasing disenchantment with the procedure due to the number of problems with which it was associated, already described earlier in this chapter.

The scope of neurostimulation for painful neuropathy is enormous. It is estimated that two-thirds of the surgical cases presently managed by spinal cord stimulation for neuropathic pain in one or two nerves in the lower extremity and almost all cases with intractable neuropathic pain of the upper extremities could be well managed by peripheral nerve stimulation. In the latter case, due to the potential instability of cervical spinal cord stimulation, this region in particular lends itself to this therapeutic modality.

At the present time, efforts are underway to develop more appropriate electrode designs, in particular to accommodate the anatomical form and the specific region and function of the nerves concerned. In spite of the fact that the surgical repair of nerves has vastly improved, particularly following the impetus of World War II, neuropathic pain still remains a problem in over 20% of cases regardless of optimal nerve repair following trauma. The other major causes of persistent neuropathy are those that develop from congenital or acquired restrictive anatomical sites (carpal tunnel, Guyon's canal, etc.) and the numerous post-infective or metabolic neuropathies that present themselves in a specific nerve region. Where pharmacological and other measures used to manage peripheral nerve pain fail, there is significant potential for both pain control and improved function with peripheral nerve stimulation. The future of the field is promising and depends on measures discussed in this and other chapters in this book.

References

Ali, J.A., Yaffee, C.S., and Serretti, C. (1981) The effect of transcutaneous electrical nerve stimulation on post-operative pain and pulmonary function. Surg., 89: 507–512.

Alo K.M., and Holsheimer J. (2001) Review. New trends in neuromodulation for the management of neuropathic pain. J. Neurosurg., 81.

Alo, K.M., Ylend, M.J., Redko, V., Feler, C., and Naumann, C. (1999) Lumbar and sacral nerve root stimulation (NRS) in the treatment of chronic pain: a novel and anatomic approach in neurostimulation techniques. Neuromodulation, 2: 23–31.

Althaus J. (1859) A treatise of medical electricity, theoretical and practical and its use in the treatment of paralysis. In: *Neuralgia and other Disease*. London, Trubner.

Andersson, S.A., Hansson, G., and Holmgren, E. (1976) Evaluation of the pain suppressant effect of different frequencies of peripheral electrical stimulation in chronic pain conditions. Acta Orthopaedica Scand., 47: 149–157.

Augustinsson, L.E., Bohlin, P., Bundsen, P., Carlsson, C.A., Forssman, L., Sjöberg, P., and Tyreman, N. (1977) Pain relief during delivery by transcutaneous nerve stimulation. Pain, 4: 59–65.

Bourke D.L., Smith B.A.C., Erickson J., Gwartz B., Lessard L. (1984) TENS reduces halothane requirement during hand surgery. Anesthesiology, 61: 769-722.

Brennan, K.R. (1976) The characterization of transcutaneous stimulating electrodes. IEEE Trans. Biomed. Eng., 23: 337–340.

Brummer, S.B. and Turner, M.J. (1977a) Electrical stimulation with Pt electrodes. I: A method for determination for 'real' electrode areas. IEEE Trans. Biomed. Eng., 24: 436.

Brummer, S.B. and Turner, M.J. (1977b) Electrical stimulation with Pt electrodes. II: Estimation of maximum surface redox (Theoretical non-gassing) limits. IEEE Trans. Biomed. Eng., 24: 440.

Brummer, S.B. and Turner, M.J. (1977c) Electrochemical considerations for safe electrical stimulation of the nervous system with platinum electrodes. IEEE Trans. Biomed. Eng., 24: 59.

Buschman, N. and Oppel, F. (1999) Periphere nervenstimulation. Schmerz, 13: 113–120.

Bütikofer, R. and Lawrence, P.D. (1979) Electrocutaneous nerve stimulation. II Stimulus waveform selection. IEEE Trans. Biomed. Eng., 26: 69–74.

Campbell, J.N. and Long, D.M. (1976) Peripheral nerve stimulation in the treatment of intractable pain. J. Neurosurg., 45: 692–699.

Cauthen, J.C. and Renner, E.J. (1975) Transcutaneous and peripheral nerve stimulation for chronic pain states. Surg. Neurol., 4: 102–104.

Chancellor, M. and Chartier-Kastler, E. (2000) Principles of sacral nerve stimulation (SNS) for the treatment of bladder and urethral sphincter dysfunctions. Neuromodulation, 3: 15–26.

Cooney, W.P. (1997) Electrical stimulation in the treatment of complex regional pain syndromes of the upper extremity. Hand Clinics. Upper extremity pain dysfunction: somatic and sympathetic disorders, 13: 519–526.

Cooney, W.P., III (1991) Chronic pain treatment with direct electrical nerve stimulation, Chapter 105. In R.H. Gelberman (Ed.), *Operative Nerve Repair and Reconstruction*, Vol. II. (pp. 1551–1561). JB Lippincott, Philadelphia.

Cooperman, A.M., Hall, B., Mikalacki, K., Hardy, R., and Sadar, E. (1977) Use of transcutaneous electrical stimulation in control of post operative pain – results of a prospective, randomized, controlled study. Am. J. Surg., 133: 185–187.

DiRosa, F., Guizzi, P., and Battistone, B. (1988) Radial nerve anatomy and vesicular arrangement. In G. Brunelli (Ed.), *Textbook of Microsurgery* (pp. 571). Masson, Milano.

Dunteman, E. (2002) Peripheral nerve stimulation for unremitting ophthalmic post-herpetic neuralgia. Neuromodulation, 5: 32–37.

Ericksson, M.B., Sjölund, B.H., and Nielzen, S. (1979) Long term results of peripheral conditioning stimulation as an analgesia measure in chronic pain. Pain, 6: 335–347.

Eriksson, M.J., Sjölund, B.H., and Sundberg, G. (1984) Pain relief from peripheral conditioning stimulation in patients with chronic facial pain. J. Neurosurg., 61: 149–155.

Goldner, J.L., Nashold, B.S., Jr., and Hendrix, P.C. (1982) Peripheral nerve electrical stimulation. Clin. Orthop., 163: 33–41.

Gybels, J. and Kupers, R. (1987) Central and peripheral electrical stimulation of the nervous system in the treatment of chronic pain. Acta Neurochirurgica. Suppl., 38: 64–75.

Hansson, P. and Ekblom, A. (1983) Transcutaneous electrical nerve stimulation (TENS) as compared to placebo-TENS for the relief of acute orofacial pain. Pain, 15: 157–165.

Harrison, R.F., Woods, T., Shore, M., Matthews, G., and Unwin, A. (1986) Pain relief in labor using transcutaneous electrical nerve stimulation (TENS). A TENS/TENS placebo controlled study in two parity groups. Br. J. Obstet. Gyn., 93: 739–746.

Hassenbusch, S.J., Stanton-Hicks, M., Schoppa, D., Walsh, J.G., and Covington, E.C. (1996) Long-term results of peripheral nerve stimulation for reflex sympathetic dystrophy. J. Neurosurg.: 415–423.

Hubbard, J.J. (1976) *The Peripheral Nervous System*, Pannum Press, New York.

Johnson, M.I., Ashton, C.H., and Thompson, J.W. (1991a) An in-depth study of long-term users of transcutaneous electrical nerve stimulation (TENS): implications for clinical use of TENS. Pain, 44: 221–229.

Johnson, M.I., Ashton, C.H., and Thompson, J.W. (1991b) The consistency of pulse frequencies and pulse patterns of transcutaneous electrical nerve stimulation (TENS) used by chronic pain patients. Pain, 44: 231–234.

Kemler, M.A., Barendse, G.A., Van Kleef, M., De Vet, H.C., Rijks, C.P., Furnee, C.A., and Van den Wildenburg, F.A. (2000) Spinal cord stimulation in patients with complex regional pain syndrome. N. Engl. J. Med., 343: 618–624.

Kirsch, W.M., Lewis, J.A., and Simon, R.H. (1975) Experiences with electrical stimulation devices for the control of chronic pain. Med. Instrum., 9: 217–220.

Law, J.T., Sweet, J., and Kirsch, W. (1981) Retrospective analysis of 22 patients with chronic pain treated by peripheral nerve stimulation. J. Neurosurg., 52: 482–485.

Linzer, M. and Long, D.M. (1976) Transcutaneous neural stimulation for relief of pain. IEEE. Trans. Biomed. Eng., 23: 341–345.

Loeser, J.D., Black, R.G., and Christman, R.M. (1975) The relief of pain by transcutaneous stimulation. J. Neurosurg., 42: 308–314.

Long, D.M. and Hagfors, N. (1975) Electrical stimulation in the nervous system: the current status of electrical stimulation of the nervous system for the relief of pain. Pain, 1: 109–123.

Long, D.M., Campbell, J.N., and Gurer, G. (1979) Transcutaneous electrical nerve stimulation for relief of chronic pain. In J.J. Bonica, J.C. Lieberskind, and D.G. Albe-fessard, (Eds.), *Advances in Pain Research and Therapy 3* (pp. 593–599). Raven Press, New York.

Long, D.M., Erickson, D., Campbell, J., and North, R. (1981) Electrical stimulation of the spinal cord and peripheral nerves for pain control: a ten year experience. Appl. Neurophysiol., 44: 207–217.

MacKay, C. (1841) *Extraordinary Popular Delusions and the Madness of Crowds*, Richard Bentley, London.

Mannheimer, C. and Carlsson, C.A. (1979) The analgesic effect of transcutaneous electrical nerve stimulation in patients with rheumatoid arthritis. A comparative study of different pulse patterns. Pain, 6: 329–334.

Mannheimer, C., Carlson, C.A., Vedin, A., and Wilhelmsson, C. (1986) Transcutaneous electrical nerve stimulation (TENS) in angina pectoris. Pain, 26: 291–300.

Mason, J.L. and MacKay, N.A.M. (1976) Pain sensations associated with electrocutaneous stimulation. IEEE Trans. Biomed. Eng., 23: 405–409.

Mayer, D.J. and Liebeskind, J.C. (1974) Pain reduction by focal electrical stimulation of the brain: an anatomical and behavioral analysis. Brain Res., 68: 73–93.

Meglio, M. (1984) Percutaneously implantable chronic electrode for radiofrequency stimulation of gasseon ganglion: a perspective in the management of trigeminal pain. Acta Neurosurch. Suppl. (Wien), 33: 521–525.

Melzack, R.A. and Wall, P.D. (1965) Pain mechanisms: a new theory. Science, 150: 971–979.

Meyer, G.A. and Fields, H.L. (1972) Causalgia treated by selective large fiber stimulation of peripheral nerves. Brain, 95: 163–167.

Meyerson, B.A. and Håkanson, S. (1980) Alleviation of atypical trigeminal pain by stimulation of the Gasserian ganglion via an implanted electrode. Acta Neurosurg., 30: 303–309.

Myers, R.A., Woolf, C.J., and Mitchell, D. (1977) Management of acute traumatic pain by peripheral transcutaneous electrical stimulation. S. African Med. J., 52: 309–312.

Nashold, B.S. and Goldner, J.L. (1975) Electrical stimulation of peripheral nerves for relief of intractable chronic pain. Medical Instrumentation, 9(5): 224–225.

Nashold, B.S., Jr., Mellen, J.B., and Avery, R. (1979) Peripheral nerve stimulation for pain relief using a multi-contact electrode system. J. Neurosurg., 51: 872–873.

Nashold, B.S., Jr., Goldner, L., Mellen, J.B., and Bright, D.S. (1982) Long-term pain control by direct peripheral nerve stimulation. J. Bone Joint. Surg. (Am), 64: 1–10.

Nathan, P.W. and Wall, P.D. (1974) Treatment of post-herpetic neuralgia by prolonged electrical stimulation. Br. Med. J., iii: 645–647.

Novak, C.B. and MacKinnon, S.V. (1999) Outcome following implantation of a peripheral nerve stimulator in patients with chronic nerve pain. Plastic Recons. Surg., 105: 1967–1972.

Ogata, K. and Naito, M. (1986) Blood flow of peripheral nerve. Effects of dissection, stretching and compression. J. Hand Surg., 11B: 10.

Peters, A., Palay, S.L., and Webster, H. de F. (1976) *The Fine Structure of the Nervous System: The Neuron and Supporting Cells*, Saunders, Philadelphia.

Picaza, J.A., Cannon, B.W., Hunter, S.E., Boyd, A.S., Guma, J., and Maurer, D. (1975) Pain suppression by peripheral nerve stimulation. II. Observations with implanted devices. Surg. Neurol., 4: 115–126.

Pike, M. (1978) Transcutaneous electrical nerve stimulation: its use in management of post-operative pain. Anesth, 33: 165–171.

Racz, G.B., Browne, T., and Lewis, R. (1988) Peripheral nerve stimulator implant for treatment of causalgia caused by electrical burns. Tex. Med., 84: 45–50.

Racz, G.B., Lewis, R., Heavner, J.E., and Scott, J. (1990) Peripheral nerve stimulator implant for treatment of causalgia. In M. Stanton-Hicks, W. Jänig, and R.A. Boas, (Eds.), *Reflex Sympathetic Dystrophy* (pp. 135–141). Kluwer, Norwell, MA.

Reynolds, D.B. (1969) Surgery in the rat during electrical analgesia induced by focal brain stimulation. Science, 164: 444–445.

Roche, P.A., Gijsbers, K., Belch, J.J.F., and Forbes, C.D. (1985) Modification of hemophiliac hemorrhage pain by transcutaneous electrical stimulation. Pain, 21: 43–48.

Seligman, L.J. (1982) Physiological stimulators: from electric fish to programmable implants. IEEE Trans. Biomed. Eng., 29: 270–284.

Shetter A.G., Racz G.B., Lewis R., Heavner J.E. (1997) Peripheral nerve stimulation. In: North, R.B. and Levi, R.N. (Eds). Neurosurgical Management of Pain. New York, NY: Springer-Verlag, pp. 261–270.

Smith, C.M., Guralnick, M.S., Gelfund, M.M., and Jeans, M.E. (1986) The effects of transcutaneous nerve stimulation on post-caesarian pain. Pain, 27: 181–194.

Smith, J.W. (1966a) Factors influencing nerve repair. 1. Blood supply of peripheral nerves. Arch. Surg., 93: 335.

Smith, J.W. (1966b) Factors influencing nerve repair. II. Collateral circulation of peripheral nerves. Arch. Surg., 93: 433.

Solomon, R.A., Viernstein, M.C., and Long, D.M. (1980) Reduction of post-operative pain and narcotic use by transcutaneous electrical nerve stimulation. Surg, 87: 142–146.

Stanton-Hicks, M. and Salamon, J. (1997) Stimulation of the central and peripheral nervous systems for the control of pain. J. Clin. Neurophysiol.: 46–62.

Strege, D.W., Cooney, W.P., Wood, M.B., Johnson, S.J., and Metcalf, B.J. (1994) Chronic peripheral nerve pain treated with direct electrical nerve stimulation. J. Hand Surg., 19a: 931–939.

Sunderland, S. (1945) The intraneural topography of the radial, median and ulnar nerves. Brain, 68: 243.

Sunderland, S. (1978) *Nerves and Nerve Injuries*. 2nd ed., Churchill Livingstone, Edinburgh.

Sweet, W.H. (1976) Control of pain by direct electrical stimulation of peripheral nerves. Clin. Neurosurg., 23: 103–111.

Sweet, W.H. and Wepsic, J.G. (1974) Stimulation of the posterior columns of the spinal cord for pain control: indications, techniques and results. Clin. Neurosurg., 21: 278–310.

Taub, E., Munz, M., and Taskar, R. (1997) Chronic electrical stimulation of the Gasserian ganglion for the relief of pain in a series of 34 patients. J. Neurosurg., 86: 197–202.

Taylor, P., Hallett, M., and Flaherty, L. (1981) Treatment of osteoarthritis of the knee with transcutaneous electrical nerve stimulation. Pain, 11: 233–246.

Thompson, J.W. (1986) The role of transcutaneous electrical nerve stimulation (TENS) for the control of pain. In D. Doyle (Ed.), *International Symposium on Pain Control. World Society of Medicine Services International Congress and Symposium Series 1, 2, 3* (pp. 27–47). World Society of Medicine Services Limited, London.

Thompson, J.W. and Filshie, E.J. (1993) Transcutaneous electrical nerve stimulation (TENS) and acupuncture. In D. Doyle, G. Hanks, and N. MacDonald, (Eds.), *Oxford*

Textbook of Palliative Medicine (pp. 229–244). Oxford University Press, Oxford.

Thorsteinsson, G., Stonnington, H.H., Stillwell, G.J., and Elveback, L.R. (1977) Transcutaneous electrical nerve stimulation: a double blind trial of its efficacy for pain. Arch. Phys. Med. Med. Rehab., 58: 8–13.

Waisbrod, H., Panhaus, C.H., Hansen, D., and Gerbershagen, H.U. (1985) Direct nerve stimulation for painful peripheral neuropathies. J. Bone Joint Surg. Br., 67: 470–472.

Wall, P.D. and Sweet, E.H. (1967) Temporary abolition of pain in man. Science, 155: 108–109.

Weiner, R.L. (2000) The future of peripheral nerve neuro-stimulation. Neurol. Res., 22: 299–303.

Weiner, R.L. and Reed, K.L. (1999) Peripheral neurostimulation for control of intractable occipital neuralgia. Neuromodulation, 2: 217–221.

Weiner R.L., Alo K.M., Fuller M.L. (1999) Peripheral neurostimulation to control intractable occipital neuraliga. 9th World Cong Pain Abs, Vienna, Austria, p. 108.

Woolf, C.J. and Thompson, J.W. (1994) Stimulation – induced analgesia: transcutaneous electrical nerve stimulation (TENS) and vibration. In P.D. Wall, and R. Melzack, (Eds.), *Textbook of Pain*. 3rd ed. (pp. 1191–1208). Churchill Livingstone, Edinburgh, London, Madrid.

Wyndaele, J., Michielsen, D., and Van Dromme, S. (2000) Influence of sacral neuromodulation on electrode sensation of the lower urinary tract. J. Urol., 163: 221–224.

Electrical Stimulation and the Relief of Pain
Pain Research and Clinical Management, Vol. 15
Edited by Brian A. Simpson

CHAPTER 5

Sacral nerve root stimulation for interstitial cystitis

Daniel S. Bennett[a],* and Daniel Brookoff[b]

[a]*Integrative Treatment Centers, 8406 Clay St.,*
Denver, CO 80031-3810, USA;
[b]*University of Tennessee College of Medicine, Comprehensive Pain Institute,*
1265 Union Avenue, Memphis, TN 38104, USA

Abstract

Interstitial cystitis (IC) is a debilitating neuropathic pain syndrome characterized by intense pain occurring with bladder distention and urination accompanied by small bladder volumes and urinary frequency. IC has been likened to 'reflex sympathetic dystrophy of the bladder'. Traditional methods of treatment have shown poor efficacy. Sacral nerve stimulation is effective in reduction of pain, normalization of bladder volumes and diminution in urinary urgency/frequency.

Keywords: Interstitial cystitis; Sacral nerve stimulation; Urge incontinence; Bladder dysfunction; Nerve root stimulation; Sacrococcygeal region; Neuromodulation

1. Introduction

Interstitial cystitis (IC) is a syndrome characterized by hypersensitivity of the urinary bladder, often progressing to debilitating hyperalgesia and allodynia. IC often starts out as 'irritable bladder' with urgency to urinate accompanied by small urinary volumes. At the extreme, patients may experience the compelling urge to urinate up to 50–80 times per day and be suffering with constant disabling pelvic pain. It is the most disabling non-malignant disorder seen by urologists and gynaecologists, affecting over 1 million people in the United States alone and contributing to an economic impact in excess of 1.7 billion US dollars (Oravisto, 1975; Held et al., 1990; Curhan et al., 1999; Kusek and Nyberg, 2001).

Even though IC has been recognized by physicians for over 150 years it has, until recently, defied definition by clinical signs or pathological findings. Its victims have been left to suffer in obscurity, often resorting to cystectomy or even suicide when the pain becomes unbearable. While IC has been characterized as a urologic disease, it may be better conceptualized as a neurologic syndrome. Indeed, it has been likened to 'reflex sympathetic dystrophy of the bladder'. As our understanding of the condition improves, we will come to see that it is an important model of visceral pain. Because of the accessibility of the bladder and its innervation, it is also likely that IC will become the model for the successful application of neuromodulation to the visceral

---

*Correspondence to: Daniel S. Bennett, MD, Integrative Treatment Centers, 8406 Clay St., Denver, CO 80031-3810, USA. Phone: + 1 (303) 487-0932; Fax: + 1 (303) 487-0934; E-mail: dbennett@denverpain.com

organs. When we study IC, we see that there are striking similarities to a wide variety of visceral diseases, such as ulcerative colitis and chronic asthma, which may also someday be controlled through neuromodulation.

2. A model of visceral hyperalgesia

In 1987, Dr. Stephen McMahon and colleagues described an important animal model for severe visceral pain (McMahon and Abel, 1987). In this model, non-destructive concentrations of a chemical irritant, turpentine oil, were instilled into the bladders of rats. With repeated episodes of chemical irritation, chemosensitive afferent fibres in the bladder wall were found to release vasoactive substances. The resulting neurogenic inflammation caused sensory and motor changes associated with hypermotility of the bladder, hypersensitivity to small volumes of urine and behaviours associated with pain and allodynia. This was correlated with increase in nerve growth factor (NGF) and substance P secretion by cells of the bladder wall into the urine. With continued irritation, sensory fibres in the bladder wall that were normally silent became activated. Ultimately, the process of neurogenic inflammation progressed to the point that it no longer depended on the instillation of the irritating chemical. The rats developed persistent allodynia of the bladder.

In a graphic demonstration of the pain caused by this irritation, after multiple instillations the affected rats would often flip themselves over on their backs and eat through their own abdominal walls, pulling out their bladders in an effort to obtain relief. Several years after his initial paper was published, Dr. McMahon was invited to lecture to a group of patients with IC and their physicians in Los Angeles. When he showed his video, the physicians hid their eyes and the patients jumped out of their chairs – many of them shouting "That's me!"

3. Clinical features

Interstitial cystitis is a clinical syndrome defined by "Chronic irritative voiding symptoms, sterile and cytologically negative urine, characteristic cystoscopic findings along with failure to find a more objective cause for this clinical picture" (Messing, 1992).

Typically, patients with IC are female (90%) and Caucasian. The female predominance is probably real but may be exaggerated by the fact that males with a symptom complex fitting IC are often considered to have chronic non-bacterial prostatitis. The syndrome begins, usually between 30 and 50 years of age, with progressive and unremitting urinary frequency and urgency, which may be the only initial presentation. Up to half of patients report dysuria, and nocturia is one of the hallmarks of IC (Leach and Raz, 1983). Male patients will often describe perineal, scrotal and groin discomfort (Badenoch, 1971). Although a combination of voiding symptoms and pelvic pain is common, in most cases one of the two symptom complexes tends to predominate (Table I). Fifty to 75% of women with IC report dyspareunia (Leach and Raz, 1983; Sant, 1991), many abstaining from sexual intercourse completely. Incontinence is rare, but when present is often of the urgency type (Parivar and Bradbrook, 1986). Gross haematuria is also uncommon though many of the patients will have microscopic haematuria. The onset of IC is often acute. Many patients can pinpoint the day that it started (Keast and De Groat, 1992). They often associate the onset with

TABLE I

Interstitial cystitis: clinical features

Dysuria
Dyspareunia
Pelvic/perineal/pubic pain (or dysaesthesias)
Urinary frequency
Urinary urgency
Haematuria
Glomerulation and/or ulcers on cystoscopic examination

---

a specific event such as a urinary tract infection or pelvic surgery (Badenoch, 1971). Most are initially treated with antibiotics for acute bacterial cystitis (Keast and De Groat, 1992). In general, patients will suffer with progressive symptoms for 3–7 years before the diagnosis is made (Koziol et al., 1993), on average seeing four physicians before the correct diagnosis is arrived at.

The onset of symptoms is often associated with potential trauma to the pelvic nerves. The majority of female IC patients have a history of pelvic surgery, most commonly hysterectomy which is already known to be a common cause of bladder dysfunction (Parys et al., 1990). In an epidemiologic study in the U.S. (Curhan et al., 1999) 44% of women with IC had undergone hysterectomy within months before onset of IC symptoms. The rate for the control group was 17%. In another study (Hanash and Pool, 1969), the majority of male IC patients had undergone transuretheral prostatectomy within months before the diagnosis of IC was made.

In a large survey of patients with IC there was a strong association with irritable bowel syndrome (64%) and a high incidence of atopia, fibromyalgia and migraine headaches; there was an excess risk in individuals of Jewish descent (Held et al., 1990). When Clauw and colleagues compared age-matched fibromyalgia and IC patients and healthy controls, a commonality of reported symptoms was seen between the fibromyalgia and IC groups, prompting speculation that similar central mechanisms in pain processing were present (Clauw et al., 1997). In a survey of symptoms, 92% reported urinary urgency, 91% urinary frequency, 70% pelvic pain, 60% dysuria, 37% pain for days after intercourse and 22% haematuria. Fifty-five percent of the patients reported daily or constant pain, with 57% of these characterizing their pain as severe or excruciating (Held et al., 1990). The pain was characteristically increased by stress, ingestion of alcohol, tomatoes, acidic or carbonated beverages, disturbances in sleep, and long car rides. The latter may be related to vibrations transmitted to the pelvis.

Interestingly, these patients do not get the same exacerbations with airplane rides. Many report that the disease has caused significant disruptions in family relationships.

There are several potential pathways for the pain. While classical neuroanatomy would implicate the pelvic nerves, fibres coming from the dome of the bladder join the hypogastric nerve which carries sympathetic preganglionic input to the pelvic ganglia and afferent input from the bladder to the thoraco-lumbar spinal cord. These bladder afferents are either lightly myelinated A-delta or unmyelinated C fibres (Gosling and Dixon, 1974). A-delta fibres are mechanoreceptors but can transmit nociceptive input to the spinal cord. There are apparently different pathways for different types of bladder pain. For example, overdistension pain may be transmitted via hypogastric nerves (with a referral pattern in dermatomes T10–12). This could explain some of the abnormal bladder sensations reported by patients with low thoracic cord transections. Mucosal irritation pain, on the other hand, may be conducted via the pelvic nerves, with referred pain to the rectum, vagina and perineum. This certainly reflects the pattern of pain that is reported by the patients with IC and often disbelieved by their physicians.

4. Pathophysiology of IC

Based on cystoscopic findings IC is classified as ulcerative or non-ulcerative (Messing, 1987). This may represent different stages of the same disease or different pathological processes (Koziol et al., 1995). Ulcers are seen in 5–20% of cases (Sant, 1991; Koziol et al., 1993). Another cystoscopic finding often regarded as characteristic of IC is the strawberry-like haemorrhages referred to as glomerulations. Typically, glomerulations are not seen on first filling of the bladder but are found on re-distension. Though widely considered to be specific and sensitive for the diagnosis of IC, they are probably neither.

4.1. A primary bladder mucosal defect?

Pathologic clues to the aetiology of IC can be elusive. There is some evidence for the presence of bladder autoantibodies but these may be non-specific and are similar to those seen in other urologic disorders (Silk, 1970). A widely-held aetiologic concept is that the bladder epithelium has become dysfunctional and leaky. Normal bladder mucosa is lined by a layer of negatively-charged sulfonated glycosaminoglycans (GAG). This GAG layer maintains the permeability barrier between urine and the bladder wall preventing the back-diffusion of water and of potassium and other solutes. When protamine sulphate (which will combine with and precipitate negatively charged GAGs) is instilled into the bladders of normal volunteers this barrier is compromised. Urinary solutes diffuse into the bladder wall and the subjects will quickly develop the symptoms of IC (Lilly and Parsons, 1990). The urinary barrier can be restored and symptoms relieved by instilling a sulphated polysaccharide (e.g. heparin) into the bladder. Based on these findings, synthetic poly-saccharides such as pentosan polysulphate (Elmiron®), an orally bioavailable heparinoid compound, have become a mainstay of treatment of IC (Parsons et al., 1994). These compounds may be more effective early on in the course of the disease but are probably not as effective once the process of continuous, self-reinforcing neurogenic inflammation has become established. There is also some evidence that pentosan polysulphate may be acting by other means, e.g. as an anti-inflammatory agent or as an inhibitor of nerve growth or angiogenesis (Liekens et al., 1997; Zugmaier et al., 1999; Sadhukhan et al., 2002). The reports of abnormalities in urinary GAG levels in IC patients are variable (Hurst et al., 1993) but may point to chemical differences in their GAG layer (Holm-Bentzen et al., 1986) which may result in increased permeability of the bladder wall (Lilly and Parsons, 1990; Parsons et al., 1991). Substance P, which is increased in the urine of IC patients, is also known to influence epithelial permeability; this has been shown to be the case in respiratory epithelium of asthmatics (Petersson and Svensjo, 1992).

Biopsies of the bladder wall in people with IC often show normal epithelium and muscularis layers with submucosal oedema and vasodilatation without a remarkable inflammatory infiltrate (Johansson and Fall, 1994). When they are found, inflammatory changes are usually limited to the lamina propria and are reminiscent of the changes seen in biopsies of the colon in ulcerative colitis. Eighty percent of biopsies will show perineural lymphocytic infiltrates. A consistent finding is marked oedema of the lamina propria with dilated vascular channels, especially venules, with some inflammatory changes in the walls of veins (Johansson and Fall, 1994). Despite severe symptoms, the histopathologic findings may be very meagre in the non-ulcerative form. This may be because the disease process actually operates proximal to the bladder wall, e.g. in nerve root.

There is indeed increasing evidence of more complex pathophysiological mechanisms. It is of note that not all inflammatory mediators are increased in the bladder in IC. Mediators associated with traumatic or immune-induced inflammation such as prostaglandins E_2, D_2, F_2, thromboxane B_2, tumour necrosis factor, leuko-trienes and interleukins 1 and 2, are found in normal or reduced levels in the urine and bladder wall of patients with IC (Fleischmann et al., 1991; Felsen et al., 1994; Martins et al., 1994). A role for inflammatory neuropeptides may explain the relief of IC symptoms after instillation of capsaicin (DeGroat et al., 1992) or resiniferatoxin (Chancellor and De Groat, 1999; March et al., 2001; Andersson and Hedlund, 2002). The decrease in pain soon after hydrodistension may also be due to depletion of neuropeptides. An increase in the number of mast cells in the bladder walls of IC patients has been described but this is not a consistent finding (Pang et al., 1995). An increase in the density of nerve fibres containing substance P has also been reported, suggesting a role for neurogenic inflammation (Hamid et al., 1988; Christmas et al., 1990).

4.2. *The role of neuropeptides*

In IC, bladder wall biopsies show increased nerve density, specifically sympathetic nerves and fibres containing substance P. While data on the density of mast cells varies, there is consistent evidence for increased mast cell degranulation in the bladder walls of patients with IC (Christmas et al., 1990; Hohenfeller et al., 1992; Pang et al., 1995; Theoharides et al., 1995; Letourneau et al., 1996). Peptide-secreting nerve fibres are often seen in close apposition to degranulating mast cells which release NGF (Messing, 1987; Woolf et al., 1996; Dines and Powell, 1997). Many of the neuropeptides found in the sensory nerve endings innervating mucosal and submucosal layers of the bladder are implicated in neurogenic inflammation. These include substance P, neurokinin A, calcitonin gene-related peptide (CGRP), vasoactive intestinal peptide (VIP), neuropeptide Y (NPY) somatostatin and enkephalin. Similar findings are commonly seen in inflammatory disease of the gastrointestinal tract such as ulcerative colitis and Crohn's disease and in other chronic inflammatory states such as psoriasis and chronic arthritis (Yonei, 1987; Hukkanen et al., 1991; Naukkarinen et al., 1991; Dvorak et al., 1992; McKay and Bienenstock, 1994).

Mast cells and sensory nerve endings maintain a mutually paracrine relationship. Mast cell secretions certainly modify nerve cell transmission (Christian et al., 1989). Certain neuropeptides released by sensory neurons, such as substance P, in turn directly activate G proteins present in mast cell membranes (Mousli et al., 1990). Close interactions between mast cells and nerve fibres are not only characteristic of the bladder wall, they are a normal feature of gastrointestinal and respiratory tissue (Bienenstock et al., 1991). Many of the products of mast cell degranulation such as histamine, prostaglandin D_2 and leukotriene C_4 can stimulate sensory neurons to release

neuropeptides such as substance P (Bjorling et al., 1994). This process may explain the relationship between IC and diseases of other organ systems – such as irritable bowel disease, asthma and fibromyalgia where mutual paracrine stimulation results in continued inflammation. Examples include: in sensitized lungs, mast cell degranulation causes excitation of vagal neurons innervating the airways (Undem et al., 1993); in the gut, mast cell activation alters ion transport and epithelial permeability (Crowe and Perdue, 1992); in the skin, mast cell degranulation can result in antidromic nerve conduction-induced vasodilatation and the neurogenic plasma extravasation which is often seen as atopy (Lembeck and Holzer, 1979).

The increased sensory innervation of the bladder wall in patients with IC is good evidence for neural plasticity within the bladder (Letourneau et al., 1996). There may be a neurotrophic effect of sustained mast cell secretion (Keast and De Groat, 1992). One of the mediators of neuritic outgrowth may be endothelin-1 (Hsu et al., 1992). Many tissue mast cells synthesize and store NGF which may not only stimulate peripheral sympathetic nerve cell growth (Kannan et al., 2000) but also can induce mast cell hyperplasia (Marshall et al., 1990). NGF supports the survival and integrity of small-fibre pain-transmitting neurons and may be responsible for some elements of nerve cell overgrowth in chronic IC. NGF is found in high concentrations in the urine of many patients with IC. It is interesting to note that in McMahon's model of chronic bladder pain (described in Section 2), antagonists to NGF blocked the development of the chronic pain syndrome that resembled IC (McMahon and Abel, 1987; Oddiah et al., 1998).

4.3. *The role of neurogenic inflammation*

Neurogenic inflammation explains many of the features of the pathophysiology of IC (Fig. 1). Neurogenic inflammation is the process by which stimulation of peripheral nerves elicits

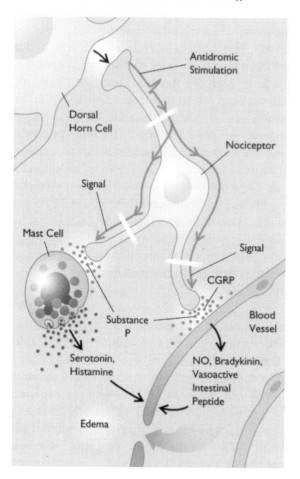

Fig. 1. Afferent signalling becomes efferent signalling. After prolonged sensitization, cells in the dorsal horn release chemicals that cause action potentials to fire backwards down the nociceptors – a dorsal root reflex. As a result of this, nociceptive dendrities release substance P and CGRP into peripheral tissues. Substance P causes degranulation of mast cells and, along with CGRP, also induces changes in vascular endothelial cells. The consequence is an outpouring of potent vasodilating and inflammatory agents (e.g. bradykinin, histamine, nitric oxide [NO], serotonin and vasoactive intestinal peptide) causing oedema and potentiating transmission of pain signals from the periphery. (From Brookoff, 2000, with permission.)

vasodilatation, plasma extravasation and other inflammatory changes in the skin and viscera (Pinter and Szolcanyi, 1995). Oedema of the bladder wall can be induced by stimulation of lumbar roots or pelvic nerves (Koltzenburg and McMahon, 1986; Pinter and Szolcanyi, 1995).

Although we think of sensory afferents as carriers of messages to the central nervous system, we now understand that they also act in the periphery through the release of neuropeptides. The histologic features of neurogenic inflammation bear a striking resemblance to the cystoscopic and pathologic findings reported in IC. Studies localizing neuropeptides in the bladder wall suggest that afferent innervation is altered in IC (Steers and Tuttle, 1997); acute neurogenic inflammation can lead to chronic changes in innervation, resulting in a persistent pain syndrome.

With increased neurogenic inflammation of the bladder wall and increased mucosal permeability (Koltzenburg and McMahon, 1986), the high concentrations of potassium in the urine will cause structural changes in the bladder wall and, ultimately, in the central nervous system. Eventually, afferent neuronal cell bodies will hypertrophy in response to chronic bladder irritation (Dupont et al., 1994a,b). NGF manufactured by bladder smooth muscle is responsible for the growth of sensory and noradrenergic nerves (Steers et al., 1991; Persson et al., 1996). Blockade of NGF can prevent hypertrophy of dorsal root ganglion cells from occurring in response to inflammation (Steers et al., 1996). Thus there is a firmly established relationship between secretion of NGF and alterations of nociceptive signalling both at peripheral and at central sites. In human and animal trials, a single systemic injection of NGF can lower nociceptive thresholds for several days and this effect can be blocked by treatments that deplete mast cells, block 5-hydroxytryptamine (5-HT) receptors or inhibit NGF (Lewin et al., 1992, 1993, 1994; Lewin and Mendell, 1993). Mast cells respond to NGF by releasing 5-HT which, in turn, causes long-lasting lowering of nociceptive thresholds promoting the inflammatory cascade (Purcell and Atterwill, 1995).

With persistent inflammation, new nerve pathways are recruited and the transmission of bladder pain is potentiated. These include sacral dorsal root ganglion neurons which carry afferent input from the bladder. These fibres are small, quiescent and normally possess high thresholds for firing (Yoshimura and DeGroat, 1992). Because of this, they are called 'silent C fibres'. With persistent bladder inflammation, these once-silent neurons become activated, expressing new sodium channels (Yoshimura et al., 1995) and new receptors for neuropeptide pain mediators (e.g. the NK-1 receptor for substance P (Lecci et al., 1994); Fig. 2). This can result in entirely new sensations. The increase in receptors for substance P leads to increased sensitivity to substance P which causes more pain and more urgency (Thompson et al., 1995). There is no known natural mechanism for deactivation of this cascade. With continued bladder inflammation, gene expression in sacral spinal cord cells is upregulated, the degree of which is related to the severity and duration of the inflammation (Lanteri-Minet et al., 1995).

4.4. Hormonal influences

Hormones may modulate nociceptive processing and may be partly responsible for the higher incidence of IC in women. Both oestrogen and progesterone affect the generation of pain signals from the bladder both peripherally and centrally (Martinez-Gomez et al., 1994). The effect of oestrogen on N-methyl D-aspartate (NMDA)

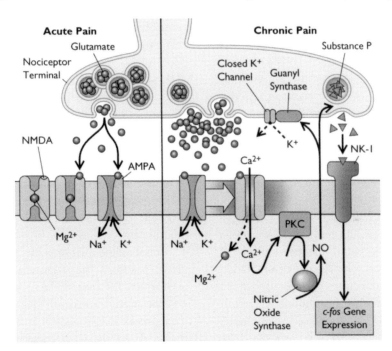

Fig. 2. Sensitization of the nociceptor – acute to chronic pain. Incoming nociceptive signals trigger the release (primarily) of glutamate from the nociceptors at the dorsal horn. In the normal state (acute pain), glutamate activates alpha-amino-3-hydroxy-5-methyl-isoxazole-4-propionic-acid (AMPA) receptors (which are G-protein coupled receptors) on Na^+/K^+ channels. With prolonged activation (i.e. sustained signal), the polarization of the membrane changes. This change of polarization causes the Mg^{2+} plug in Ca^{2+} channels to dissociate, priming these N-methyl-D-Aspartate (NMDA) receptors of the channel complex for glutamate activation. The increasing intracellular Ca^{2+} activates protein kinase C (PKC), a key coenzyme necessary for nitric oxide (NO) synthase production of NO. NO diffuses out of the dorsal cell membrane, through the synaptic cleft and into the nociceptors, stimulating guanyl sythase-induced closure of K^+ channels. The closure of these K^+ channels induces enkephalin and endorphin resistance, as these endogenous substances inhibit pain by opening these channels. The presence of NO stimulates the release of substance P which binds to neurokinin-1 (NK-1) receptors in the dorsal horn membrane triggering c-fos gene expression and promotes neural remodelling and hypersensitization. (From Brookoff with permission.)

receptors may cause less noxious stimuli to elicit more pain in women (Smith, 1994).

5. A legacy of neurodestruction

While the bladder in IC provides a promising target for neuromodulation, the history of the treatment of this condition chronicles more than 100 years of neurodestruction. The first medical reference to IC was published in France in 1836 (Mercier, 1836). The use of intravesicular caustic silver nitrate was described relatively soon thereafter (Tait, 1870). Silver nitrate bladder instillations continue to be used to this day, although the benefit is questionable. The term IC dates to a 19th century textbook by Skene (Skene, 1887). Guy Hunner described the 'characteristic ulcer' in 1914, which bears his name (Hunner, 1915). At first, Hunner advocated the resection of the ulcerated tissue (which is now known to occur in less than 10% of cases) but the high recurrence rate led him to abandon the surgical approach which he detailed in a paper with the interesting title of 'Neurosis of the Bladder' (Hunner, 1930). Actually, Hunner's ulcer is not an ulcer but rather an area of inflamed granulation tissue that is probably better referred to as 'Hunner's patch'.

With the turn of the 20th century, IC was noted to be associated with dental infections (Bidgood, 1928). The association between flares of bladder pain and distant infections (especially dental infections) persists to this day though it remains unexplained. Female predominance was noted early on (Baumrucker, 1955) and soon thereafter came the association of IC with psychiatric and emotional disturbance. A paper from 1958 entitled 'Masochism and Interstitial Cystitis' (Bowers et al., 1958) discussed the aetiology of IC as being repressed hostility toward parental figures handled masochistically via bladder symptoms. Interestingly, while many urologists subscribed to the psychosomatic aetiology of IC they continued to advocate surgical treatment (Gil-Vernet et al., 1960). One urology textbook, which strongly

recommended early cystectomy, described the syndrome as 'the end-stage of a bladder that has been made irritable by emotional disturbance – a pathway for the discharge of unconcious hatreds' (Walsh, 1978). It is important to point out that psychological studies have shown a link between pelvic pain (in general) and a history of sexual victimization (Haber and Roos, 1985; Walker et al., 1992, 1995; Walling et al., 1994; Harrop-Griffiths et al., 1998).

Some of the early treatments for IC can be seen as primitive attempts at neuromodulation. In the 1930s cystodistension under general anaesthesia came into vogue (Bumpus, 1930). Hydrodistension is still a standard treatment for IC which may work by temporarily disrupting nociceptive afferent fibres in the bladder wall. This may also explain the temporary effectiveness of the instillation of solvents (such as dimethyl sulfoxide – DMSO – which was approved for use in the U.S. in 1978) or caustics (such as silver nitrate). In the 1940s, instillation of caustic chemical agents was found to cause irritation then temporary relief (Higgins, 1941; Pool and Rives, 1944). Unfortunately, in most cases the symptoms returned in weeks to months and they returned with greater intensity. The irritation not only brought temporary relief, it probably also sparked neural remodelling.

Presacral neurectomy for the pain of IC was first described in 1926 and was commonly performed for over 40 years though any positive results were transient (Pieri, 1930). Another neurosurgical approach to the pain (and 'sympathetic overactivity') recommended in 1934 was surgical excision of the superior hypogastric plexus (Douglass, 1934). In 1937, urinary diversion via bilateral ureterosigmoidostomies was recommended for refractory IC despite a greater than 20% operative mortality (Counsellor, 1937). In 1951, more selective neurectomies were described (Bourque, 1951). In the 1950s steroids were used with disappointing results despite the association of IC with colitis, gastritis, arthralgias, and atopy (Burke and Vernon, 1952; Hoyt, 1952;

Franksson, 1957). By the late 1950s, the increase in mast cells in the bladder walls of patients with IC (now understood to be a hallmark of neurogenic inflammation) led to treatment with antihistamines (Simmons and Bunce, 1958). Several investigators have noted increased sympathetic activity in the lower extremities of IC patients compared to controls (Irwin et al., 1993a). Lumbar sympathetic blocks have been reported to ease the pain in rare cases, probably indicating other more centralized pathways (Irwin et al., 1993b). Overall, during more than a century since the initial description by Skene, there have been few major therapeutic advances for patients with IC.

6. Neuromodulation in IC

6.1. Rationale

While most current therapies for IC are directed at the lining of the bladder, some of the stimuli eliciting neurogenic inflammation of the bladder may act outside the bladder itself. For example, in some cases symptoms of IC have been attributed to lumbar disc disease or pelvic surgery. Oedema of the bladder wall can be generated by direct stimulation of lumbar roots (Pinter and Szolcanyi, 1995) or pelvic nerves (Koltzenburg and McMahon, 1986). In animal models, isolated central nervous system lesions (e.g. due to viral infection) can produce a clinical picture very similar to IC (Jasmin et al., 1998). A common cause of bladder dysfunction in women is neural damage following hysterectomy (Parys et al., 1990). It is striking that approximately 40% of women with IC had undergone recent hysterectomy prior to the onset of symptoms (Koziol, 1994; Curhan et al., 1999).

If chronic neurogenic inflammation is altering innervation and central processing of pain signals this suggests that therapy for advanced stages of IC will have to be targeted beyond the level of the bladder. Most of the commonly-used therapies are aimed at silencing nociceptive afferents in the

bladder (DMSO, caustics and hydrodistension); these work only temporarily, however. These treatments can cause injuries to the bladder wall which promote further sensory re-modelling and can augment and ingrain the pain. This is certainly what has been observed clinically. Even cystectomy fails to abolish the pain in most of the patients who opt for this mutilating procedure (Baskin and Tanagho, 1992); this also indicates that more proximal pathways of pain transmission or generation have been induced.

There is published evidence that electrical modulation of sacral nerves entering the dorsal horn of the spinal cord can affect the course of IC. In animal studies, antidromic stimulation of dorsal sacral nerve roots results in plasma extravasation and neurogenic inflammation of the bladder (Pinter and Szolcanyi, 1995). This implies that sensory nerves can take on an 'efferent function' which may underlie the neuropathology of IC. By blocking these aberrant inputs through the use of neuromodulation, it should be possible to disrupt the neural circuits that maintain neurogenic inflammation.

Selectively stimulating large-diameter sensory axons should inhibit transmission in C fibre nociceptors and not only relieve pain but possibly promote healing. This has already been suggested by early studies. In addition to improving clinical parameters such as pain and urgency of micturition, stimulation of the S3 nerve roots was also associated with increases in the urinary concentrations of heparin-binding epidermal growth factor and reduced concentrations of anti-proliferative factor, urinary markers correlated with symptoms of IC (Chai et al., 2000).

6.2. Clinical outcomes

In human trials, stimulation of sacral nerve roots has already been proven to be of benefit in sensory disorders of the bladder. All bladder motor function is ultimately regulated through the S2–S4 nerve roots. S3 neuromodulation is able to change sensory parameters in patients with urge incontinence. Sacral nerve stimulation can increase the urinary volume at which the urge to void is triggered (Bosch and Groen, 1995). This is similar to the therapeutic goals of neuromodulation in IC.

The FDA (Food and Drug Administration) has already approved a device (Interstim®, Medtronic, Minneapolis MN) to stimulate sacral nerve roots transforaminally for the syndrome of urge incontinence (a symptom complex that probably includes some cases of IC). The device that is currently marketed in the U.S. is reported to have a 40% success rate. Some of the treatment failures have been attributed to migration of the neurostimulator leads, which commonly occurs with the device that is currently commercially available (Siegel, 1992). A recently published study of the long-term use of this device showed sustained clinical benefit in patients with urgency–frequency syndrome which is probably a form of IC (Siegel et al., 2000)

Electrical stimulation of sacral nerves has become an acceptable and promising modality for controlling various forms of voiding dysfunction. Sacral nerve stimulation has already been shown in European studies to reduce pain related to voiding and other forms of pelvic pain (Koldewijn et al., 1994). Maher prospectively studied 15 women with refractory IC, having a mean duration of symptoms of 5.2 years, for the efficacy of S3 stimulation in relief of pain and other symptoms. Mean voiding volume increased from 90 to 143 cm^3 ($P < 0.001$), mean daytime frequency decreased from 20 to 11 ($P = 0.012$) and nocturnal frequency decreased from 6 to 2 ($P = 0.007$). Mean numeric pain scoring (scale 0–10) decreased from 8.9 to 2.4 ($P < 0.001$; Maher et al., 2001). Permanently implanted sacral nerve stimulators have already been used on a long-term basis in patients with IC with good results (Kerrebroeck and Philip, 1997). The initial devices generated low frequency (10–50 Hz) and a pulse width of 200 ms. At these settings they stimulated pelvic floor muscles and may have been most effective in patients with associated detrusor instability, although long term data on the frequencies necessary for neuropathic pain control

are not available. Long term stimulation at the intensity needed to alleviate voiding symptoms did not induce neural damage (Elabbady et al., 1994). This has been the case even when the stimulators have been implanted in childhood and have been operating for many years. In patients with urinary symptoms due to detrusor instability, sacral nerve root stimulation can obviate the need for more invasive surgery. The same may be true for patients with IC with intractable pain who are facing the prospect of cystectomy.

Using a retrograde lumbar approach, Feler and colleagues reported significant reduction of pelvic pain by stimulating bilateral S2 and S3 roots in 15 of 17 patients with IC who had failed aggressive pain treatment and were facing cystectomy (Feler et al., 1999). They have since carried out this procedure in over 100 patients and, using relatively high frequencies (200–1000 Hz), they have maintained a 75% success rate (unpublished data).

A peripherally placed neuromodulation system has been developed which delivers low frequency S3 stimulation via the tibial nerve. The leads are inserted near the ankle or lower tibia. This device has shown some success in the treatment of urge incontinence. The device, which is not available in the U.S., does not have an implanted pulse generator but rather it is used in 30 min sessions once per week (Klingler et al., 2000).

6.3. Technique of sacral nerve stimulation: transforaminal versus retrograde

Dorsal column stimulation and conus stimulation have not shown adequate long term coverage for sacral mediated pain. This is probably due to the variability of sacral rootlet contact with the active cathode(s) (in conus stimulation) and to the depth of sacral fibres (in dorsal column stimulation) which results in the production of painful dysaesthesias in more proximal neural structures during stimulation.

Sacral nerve stimulation has been described using a transforaminal approach, limiting the targets to one nerve root or pair of nerve roots

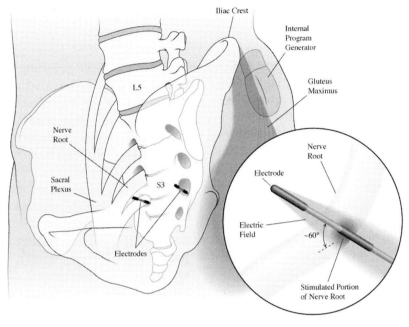

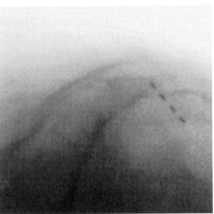

Fig. 3. Transforaminal sacral nerve stimulation (classical approach). (a) In the traditional or 'classic' approach, a linear electrode array (stimulation lead) is inserted at a nearly perpendicular angle to the exiting sacral nerve through a transforaminal approach. The lead (in this case an Interstim® device; Medtronic Inc.) is then secured to the fascia overlying the os sacrum and then connected to either a RF-receiver or IPG which is placed in the subdermal tissues. (b) Radiographic appearance.

(S2 or S3). Utilizing this approach, the implanter passes an electrode array directly into the foramen of the desired nerve root (Fig. 3). The anatomy makes this approach problematic: the nerve is exiting perpendicular to the electrode array. This probably explains the variable paraesthesia coverage experienced by patients with this form of implant, as well as the 'shocking' phenomenon that some patients describe.

Unilateral stimulation of sacral nerve roots (typically S3 in the case of transforaminal stimulation) has been advocated for urge–incontinence and pelvic pain, although there is some evidence for increased efficacy when bilateral stimulation is employed (Koldewijn et al., 1994; Hohenfellner et al., 1998; Braun et al., 2000). In IC we have found it beneficial to place bilateral electrode arrays (leads), although in a parallel position relative to the nerve (in distinction to perpendicular to the nerve), with establishment of an electrical field across the sacrum (multiple sacral nerve roots). This is possible as the amount of cerebral spinal fluid (CSF) is essentially negligible (i.e. distance from dura to nerve target is less than 1 mm); an electrical field is therefore easily established which affects multiple nerve roots (as determined by areas of paraesthesia fields reported by patients).

A more recent advance has been the introduction of lumbar retrograde sacral nerve stimulation (Alo and Zidan, 2000; Alo and McKay, 2001; Alo et al., 2001). This technique, both percutaneously applied as described by Alo and via S1/S2 laminectomy, has shown consistent coverage with limited electrode migration. In addition, unlike transforaminal systems, this approach is easily able to cover S2–S4 (Fig. 4). This is important in that approximately 70% of IC is thought to be mediated by S3, while the remainder of these patients require S2 and/or S4 coverage.

In the percutaneous approach, the patient is positioned prone in a flexed position with appropriate padding to 'break' the L5/sacrum angle (i.e. to lessen the angular degree to promote passage from the lumbar space into the sacral space). An advantage of this technique is that the anatomy of

the yellow ligament (ligamentum flavum), which runs rostral-caudal, helps to guide the electrode array caudally. This author (Bennett) employs a paravertebral block involving the segment proximal and distal in addition to the planned entry site; this serves to densely anaesthetize the laminar ridges which are quite painful when encountered during rostral-caudal (retrograde) epidural access (Fig. 5). Anaesthesia of the dura is always avoided, as this would remove an effective safeguard to unwanted nerve root trauma. Entry is made proximal to the L5/S1 junction, preferably at L3/L4, to allow steering of the array in a caudal fashion. Entry into the epidural space is made via a paramedian approach, usually 1½–2 levels proximal to the desired entry point, aiming the insertion cannula toward the midline. Once entry is made (usually using a standard loss of resistance technique), the electrode array is guided through the cannula and midline until it passes the L5/S1 junction. Assuming normal sacral anatomy (the reader is reminded of the variability of sacral architecture), the electrode array is guided in the midline, with turning toward the desired sacral foramen at the level proximal (i.e. if one wishes to place the array at the S3 foramen, then turning occurs at S2). Each array is guided to, but not through, the foramen to prevent ventral placement

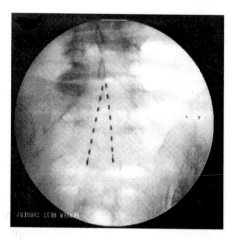
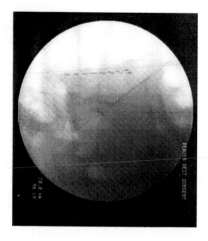

Fig. 4. Retrograde percutaneous sacral stimulation. Placement of bilateral linear arrays (stimulation leads) which run parallel with the exiting nerve rootlets, allows the establishment of an electric field across the sacral region. This field affects multiple nerve rootles as they transit the sacrum toward their respective foramina.

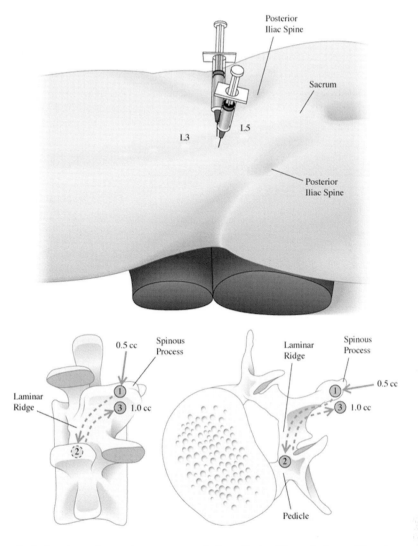

Fig. 5. Periosteal anaesthesia for retrograde percutaneous approach. Anaesthesia of the periosteum of the spinous process and laminar ridge is recommended in the retrograde percutaneous approach. As cannula insertion is necessary under the inferior ridge of the intralaminar space, periosteal abutment can lead to significant pain for the patient. Ablation of the periosteal sensitivity allows for easier insertion without undue movement by the patient, thereby facilitating a more controlled entry into the epidural space. One places a 22G or 25G needle in midline until contact with the posterior portion of the spinous process superior to the intralaminar space and deposits 0.5 cc of 0.5% bupivacaine with 1:200,000 epinephrine solution. Slight retraction of the needle then allows advancement of the needle laterally to the pedicle/laminar ridge with 1 cc of the solution being deposited as the needle is brought from the pedicle/laminar ridge upward to the spinous process; this manoeuvre is repeated on the opposite site. One then performs the entire procedure again for the spinous process/laminar ridge of the segment inferior to the intralaminar space. This can be performed at an additional level above to allow pre-procedural anaesthesia of two intralaminar spaces.

of the array which will give unpleasant motor or mixed stimulation patterns (Fig. 6).

Anchoring the electrode array is paramount to prevent displacement. A paramedian entry assists in preventing movement, as placement is off centre for the fulcrum (midline spinal ligament) of spine movement. Dissection of the ligament on the side of exiting electrode array provides a place to securely anchor the array with a strain relief boot (Fig. 7). The paraspinal muscles are then reattached.

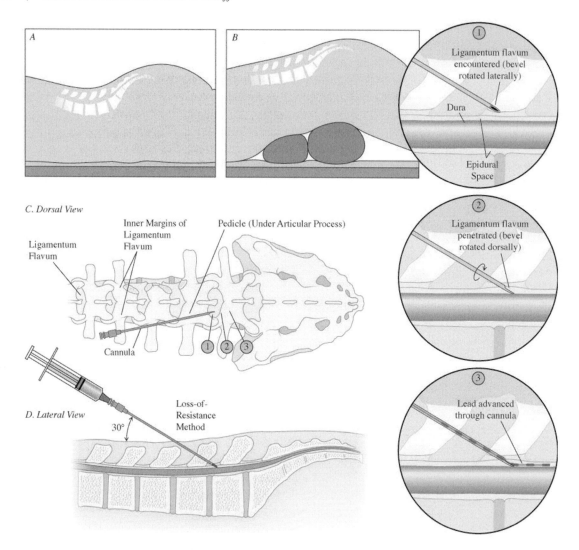

Fig. 6. Approach/advancement in percutaneous retrograde stimulation. Padding is used to reduce the lumbo-sacral angle (A,B). For cannulation of the epidural space, a 14G cannula (needle) is positioned $1\frac{1}{2}$ segments proximal to the planned entry point (intralaminar space) (C) and guided in a paramedian direction caudally, aiming the point toward midline with the bevel rotated to point laterally. This should allow entry into the spinal ligament/ligamentum flavum interface at or near midline. Loss of resistance technique is then utilized for entry into the epidural space (D); entry is followed by rotation of the bevel dorsally to void inadvertent puncture of dura with patient movement. Once entry into the space has been accomplished, the linear array (stimulation lead) is inserted and *gently* and *slowly* advanced caudally (note: advancement caudally allows the lead to follow the direction of the fibres of the ligamentum flavum (yellow ligament)) until passage past the acute angle of the L5/S1 junction. At this point, the tip of the lead can be turned and directed toward the desired foramen. This technique allows the placement of four quadrapolar arrays (an issue can be made for an array in the direction of the S2 exiting nerve and one in the direction of the S3 exiting nerve [S3 and S4 run in the same plane, whereas S1 and S2 divert laterally in different planes]) or two octapolar arrays (the upper electrodes can be configured to capture S2).

The necessity of intraoperative testing is in debate. This author (Bennett) prefers intraoperative testing to ensure that motor recruitment is not occurring (in the percutaneous approach where the electrode array can turn ventrally if passed through the foramen; intraoperative testing is unnecessary in laminectomy approaches). Programming of the array is performed using

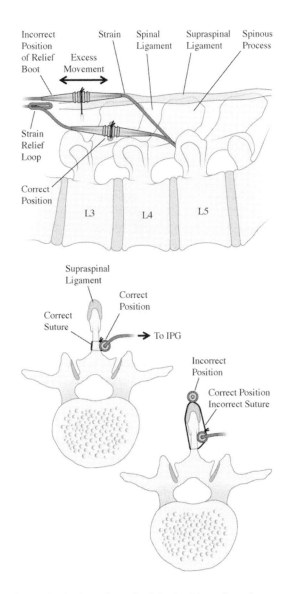

Fig. 7. Anchoring of proximal lead with anchor sleeve to reduce movement. Because the fulcrum of the lumbar spine is along the midline (spinous process), anchoring of the proximal portions of the stimulation lead(s) should occur lateral to the spinal ligament; a strain relief anchor sleeve is recommended. Exposure of the spinal ligament is accomplished with exposure at least half the distance to the respective lamina. The lead can be attached to ligament or bone, with the use of a braided non-absorbable suture.

a 'flayed cathodal' approach (Fig. 8). As the amount of CSF is negligible, the array is essentially being utilized as a peripheral nerve stimulator. The rule of thumb is low pulse width

and low amplitude (depending upon the amount of CSF, amplitudes can be under 1.0 V).

Until summary data are analysed in a large subset, it is unclear whether S3 alone is the appropriate neural target in IC. Therefore, it is recommended that S2–S4 be covered. Because S3 and S4 are in a linear plane as they exit the sacrum, one usually captures S4 with a S3 positioned array. Therefore, coverage of S2 is undertaken with an extra array, placed proximal to the S2 foramen or with octapolar arrays. In our experience, the majority of patients respond with S3, S4 stimulation.

The retrograde laminectomy technique is carried out under general anaesthesia (it is difficult to anaesthetize the sacral region locally, unlike the lumbar region). A laminotomy is made at S1/S2 to allow passage of a paddle array (a dual four contact system is preferred at our centres as this provides significant programming control, obviating the need for surgical revision) until the tip is between S3 and S4 (Fig. 9). Anchoring the paddle to the dura is optional, but recommended if the sacral space is wide (to prevent displacement). The only unique aspect of programming for sacral paddles is a significantly lower stimulus amplitude, as paddle electrode arrays displace dura, which positions the active cathodes extremely close to the neural structure. It remains unclear as to whether percutaneous or paddle arrays will prove more stable with time.

Whether one chooses a percutaneous or laminectomy approach, delay in pain relief can be up to 3 days. Initially, patients note a reduction in the 'burning' dysaesthesias while complaining of a 'deep ache' which can persist. It is postulated that this phenomenon is similar to the effect of neuromodulation in vasculopathies, where lactate 'washout' takes place over several days producing a delayed onset of optimal pain control. In addition, instrumentation in a retrograde fashion (noted primarily with percutaneously applied arrays), can produce significant post-operative low back pain; this should be anticipated in the perioperative period as it can produce significant

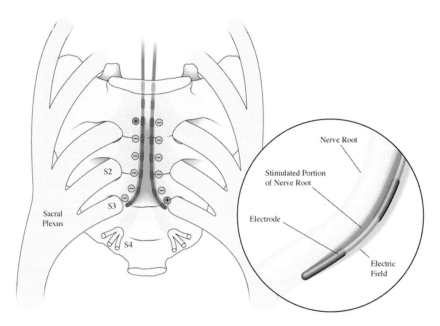

Fig. 8. Programming of retrograde sacral electrode arrays. Because the distance from dura to nerve is small (generally the CSF layer is 1 mm or less) in the sacrum, the neural target is extremely close to the active cathode(s). Stringing the cathodes or 'flaying' the cathodes will reduce the depth of the field to avoid dysaesthesias or motor recruitment. In addition, because the CSF is an excellent conducting medium, a trans-sacral field can be established to 'capture' multiple sacral nerves (S2–S4). Electrodes illustrated are Orctrodes® (Advanced Neuromodulation Systems Inc.)

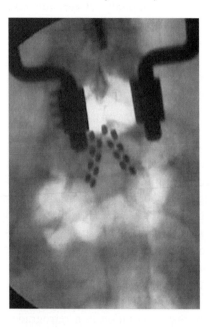

Fig. 9. Retrograde paddle arrays for sacral stimulation. Placement of paddle arrays is done via a laminotomy of the os sacrum at S1/S2, with straightforward anatomic placement. As a rule, extremely low amplitude (often < 0.5 V) and pulse width is needed as the dura to nerve distance is small.

distress to the patient. Treatment usually consists of systemic opioids and muscle relaxants (such as diazepam). Instillation of epidural anaesthetics has been suggested by some to mitigate post-operative low back pain, although this can (theoretically) increase the incidence of post-operative infection.

6.4. IC versus pelvic floor dysfunction

Stimulation parameters for predominant neuropathic pain in IC differ from those for cases in which pelvic floor dysfunction predominates. Data at our centres have shown that, for neuropathic pain in IC, increases in stimulation frequency (ranging from 150 to 1025 Hz) are required and are sustained whereas in pelvic floor dysfunction, low frequencies (10–50 Hz) are the rule. When attempting to differentiate the requirements for an individual patient, trialling (i.e. externalizing an extension lead from permanently positioned electrode arrays) is recommended. The duration of the trial depends upon the skill and experience of the implanter; it is suggested that trials occur for a minimum of 1 week to allow documentation of significant pain relief. In addition, trialling can allow a determination as to whether a radio-frequency based system (for those patients who require frequencies higher than 200 Hz) or an implantable pulse generator (IPG) should be employed (it is important to note that currently available IPG systems are limited to eight contacts; single eight or dual four configurations).

7. Conclusions

Interstitial cystitis is a neuropathic syndrome characterized by hypersensitivity of the bladder associated with low bladder volumes, severe urinary frequency/urgency, and often associated with debilitating hyperalgesia and allodynia. Sacral nerve stimulation involves electrical stimulation of somatic afferent nerves with consequential inhibition of aberrant sensory processing in the spinal cord/brainstem loop, in part via C fibre afferents. Sacral nerve stimulation is effective in reducing painful dysaesthesias while promoting normalization of bladder volumes, and should be considered as a viable treatment option in patients suffering from this debilitating syndrome.

References

Alo, K.M. and McKay, E. (2001) Selective nerve root stimulation (SNRS) for the treatment of intractable pelvic pain and motor dysfunction: a case report. Neuromodulation, 4(1): 19.

Alo, K.M. and Zidan, A.M. (2000) Selective nerve root stimulation (SNRS) in the treatment of end-stage, diabetic, peripheral neuropathy: a case report. Neuromodulation, 3(4): 201.

Alo, K.M., Gohel, R., and Corey, C.L. (2001) Sacral nerve root stimulation for the treatment of urge incontinence and detrusor dysfunction utilizing a cephalocaudal intraspinal method of lead insertion: a case report. Neuromodulation, 4(2): 53.

Andersson, K.E. and Hedlund, P. (2002) Pharmacologic perspective on the physiology of the lower urinary tract. [Review] Urology, 60(5 Suppl. 1): 13–21.

Badenoch, A.W. (1971) Chronic interstitial cystitis. Br. J. Urol., 43: 718–721.

Baskin, L.S. and Tanagho, E.A. (1992) Pelvic pain without pelvic organs. J. Urol., 147: 683–686.

Baumrucker, G.O. (1955) An experimental study of elusive bladder ulcer of Hunner. J. Int. Coll. Surg., 23: 221–225.

Bidgood, C.Y. (1928) Tissue cultures in two cases of interstitial cystitis. Am. J. Surg., 4: 140–142.

Bienenstock, J., MacQueen, G., Sestini, P., Marshall, J.S., Stead, R.H., and Perdue, M.H. (1991) Mast cell/nerve interactions in vitro and in vivo. Am. Rev. Respir. Dis., 143: S55–S58.

Bjorling, D.E., Saban, M.R., and Saban, R. (1994) Neurogenic inflammation of guinea pig bladder. Mediators Inflamm., 3: 189–197.

Bosch, J.L.H.R. and Groen, J. (1995) Sacral (S3) segmental nerve stimulation as a treatment for urge incontinence in patients with detrusor instability: results of chronic electrical stimulation using an implantable neural prosthesis. J. Urol., 154: 504–507.

Bourque, J.P. (1951) Surgical management of the painful bladder. J. Urol., 65: 25–35.

Bowers, J.E., Schwarz, B.E., and Leon, M.J. (1958) Masochism and interstitial cystitis. Psychosom. Med., 20: 296–302.

Braun, P.M., Bross, S., Scheepe, J.R., Sief, C., Alken, P., Juenemann, P. (2000) Chronic bilateral sacral neuromodulation in patients with bladder dysfunction. Abstract 415. The International Continence Society (ICS) Annual Meeting. Tampere, Finland.

Brookoff, D. (2000) Chronic pain: 1. A new disease? Hosp. Pract., 35(7): 45–52, 59.

Bumpus, H.C. (1930) Interstitial cystitis: its treatment by over-distension of the bladder. Med. Clin. North Am., 13: 1495–1498.

Burke, J. and Vernon, H.K. (1952) Effects of ACTH on Hunner's ulcer of the urinary bladder. Br. Med. J., 2: 477.

Chai, T.C., Zhang, C., Warren, J.W., and Keay, S. (2000) Percutaneous sacral third nerve root neurostimulation improves symptoms and normalizes urinary HB-EGF levels and antiproliferative factor in patients with interstitial cystitis. Urology, 55: 643–646.

Chancellor, M.B. and De Groat, W.C.. (1999) Intravesical capsaicin and resiniferatoxin therapy: spicing up the ways to treat the overactive bladder. J. Urol., 162(1): 3–11.

Christian, E.P., Undem, B.J., and Weinreich, D. (1989) Endogenous histamine excites neurones in the guinea pig superior cervical ganglion. J. Physiol. (Lond.), 409: 297–312.

Christmas, T.J., Rode, J., Chapple, C.R., Milroy, E.J.G., and Turner-Warwick, R.T. (1990) Nerve fibre proliferation in interstitial cystitis. Virchows Arch. Pathol. Anat. Histopathol., 416: 447–451.

Clauw, D.J., Schmidt, M., Radulovic, D., Singer, A., Katz, P., and Bresette, J. (1997) The relationship between fibromyalgia and interstitial cystitis. J. Psychiatr. Res., 31(1): 125–131.

Counsellor, V.S. (1937) Bilateral transplantation of ureters in the female. Am. J. Obstet. Gynecol., 33: 234–249.

Crowe, S.E. and Perdue, M.H. (1992) Functional abnormalities in the intestine associated with mucosal mast cell activation. Reg. Immunol., 4: 113–117.

Curhan, G.C., Speizer, F.E., Hunter, D.J., Curhan, S.G., and Stampfer, M.J. (1999) Epidemiology of interstitial cystitis: a population based study. J. Urol., 161: 549–552.

DeGroat, W.C., Fowler, C.J., Jewkes, D., McDonald, W.I., and Lynn, B. (1992) Intravesicular capsaicin for neurogenic bladder dysfunction. Lancet, 339: 1239.

Dines, K.C. and Powell, H.C. (1997) Mast cell interactions with the nervous system: relationship to mechanisms of disease. J. Neuropathol. Exp. Neurol., 56(6): 627–640.

Douglass, H.L. (1934) Excision of the superior hypogastric plexus in the treatment of intractable interstitial cystitis, report of five cases. Am. J. Surg., 25: 249–257.

Dupont, M.C., Steers, W.C., and Tuttle, J.B. (1994a) Inflammation induced neural plasticity in autonomic pathways supplying the bladder may depend on NGF. Soc. Neurosci. Abstr., 20: 53.1.

Dupont, M., Steers, W.D., McCarty, R., and Tuttle, J.B. (1994b) Neural plasticity and alterations in nerve growth factor and norepinephrine in response to bladder inflammation. J. Urol., 151: 284.

Dvorak, A.M., McLeod, R.S., and Onderdonk, A.B. (1992) Human gut mucosal mast cells: ultrastructural observations and anatomic variations in mast cell-nerve associations. Int. Arch. Allergy Immunol., 98: 150–168.

Elabbady, A.A., Hassouna, M.M., and Ethilali, M.M. (1994) Neural stimulation for chronic voiding dysfunctions. J. Urol., 152: 287–291.

Feler, C.A., Whitworth, L.A., Brookoff, D., and Powell, R. (1999) Recent advances: sacral nerve root stimulation using a retrograde method of lead insertion for the treatment of pelvic pain due to interstitial cystitis. Neuromodulation, 2: 211–216.

Felsen, D., Frye, S., Trimble, L.A., Bavendam, T.G., Parsons, C.L., Sim, Y., and Vaughan, E.D., Jr. (1994) Inflammatory mediator profile in urine and bladder wash fluid of patients with interstitial cystitis. J. Urol., 152: 355–361.

Fleischmann, J.D., Huntley, H.N., Shingleton, W.B., and Wentworth, D.B. (1991) Clinical and immunological response to nifedipine for the treatment of interstitial cystitis. J. Urol., 146: 1235–1239.

Franksson, C. (1957) Interstitial cystitis: a study of fifty-nine cases. Acta Chir. Scand., 113: 51–62.

Gil-Vernet, J.M., Gonzalez, V., and Fernandez, E. (1960) Etiopathogenie et traitement de la cystite interstitielle. Acta Urol. Belg., 28: 425–440.

Gosling, J.A. and Dixon, J.S. (1974) Sensory nerves in the mammalian urinary tract. An evaluation using light and electron microscopy. J. Anat., 117: 133–144.

Haber, J. and Roos, C. (1985) Effects of spouse and/or sexual abuse and the development and maintenance of chronic pain in woman. Adv. Pain Res. Ther., 9: 890–895.

Hamid, Q.A., Rode, J., and Flanagan, A.M. (1988) Endocrine differentiation in inflamed urinary bladder epithelium with metaplastic changes. Virchows Arch. Pathol. Anat. Histopathol., 412: 267–272.

Hanash, K.A. and Pool, T.L. (1969) Interstitial cystitis in men. J. Urol., 102: 427–428.

Harrop-Griffiths, J., Katon, W., Walker, E., Holm, L., Russo, J., and Hickok, L. (1998) The association between chronic pelvic pain, psychiatric diagnoses, and childhood sexual abuse. Obstet. Gynecol., 71: 589–594.

Held, P.J., Hanno, P.M., Wein, A.J., Pauly, M.V., and Cann, M.A. (1990) Epidemiology of interstitial cystitis. In: P.M. Hanno, D.R. Staskin, R.J. Krane, and A.J. Wein, (Eds.), *Interstitial Cystitis* (pp. 29–48). Springer-Verlag, New York.

Higgins, C.C. (1941) Hunner ulcer of the bladder (review of 100 cases). Ann. Int. Med., 15: 708–715.

Hohenfeller, M., Nunes, L., Schmidt, R.A., Lampel, A., Thuroff, J.W., and Tanagho, E.A. (1992) Interstitial cystitis: increased sympathetic innervation and related neuropeptide synthesis. J. Urol., 147: 587–591.

Hohenfellner, M., Schultz_Lampel, D., Dahms, S., Klaus, M., and Thuroff, J.W. (1998) Bilateral chronic sacral neuromodulation for treatment for lower urinary tract dysfunction. J. Urol., 160: 821–824.

Holm-Bentzen, M., Ammitzboll, T., and Hald, T. (1986) Glycosaminoglycans on the surface of the human urothelium: a preliminary report. Neurourol. Urodyn., 5: 519–523.

Hoyt, H.S. (1952) Cortisone in urological conditions with report of a trial in interstitial cystitis. J Urol., 67: 889–893.

Hsu, L., Savage, P., and Jeng, A.Y. (1992) Dual effects of endothelin-1 on neurite outgrowth induced by 12-0-tetradecanoylphorbol-13-acetate. Neurosci. Lett., 136: 219–222.

Hukkanen, M., Gronblad, M., and Rees, R. (1991) Regional distribution of mast cells and peptide containing nerves in normal and adjuvant arthritic rat synovium. J. Rheumatol., 18: 177–183.

Hunner, G.L. (1915) A rare type of bladder ulcer in women: report of cases. Trans. South Surg. Gynecol. Assoc., 27: 247–292.

Hunner, G.L. (1930) Neurosis of the bladder. J. Urol., 24: 567–585.

Hurst, R.E, Parson, C.L, Roy, J.B., and Young, J.L. (1993) Urinary glycosaminoglycan excretion as a laboratory marker in the diagnosis of interstitial cystitis. J. Urol., 149: 31–35.

Irwin, P., James, S., Watts, L., Fleming, L.L., and Galloway, N.T.M. (1993a) Abnormal pedal thermoregulation in interstitial cystitis. Neurourol. Urodyn., 12: 139–144.

Irwin, P., Hammonds, W.D., and Galloway, N.T.M. (1993b) Lumbar epidural blockade in the management of pain in interstitial cystitis. Br. J. Urol., 71: 413–416.

Jasmin, L., Janni, G., Manz, H.J., and Rabkin, S.D. (1998) Activation of CNS circuits producing a neurogenic cystitis: evidence for centrally induced peripheral inflammation. J. Neurosci., 18(23): 10,016–10,029.

Johansson, S.L. and Fall, M. (1994) Pathology of interstitial cystitis. Urol. Clin. North Am., 21: 55–62.

Kannan, Y., Moriyama, M., Sugano, T., Yamate, J., Kuwamura, M., Kagaya, A., and Kiso, Y. (2000) Neurotrophic action of interleukin 3 and granulocyte-macrophage colony-stimulating factor on murine sympathetic neurons. Neuroimmunomodulation, 8(3): 132–141.

Keast, J.R. and De Groat, W.C. (1992) Segmental distribution and peptide content of primary afferent neurons innervating the urogenital organs and colon of male rats. J. Comp. Neurol., 319: 615–623.

Kerrebroeck, V. and Philip, E.V. (1997) Electrical stimulation in the management of interstitial cystitis. In: G.R. Sant (Ed.), *Interstitial Cystitis* (pp. 219–221). Lippincott-Raven Publishers, Philadelphia.

Klingler, H.C., Pycha, A., Schmidbauer, J., and Marberger, M. (2000) Use of peripheral neuromodulation of the S3 region for treatment of detrusor overactivity. Urology, 56: 766–771.

Koldewijn, E.L., Rosier, P.F.W.M., and Meuleman, E.J.H. (1994) Predictors of success with neuromodulation in lower urinary tract dysfunction: results of trial stimulation in 100 patients. J. Urol., 152: 2071–2075.

Koltzenburg, M. and McMahon, S.B. (1986) Plasma extravasation in the rat urinary bladder following mechanical, electrical and chemical stimuli: evidence for a new population of chemosensitive primary sensory neurons. Neurosci. Lett., 72: 352–356.

Koziol, J.A. (1994) Epidemiology of interstitial cystitis. Urol. Clin. North Am., 21: 7–20.

Koziol, J.A., Clark, D.C., Gittes, R.F., and Tan, E.M. (1993) The natural history of interstitial cystitis – a survey of 374 patients. J. Urol., 149: 465–469.

Koziol, J.A., Adams, H.P., and Frutos, A. (1995) Discrimination between the ulcerous and the non-ulcerous forms of interstitial cystitis by non-invasive findings. J. Urol., 155: 87–90.

Kusek, J.W. and Nyberg, L.M. (2001) The epidemiology of interstitial cystitis: is it time to expand our definition? Urology, 57(6 Suppl. 1): 95–99.

Lanteri-Minet, M., Bon, K., De Pommery, J., Michiels, J.F., and Menetrey, D. (1995) Cyclophosphamide cystitis as a model of visceral pain in rats: model elaboration and spinal structures involved as revealed by the expression of c-Fos and Krox-24 proteins. Exp. Brain Res., 105: 220–232.

Leach, G.E. and Raz, S. (1983) Interstitial cystitis. In: S. Raz (Ed.), *Female Urology* (pp. 351–356). WB Saunders, Philadelphia.

Lecci, A., Guiliani, S., Santicioli, P., and Maggi, C.A. (1994) Involvement of spinal tachykinin NK1 and NK2 receptors in detrusor hyperreflexia during chemical cystitis in anesthetized rats. Eur. J. Pharmacol., 259: 129–135.

Lembeck, F. and Holzer, P. (1979) Substance P as neurogenic mediator of antidromic vasodilatation and neurogenic plasma extravasation. Naunyn Schmiedebergs Arch. Pharmacol., 310: 175–183.

Letourneau, R., Pang, X., Sant, G.R., and Theoharides TC. (1996) Intragranular activation of bladder mast cells and their association with nerve processes in interstitial cystitis. Br. J. Urol., 77: 41–54.

Lewin, G.R. and Mendell, L.M. (1993) Nerve growth factor and nociception. Trends. Neurosci., 16: 353–359.

Lewin, G.R., Ritter, A.M., and Mendell, L.M. (1992) On the role of nerve growth factor in the development of myelinated nociceptors. J. Neurosci., 12: 1896–1905.

Lewin, G.R., Ritter, A.M., and Mendell, L.M. (1993) Nerve growth factor induced hyperalgesia in the neonatal and adult rat. J. Neurosci., 13: 2136–2148.

Lewin, G.R., Rueff, A., and Mendell, L.M. (1994) Peripheral and central mechanisms of NGF induced hyperalgesia. Eur. J. Neurosci., 6: 1903–1912.

Liekens, S., Neyts, J., Degreve, B., and De Clercq, E. (1997) The sulfonic acid polymers PAMPS [poly(2-acrylamido-2-methyl-1-propanesulfonic acid)] and related analogues are highly potent inhibitors of angiogenesis. Oncol. Res., 9(4): 173–181.

Lilly, J.D. and Parsons, C.L. (1990) Bladder surface glycosaminoglycans is a human epithelial permeability barrier. Surg. Gyn. Obstet., 171: 143–145.

Maher, C.F., Carey, M.P., Dwyer, P.L., and Schlucter, P.L. (2001) Percutaneous sacral nerve root neuromodulation for intractable interstitial cystitis. J. Urol., 165: 884–886.

March, P., Teng, B., Westropp, J., and Buffington, T. (2001) Effects of resiniferatoxin on the neurogenic component of feline interstitial cystitis. Urology, 57(6 Suppl. 1): 114.

Marshall, J.S., Stead, R.H., McSharry, C., Nielsen, L., and Bienenstock, J. (1990) The role of mast cell degranualtion products in mast cell hyperplasia. Mechanism of action of nerve growth factor. J. Immunol., 144: 1886–1892.

Martinez-Gomez, M., Cruz, Y., Salas, M., Hudson, R., and Pacheco, P. (1994) Assessing pain threshhold in the rat: changes with estrus and time of day. Physiol. Behav., 55: 651–657.

Martins, S.M., Darlin, D.J., Lad, P.M., and Zimmern, P.E. (1994) Interleukin-1beta: a clinically relevant urinary marker. J. Urol., 151: 1198–1201.

McKay, D.M. and Bienenstock, J. (1994) The interaction between mast cells and nerves in the gastrointestinal tract. Immunol. Today, 15: 533–538.

McMahon, S.B. and Abel, C. (1987) A model for the study of visceral pain states: chronic inflammation of the chronic decerebrate rat urinary bladder by irritant chemicals. Pain, 28(1): 109–127.

Mercier, L.A. (1836) Memoire sur certaines perforations spontanées de la vessie non decrites jusqu'a ce jour. Gaz. Med. Paris, 4: 257–263.

Messing, E.M. (1987) The diagnosis of interstitial cystitis. Urology, 29(Suppl. 4): 4–7.

Messing, E.M. (1992) Interstitial cystitis and related syndromes. In: P.C. Walsh, A.B. Retik, T.A. Stamey, and Darracott-Vaughan, E., Jr., (Eds.), *Campbell's Urology*. 3rd ed. (pp. 982–1005). W.B. Saunders, Philadelphia.

Mousli, M., Bueb, J.L., Bronner, C., Rouot, B., and Landry, Y. (1990) G protein activation: a receptor-independent mode of action for cationic amphiphilic neuropeptides and venom peptides. Trends Pharmacol. Sci., 11: 358–362.

Naukkarinen, A., Harvima, I.T., Aalto, M.L., Harvima, R.J., and Horsmanheimo, M. (1991) Quantitative analysis of contact sites between mast cells and sensory nerves in cutaneous psoriasis and lichen planus based on a double staining technique. Arch. Dermatol. Res., 283: 433–437.

Oddiah, D., Anand, P., McMahon, S.B., and Rattray, M. (1998) Rapid increase of NGF, BDNF and NT-3 mRNAs in inflamed bladder. Neuroreport, 9: 1455–1488.

Oravisto, K.J. (1975) Epidemiology of interstitial cystitis. Ann. Chir. Gynecol. Fenn., 64: 75–77.

Pang, X., Marchand, J., Sant, G.R., Kream, R.M., and Theoharides, T.C. (1995) Increased number of substance P positive nerve fibres in interstitial cystitis. Br. J. Urol., 75: 744–750.

Parivar, F. and Bradbrook, R.A. (1986) Interstitial cystitis. Br. J. Urol., 58: 239–243.

Parsons, C.L., Lilly, J.D., and Stein, P. (1991) Epithelial dysfunction in nonbacterial cystitis. J. Urol., 145: 732–735.

Parsons, C.L., Housley, J.D., Schmidt, J.D., and Lebow, D. (1994) Treatment of interstitial cystitis with intravesical heparin. Br. J. Urol., 73: 504–507.

Parys, B.T., Woolfenden, K.A., and Parsons, K.F. (1990) Bladder dysfunction after simple hysterectomy: urodynamic and neurological evaluation. Eur. Urol., 17: 129–133.

Persson, K., Sando, J., Tuttle, J.B., and Steers, W.D. (1996) Protein kinase C in cyclic stretch-induced nerve growth factor production by urinary tract smooth muscle cells. Am. J. Physiol., 269: C1018–C1024.

Petersson, G. and Svensjo, E. (1992) Nasal mucosal permeability after methacholine, substance P and capsaicin challenge in the rat. Int. J. Microcirc. Clin. Exp., 9: 205–212.

Pieri, G. (1930) Clinical contributions on the surgery of the sympathetic nervous system. The treatment of tuberculous cystitis. Arch. Ital. Chir., 27: 454–482.

Pinter, E. and Szolcanyi, J. (1995) Plasma extravasation in the skin and pelvic organs evoked by antidromic stimulation of the lumbosacral dorsal roots in the rat. Neuroscience, 68: 603–614.

Pool, T.L. and Rives, H.F. (1944) Interstitial cystitis: treatment with silver nitrate. J. Urol., 51: 520–525.

Purcell, W.M. and Atterwill, C.K. (1995) Mast cells in neuroimmune function: neurotoxicological and neuropharmacological perspectives. Neurochem. Res., 20: 521–532.

Sadhukhan, P., Tchetgen, M., Rackley, R., Vasavada, S., Liou, L., and Bandyopadhyay, S. (2002) Sodium pentosan polysulfate reduces urothelial responses to inflammatory stimuli via an indirect mechanism. J. Urol., 168(1): 289–292.

Sant, G.R. (1991) Interstitial cystitis. Monogr. Urol., 12: 37–63.

Siegel, S. (1992) Management of voiding dysfunction with an implantaable neuroprosthesis. In The Craft of Urologic Surgery, 19(1): 163–170.

Siegel, S.W., Catanzaro, F., and Dijkema, H.E. (2000) Long-term results of a multicenter study on sacral nerve stimulation for treatment of urinary urge incontinence, urgency-frequency and retention. Urology, 56(Suppl. 6A): 87–91.

Silk, M.R. (1970) Bladder antibodies in interstitial cystitis. J. Urol., 103: 307–309.

Simmons, J.L. and Bunce, P.L. (1958) On the use of antihistamine in the treatment of interstitial cystitis. Am. Surg., 24: 664–667.

Skene, A.J.C. (1887) *Diseases of the Bladder and Urethra in Women* (p. 167). Wm Wood, New York.

Smith, S.S. (1994) Female sex steroid hormones: from receptors to networks to performance-actions on the somatosensory system. Prog. Neurobiol., 44: 55–86.

Steers, W.D. and Tuttle, J.B. (1997) Chapter 8: Neurogenic inflammation and nerve growth factor: possible roles in IC. In: G.R. Sant (Ed.), *Interstitial Cystitis* (pp. 67–75). Lippincott-Raven, Philadelphia.

Steers, W.D., Kolbeck, S., Creedon, D., and Tuttle, J.B. (1991) Nerve growth factoring the urinary bladder of the adult regulates neuronal form and function. J. Clin. Invest., 88: 1709–1715.

Steers, W.D., Creedon, D., and Tuttle, J.B. (1996) Immunity to NGF prevents afferent plasticity following hypertrophy of the urinary bladder. J. Urol., 155: 379–386.

Tait, L. (1870) Cure of the chronic perforating ulcer of the bladder by the formation of an artificial vesico-vaginal fistula. Lancet, 2: 738.

Theoharides, T.C., Sant, G.R., El-Mansoury, M., Letourneau, R., Ucci, A.A., Jr., and Meares, E.R., Jr. (1995) Activation of bladder mast cells in interstitial cystitis: a light and electron microscopic study. J. Urol., 153: 629–636.

Thompson, S.W.N., Dray, A., McCarson, K.E., Krause, J.E., and Urban, L. (1995) Nerve growth factor induces mechanical allodynia associated with novel A fibre-evoked spinal reflex activity and enhanced neurokinin-1 receptor activation in the rat. Pain, 62: 219–231.

Undem, B., Weinreich, D., Ellis, J., Meyers, A. (1993) Neuronal consequences of the allergic response in airways. In: F.T. Holgate, K.F. Austin, L.M. Lichtenstein, A.B. Kay (Eds.) *Asthma: Physiology, Immunopharmacology and Treatment.* Fourth International Symposium. London: Academic Press. pp. 275–286.

Walker, E.A, Katon, W.J., Neraask, Jemelka, R.P., Massoth, D. (1992) Dissociation women with chronic pelvic pain, Am. J. Psych. 149(4): 534–537.

Walker, E.A., Katon, W.J., Hansom, J., Harrop-Griffith, J., Holm, L., Jones, M.L., Hickok, L.R., and Russo, J. (1995) Psychosomatic diagnoses and sexual victimization in women with chronic pelvic pain. Psychosomatics, 36(6): 531–540.

Walling, M.K., O'Hara, M.W., Reiter, R.C., Milburn, A.K., Lilly, G., and Vincent, S.D. (1994) Abuse history and chronic pain in women: II. A multivariate analysis of abuse and psychological morbidity. Obstet. Gynecol., 82(2): 200–206.

Walsh, A. (1978) Interstitial cystitis. In: J.H. Harrison, R.F. Gittes, and A.D. Perlmutter, (Eds.), *Campbell's Urology*. 4th ed., WB Saunders, Philadelphia, pp. 693–707.

Woolf, C.J., Ma, Q.P., Allchorne, A., and Poole, S. (1996) Peripheral cell types contributing to the hyperalgesic action of nerve growth factor in inflammation. J. Neurosci., 16(8): 2716–2723.

Yonei, Y. (1987) Autonomic nervous alterations and mast cell degranulation in the exacerbation of ulcerative colitis. Jpn. J. Gastroenterol., 84: 1045–1056.

Yoshimura, N. and DeGroat, W.C. (1992) Patch clamp analysis of afferent and efferent neurons that innervate the urinary bladder of the rat. Soc. Neurosci. Abstr., 18: 127.

Yoshimura, N., Yoshida, O., and De Groat, W.C. (1995) Regional differences in plasticity of membrane properties of rat urinary bladder afferent neurons following spinal cord injury. J. Urol.: 153–262.

Zugmaier, G., Favoni, R., Jaeger, R., Rosen, N., and Knabbe, C. (1999) Polysulfated herarinoids selectively inactivate heparin-binding angiogenesis factors. Ann. N.Y. Acad. Sci., 886: 243–248.

Electrical Stimulation and the Relief of Pain
Pain Research and Clinical Management, Vol. 15
Edited by Brian A. Simpson

CHAPTER 6

Spinal cord stimulation for back pain

Giancarlo Barolat*, Ashwini Sharan, and Joseph Ong

Department of Neurosurgery, Thomas Jefferson University Hospital, 1015 Chestnut Street,
Philadelphia, PA 19107, USA

Abstract

Spinal cord stimulation (SCS) has been shown to be an effective treatment modality for managing intractable leg and, to a lesser extent, low back pain. Prospective and retrospective studies show that between 50 and 70% of patients with failed back syndrome treated with SCS obtain greater than 50% pain relief. Complex pain patterns, such as those of patients who have pain in the low back and in one or both lower extremities, are more difficult to cover satisfactorily with SCS. They might require a higher voltage and a more complex implanted system. While the ability to direct paraesthesiae and to relieve pain in the lower extremities can be accomplished in a large percentage of patients, relief of low back pain remains challenging and far from being uniformly achieved.

Keywords: Failed back syndrome; Lumbar spine; Spinal cord stimulation; Neurostimulation; Radicular pain; Arachnoiditis

1. Background

Chronic low back pain represents one of the most widespread and costly medical problems today; it also is a major cause of absenteeism from the workplace. Past analyses have demonstrated that over 5 million people in the United States are afflicted with chronic low back pain. Conservative estimates place the annual cost of treatment at 25 billion dollars (Frymoyer and Cats-Baril, 1991). A significant fraction of these dollars is attributable to the more than 200,000 US patients yearly who elect for lumbosacral surgery to relieve their pain. Unfortunately, 20–40% of surgical patients will experience persistent or recurrent pain (Wilkinson, 1991).

One important subset of patients includes those with the so-called 'failed back surgery syndrome'

(FBSS). In the literature this multidimensional syndrome has been used to describe various types of pain, including centrally located lumbosacral pain, buttock pain and even diffuse lower extremity pain. Many published series emphasize the distinction between back and leg pain; however details of the pain syndromes are usually lacking. The aetiology of this syndrome has included the following: wrong diagnosis, wrong level of surgery, psychological illness, arachnoiditis, lumbosacral epidural fibrosis, radiculitis, vertebral microinstability and recurrent disc herniations. A significant number of patients with FBSS are so debilitated that they are unable to return to work and often require analgesics.

Spinal cord stimulation (SCS) has been available for over 30 years and is currently accepted in

*Correspondence to: Dr. Giancarlo Barolat, 717 Canterbury Lane, Villanova, PA 19085, USA. Phone: +1 (215) 955 2364; Fax: +1 (215) 955 1113; E-mail: gbr@bellatlantic.net

the treatment of leg pain. In contrast, its use for pain relief in the lower lumbar area still remains to be defined. Moreover, these studies have not consistently reported on how effective the overlap of the paraesthesia and the pain regions have been. Finally, to the authors' knowledge, no group has compared SCS against a placebo treatment.

2. Selection criteria

Several studies emphasize that proper patient selection is crucial to maximizing the proportion of patients with FBSS who achieve adequate pain relief with SCS (Dumoulin et al., 1996; Segal et al., 1998). Rainov and colleagues concluded that careful selection of SCS candidate patients with a rigid selection protocol can lead to shorter trial stimulation periods; as a result, therapeutic failures, infection risk and overall cost may be reduced (Rainov et al., 1996). Burchiel and colleagues deduced that certain factors including patient age, Minnesota Multiphasic Personality Inventory depression subscale, and McGill Pain Questionnaire (MPQ) may be clinically useful in the prediction of pain status after 3 months of SCS (Burchiel et al., 1996). Their results underscore the fact that psychosocial influences exist in certain patients with FBSS. Van De Kelft and De La Porte (1994) observed 78 patients with FBSS during a trial stimulation period and discovered that, interestingly, these patients responded more positively than the SCS patients with other diagnoses.

3. Retrospective studies

Multiple well-conducted retrospective reviews on SCS for FBSS exist (Nielson et al., 1975; Erickson and Long, 1983; Leibrock et al., 1984; Daniel et al., 1985; Kumar et al., 1986; Koeze et al., 1987; Meglio et al., 1989; Meilman et al., 1989; North et al., 1991a,b, 1993; De La Porte, 1993; De La Porte and Van De Kelft, 1993; Meglio and Cioni, 1994; Devulder et al., 1997; Alo et al., 1999).

Longitudinal studies by North showed that in patients with post-surgical lumbar arachnoid or epidural fibrosis without surgically remediable lesions, SCS is superior to repeated surgical interventions on the lumbar spine, for back and leg pain (North et al., 1991a,b) and others have shown its superiority to dorsal ganglionectomy for leg pain (Fiume et al., 1995). Turner and colleagues (1995) exhaustively reviewed 41 articles from 1966 to 1994. With a mean follow-up of 16 months, they found that approximately 50–60% of patients with FBSS reported > 50% pain relief from the use of SCS. Hieu obtained comparable results after reviewing 77 patients treated for chronic, refractory, low back and radicular pain with SCS, with a mean follow-up of 42 months. Long-term efficacy was good in 63.6% and fair in 22% (Hieu et al., 1994). De La Porte and Van De Kelft (1993) studied 64 patients with FBSS treated with SCS. The mean follow-up period was 4 years. Thirty-five patients (55%) had more than 50% pain relief, 90% reduced their medication, and 61% reported a significant improvement in their ability to carry out activities of daily living.

Whether SCS, or for that matter any procedure that treats patients with chronic low back pain, can increase the return to work status of an individual is undecided. However, a few studies to date have shown promise. In 1991 North examined 50 disabled FBSS patients and discovered that 25% of this population returned to work after SCS. Greater than 50% sustained relief of pain was noted in 53% of patients at 2.2 years and 47% of patients at 5.0 years (North et al., 1991b). From 1982 to 1992 Fiume's group used SCS to treat 34 patients with FBSS secondary to lumbosacral fibrosis, and 56% reported better than 50% pain relief. Moreover, 10 of 34 patients (29.4%) were able to return to work (Fiume et al., 1995)

Unfortunately, there are many factors which cloud these issues. The worker compensation system does not encourage an injured labour worker to return to his or her previous occupation. Litigation further compounds the issue as individuals who are benefiting from SCS may not be encouraged to declare such success. The authors' experience is such that very few patients who are disabled at the time of implant will actually return to become part of the workforce. It is possible that the most significant benefit of SCS lies in maintaining within the workforce patients who are, at the time of implant, gainfully employed. Additional studies will hopefully provide more data on this increasingly important issue.

4. Prospective studies

In recent times, there have been four prospective series aimed at studying the effects of SCS on FBSS. Barolat's group prospectively enrolled patients with low back pain or low back pain greater than or equal in severity to the leg pain (Barolat et al., 2001). These patients underwent implantation with a multilead paddle electrode manufactured by ANS (Advanced Neuromodulation Systems, Inc., Plano, TX) and were followed using a visual analog scale (VAS), Oswestry Questionnaire and Sickness Impact Profile (SIP) (Bergner et al., 1976; Fairbanks, 1980; Carlsson, 1993; De Bruin, 1994). The study demonstrated a 69% successful reduction in back pain and 88% successful reduction in leg pain at 1 year follow-up; there was significant improvement in VAS, Oswestry and SIP scores. In 1996, Burchiel demonstrated similar results (Burchiel et al., 1996), with successful management of pain in 55% of 70 patients after 1 year. Medication usage and work status were unchanged in this study. In a recent cohort study from Italy, patients with FBSS treated unsuccessfully with medical therapy were given SCS after a trial of stimulation and compared with a group who continued to receive successful medical therapy (Dario et al., 2001). With SCS there was a small but statistically significant improvement in VAS for back pain but only 40% of the SCS group had back pain and although the study was prospective and controlled, interpretation of the results is not straightforward. Lastly, North conducted the first prospective,

randomized comparison of SCS with any other treatment modality, in this case re-operation, with a 6 month cross-over arm in the study. In that study, 51 patients with FBSS consented to randomization (North et al., 1994, 1995). The study demonstrated a significant difference between the patients who opted for crossover from SCS to re-operation versus the opposite and concluded that SCS is a viable alternative to re-operation for FBSS.

5. Cost-effectiveness

A few studies have reported on the cost-effectiveness of SCS in FBSS. In 1997 Bell and colleagues compared the costs of SCS with surgeries and alternative treatments (Bell et al., 1997). They calculated the estimated cost of therapy for each group over a 5-year period without quantifying the improvements offered by successful SCS. The authors found that by reducing the demand for medical care made by patients with the failed back syndrome, SCS therapy can lead to medical costs saving. They reported that in patients who responded favourably to SCS, the therapy would pay for itself within 2.1 years. In the same year Devulder calculated that on average SCS costs 3660 dollars per patient per year, which may be cost-effective if other therapeutic modalities fail (Devulder et al., 1997).

6. SCS for axial low back pain

6.1. Why is it so difficult to stimulate the low back fibres?

The dorsal column fibres to the lower lumbar region are located, in the thoracic spinal cord, lateral to the fibres to the lower extremities (Fig. 1). Their location places them adjacent to the dorsal root entry zone (DREZ). This is the area where the dorsal rootlets enter the dorsal horn. The studies by Holsheimer have demonstrated that the DREZ

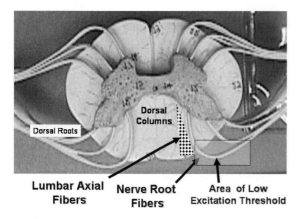

Fig. 1. Transverse section of spinal cord showing the location of afferent lumbar fibres in the dorsal columns.

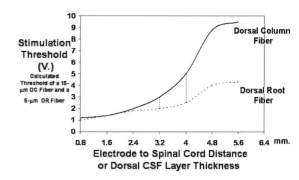

Fig. 2. Dorsal column and dorsal root fibres behave differently with varying distances between the electrode and the spinal cord. (After Holsheimer, 1997.)

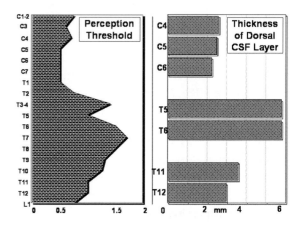

Fig. 3. Relationship between the thickness of the dorsal (posterior) CSF space and stimulation perception thresholds.

is uniquely situated at the junction of a high conductor (the CSF) and low conductor (the spinal cord) (Holsheimer and Struijk, 1991). This fact substantially lowers the excitation threshold of the segment where the rootlets enter the spinal cord. An electrical field generated by a dorsally placed epidural electrode will therefore stimulate preferentially the dorsal rootlets, rather than the dorsal column fibres to the lumbar area. This explains the fact that often stimulation in the low back is perceived only in conjuction with segmental thoracic or abdominal wall stimulation (dorsal root activation). An increasing amount of CSF between the electrode and the neural structures greatly favours the activation of the dorsal rootlets (Fig. 2; Holsheimer, 1997). The difficulty with thoracic SCS is therefore further compounded by the anatomy of the CSF space in the mid-thoracic region. The dorsal CSF space is at its thickest between T4 and T8 (Fig. 3). This is due to the narrowness of the spinal cord and the thoracic kyphosis (which causes the spinal cord to lie in a ventral location in the spinal canal). At the T9–10 levels, the dorsal CSF space becomes narrower due in part to the lumbar enlargement and to the reduction of the thoracic kyphosis. An electrode placed below the T10 level is unlikely to stimulate the lumbar region dorsal column fibres, being too low. Electrodes placed above T9, where the dorsal CSF becomes thicker, are more likely to

stimulate only the dorsal rootlets at their entrance in the spinal cord. To make the situation even more treacherous, selective and exclusive activation of the dorsal rootlets might not take place until a few weeks following the implant. This might make it difficult to predict with certainty the extent of extraneous segmental stimulation that will occur in the months following the implant. Personal experience has demonstrated that, for the previously mentioned reasons, an electrode placement above T8 is much more likely to result in such an undesirable stimulation. This also stresses the importance of complex array designs, to try to obviate electronically the somewhat unpredictable anatomical and physiological electrical responses of the intraspinal structures in the mid-thoracic region (see below).

Experience with SCS for intractable leg/low back pain has been reported in several publications (Nielson et al., 1975; Erickson and Long, 1983; Leibrock et al., 1984; Daniel et al., 1985; Kumar et al., 1986; Koeze et al., 1987; Meglio et al., 1989; Meilman et al., 1989; North et al., 1991a,b, 1993; De La Porte, 1993; De La Porte and Van De Kelft, 1993; Meglio and Cioni, 1994; Devulder et al., 1997; Alo et al., 1999). While it is relatively easy to obtain stimulation in the lower extremities and buttocks with single electrode technology, extending and maintaining the paraesthesia into the lower lumbar area has proven to be a formidable task. Further, there is only limited information regarding the ability to stimulate the low back over an extended period of time.

A previous study showed that the ideal location for stimulation of the lower lumbar area is at T9–10 with two quadripolar electrodes placed parallel to, and a few millimeters on each side of, the physiological midline (Law, 1987). It was noted that low back stimulation could also be achieved with electrodes placed at more cephalad vertebral levels but the introduction of unpleasant band-like abdominal and chest wall stimulation, probably due to dorsal root stimulation, precluded electrode placement at these levels. The results of a multicentre study on a group of patients who responded successfully to SCS for low back pain confirm these findings (Barolat et al., 2001; Sharan et al., 2002). While the electrodes were commonly placed with the tip at the middle of T8, the majority of cathodes were initially positioned at T9. More interestingly, the data revealed that by 6 months post-operatively, the majority of patients were using a rostral cathode positioned at T10. Law showed that the low back fibres may be more selectively activated by a matrix of closely spaced electrodes at the T9–10 spine level (Law, 1983, 1987).

It is commonly observed that, even if one is able to achieve direct stimulation of the low back, after a few weeks or months this pattern of paraesthesia is often replaced by an unpleasant segmental band of stimulation, thereby negating the benefits of the procedure. In addition, observation has found that the pattern of stimulation changes over time. This is seldom due, at least with implanted plate electrodes, to migration of the electrode. The reason is unknown, but it is most likely secondary to changes in the distribution of the electrical fields within the spinal canal. The changes in the paraesthesia distribution, as perceived by the patients, can be dramatic and can result in complete loss of coverage of the painful area. Even if initially one were able to perfectly target the physiological midline, it is unlikely, due to both the changing pain patterns and changing paraesthesia coverage, that this can be maintained over a long period of time. Sometimes the painful area changes in time, usually with further body regions becoming sources of chronic pain.

North has recently challenged the advantage of dual quadripolar percutaneous electrodes compared with a single quadripolar electrode in the midline (see Chapter 12). His data, applied in the context of relatively short-term SCS, showed no significant difference in the ability to generate paraesthesia in the lumbar area between dual percutaneous electrodes and a single quadripolar electrode in the midline. Although initially this may be possible, a number of issues are apparent: obtaining implantation at the physiological midline can be problematic and the changing nature of pain may not allow adequate recapture of the paraesthesia with a single quadripolar electrode. The observed change in electrical requirements noted in this study may not be appropriately addressed by a single quadripolar electrode.

The study by Sharan demonstrates the usefulness of more complex implantable systems (Sharan et al., 2002). In this study, shortly after implantation, an equal number of patients utilized either one or two columns of contacts; however, over the 2 year follow-up period, 75% of the patients required the use of two columns to continue to provide adequate paraesthesia coverage to their painful area. Besides the need to activate electrical contacts on both columns, patients also more often required multiple cathodes to configure the electrical field in a manner which could achieve low back coverage. Less than 20% of all the patients used only two contacts, with the majority of them eventually requiring more than four activated contacts. The study also showed that 88% of the patients required a change in the cathode location at each assessment although some degree of stabilization did eventually occur. This argues for more complex electrodes and arrays driven by pulse generators capable of activating multiple cathodes and anodes providing multiple programming capabilities, including dual channel systems that permit electronic steering of the electrical field medio-laterally.

Even though definitive data do not exist in the literature, most implanting physicians share the experience that SCS is far more effective for radicular pain than for axial low back pain. Nevertheless, SCS does provide patients with FBSS a real alternative, which may be equivalent to or better than any other treatment modality and may even be cost-effective. Even though stimulation in the lower lumbar area can occasionally be achieved with a single quadripolar electrode, we recommend that SCS for the failed back syndrome should be undertaken only by physicians who have familiarity with the implantation and programming of complex stimulation systems.

6.2. *Paddle versus catheter-type electrodes*

Paddle electrodes seem to have an advantage over catheter-type electrodes in the long-term implementation of SCS. Preliminary data by North have shown a broader stimulation pattern and lower stimulation requirements with paddle electrodes (North et al., 2002). Villavicencio studied the long-term clinical outcome of 27 patients who had undergone permanent SCS utilizing percutaneous or paddle electrodes (Villavicencio et al., 2000). Patients were implanted only after a successful percutaneous trial. Although patients were not prospectively randomized to each of the two

treatment arms, paddle electrodes appeared to be associated with improved long-term effectiveness over those placed percutaneously. One hundred percent of the 12 patients who underwent paddle electrode implantation for SCS in the thoracic region had more than 50% pain relief at long-term follow-up; 90% of these patients did not require the use of narcotics. No patient in this group had what was defined as a poor outcome. Percutaneous electrodes were associated with a good or excellent outcome in 53% of patients, fair in another 27% and poor in 21%. Paddle electrodes exhibited significantly greater pain relief at long-term follow-up when compared to percutaneous electrodes as measured by a four-tier outcome grading scale ($P = 0.02$).

Other considerations greatly favour the use of paddle electrodes particularly for the management of low back pain. These patients typically have high power requirements, often over 5 V. By lowering the power requirements, paddle electrodes increase battery life. Several expert implanters have also observed that high voltage stimulation with percutaneous electrodes placed in the mid-thoracic area often results in a painful sensation located in the low back at the level of the electrode. This has been attributed to painful stimulation of the ligamentum flavum by the current that spreads circumferentially (author's observation). This problem has not been observed with the utilization of paddle electrodes, since the current only spreads toward the intradural structures.

For this specific indication radio-frequency coupled systems have a particular advantage. In the authors' experience, the currently available lithium-powered implantable systems cannot consistently deliver enough power to satisfactorily stimulate the low back, particularly in instances requiring stimulation voltage greater than 4–5 V. High-voltage stimulation cannot be sustained long-term by lithium-powered fully implantable systems without requiring unacceptably frequent surgical replacements of the pulse generators. The ability to cyclically alternate through different stimulation patterns is also of great benefit.

As many of these patients have pain in the low back as well as in both lower extremities, dual channel stimulation without the ability to automatically switch among multiple programmes might not be sufficient to deliver optimal stimulation.

7. Complications

Various authors have previously commented on the complications of SCS implantation, including neurological damage (< 1%), electrode migration (1–15%), hardware failure (< 2%), and infection (0.5–15%). In particular, electrode migration was reported by at least one group to be the most common complication of SCS for FBSS (LeDoux and Langford, 1993). Further investigation is required to definitively state the relative complication rates for FBSS patients versus those who receive SCS for other reasons.

8. Conclusions

(1) SCS has been shown to be an effective treatment modality for managing intractable leg and, to a lesser extent, low back pain.

(2) Prospective and retrospective studies show that between 50 and 70% of FBSS patients treated with SCS have greater than 50% pain relief.

(3) Complex pain patterns, such as those of patients who have pain in the low back and in one or both lower extremities, require a high degree of flexibility in the implanted SCS system. The system must provide the capability to redirect the current electronically over at least two segments of the spinal canal, to electronically steer the current in a medio-lateral direction and to activate multiple electrical contacts simultaneously.

(4) The willingness and ability of the physician and his team to provide extensive reprogramming in the long-term follow-up is also of utmost importance. The pain of FBSS and its treatment with SCS is a dynamic process.

(5) While the ability to direct paraesthesiae and to relieve pain in the lower extremities can be accomplished in a large percentage of patients, relief of low back pain remains challenging and far from being uniformly achieved.

References

Alo, K.M., Yland, M.J., Charnov, J.H., and Redko, V. (1999) Multiple program spinal cord stimulation in the treatment of chronic pain: follow-up of multiple program SCS. Neuromodulation, 2(4): 266–272.

Barolat, G., Oakley, J.C., Law, J.D., North, R.B., Ketcik, B., and Sharan, A. (2001) Epidural spinal cord stimulation with multiple electrode paddle leads is effective in treating intractable low back pain. Neuromodulation, 4(2): 59–66.

Bell, G.K.K., Kidd, D.H., and North, R.B. (1997) Cost-effectiveness analysis of spinal cord stimulation in treatment of failed back surgery syndrome. J. Pain Symptom Manage., 13(5): 286–295.

Bergner, M., Bobbit, R.A., and Pollard, W.E. (1976) The sickness impact profile: validation of a health status measure. Med. Care, 14: 56–67.

Burchiel, K.J., Anderson, V.C., Brown, F.D., Fessler, R.G., Friedman, W.A., Pelofsky, S., Weiner, R.L., Oakley, J., and Shatin, D. (1996) Prospective, multicenter study of spinal cord stimulation for relief of chronic back and extremity pain. Spine, 21(23): 2786–2794.

Carlsson, A.M. (1993) Assessment of chronic pain. I Aspects of the reliability and validity of the visual analog scale. Pain, 16: 87–101.

Daniel, M.S., Long, C., Hutcherson, W.L., and Hunter, S. (1985) Psychological factors and outcome of electrode implantation for chronic pain. Neurosurgery, 17: 773–777.

Dario, A., Fortini, G., Bertollo, D., Bacuzzi, A., Grizzetti, C., and Cuffare, S. (2001) Treatment of failed back surgery syndrome. Neuromodulation, 4: 105–110.

De Bruin, A.F., Diederiks, L.P., and De Witte, L.P. (1994) The development of a short generic, version of the sickness impact profile. J. Clin. Epidemiol., 47: 407–418.

De La Porte, C.V. (1993) Spinal cord stimulation in failed back surgery syndrome. Pain, 52(1): 55–61.

De La Porte, C. and Van De Kelft, E. (1993) Spinal cord stimulation in failed back surgery syndrome. Pain, 52(1): 55–61.

Devulder, J., De Laat, M., and Van Bastelaere, M. (1997) Spinal cord stimulation: a valuable treatment for chronic failed back surgery patients. J. Pain Symptom Manage., 13(5): 296–301.

Dumoulin, K., Devulder, J., Castille, F., De Laat, M., Van Bastelaere, M., and Rolly, G.A. (1996) Psychoanalytic investigation to improve the success rate of spinal cord stimulation as a treatment for chronic failed back surgery syndrome. Clin. J. Pain, 12(1): 43–49.

Erickson, D.L. and Long, D.M. (1983) Ten-year follow-up of dorsal column stimulation. In J.J. Bonica, U. Lindblom, and A. Iggo, (Eds.), *Advances in Pain Research and Therapy*, Vol. 5. (pp. 583–589). Raven Press, New York.

Fairbanks, J.C., Cooper, J., and Davies, J.B. (1980) The Oswestry low back pain disability questionnaire. Physiotherapy, 66: 271–272.

Fiume, D., Sherkat, S., Callovini, G.M., Parziale, G., and Gazzeri, G. (1995) Treatment of the failed back surgery syndrome due to lumbo-sacral epidural fibrosis. Acta Neurochir. Suppl. (Wien), 64: 116–118.

Frymoyer, J.W. and Cats-Baril, W.L. (1991) An overview of the incidences and costs of low back pain. Orthop Clin. North Am., 22: 263–271.

Hieu, P.D., Person, H., Houidi, K., Rodriguez, V., Vallee, B., and Besson, G. (1994) Treatment of chronic lumbago and radicular pain by spinal cord stimulation. Rev. Rhum. Ed. Fr., 61(4): 271–277.

Holsheimer, J. (1997) Effectiveness of spinal cord stimulation in the management of chronic pain: analysis of technical drawbacks and solutions. Neurosurgery, 40: 990–999.

Holsheimer, J. and Struijk, J.J. (1991) How do geometric factors influence epidural spinal cord stimulation? A quantitative analysis by computer modeling. Stereotact. Funct. Neurosurg., 56: 234–249.

Koeze, T.H., Williams, A.C., and Reiman, S. (1987) Spinal cord stimulation and the relief of chronic pain. J. Neurol. Neurosurg. Psych., 50: 1424–1429.

Kumar, K., Wyant, G.M., and Ekong, C.E.U. (1986) Epidural spinal cord stimulation for relief of chronic pain. The Pain Clinic, 1: 91–99.

Law, J. (1983) Spinal stimulation: statistical superiority of monophasic stimulation of narrowly separated, longitudinal bipoles having rostral cathodes. Appl. Neurophys., 46: 129–137.

Law, J.D. (1987) A new method for targeting a spinal stimulator: quantitatively paired comparisons. Appl. Neurophys., 50: 436.

LeDoux, M.S. and Langford, K.H. (1993) Spinal cord stimulation for the failed back syndrome. Spine, 18(2): 191–194.

Leibrock, L.G., Meilman, P., and Green, C. (1984) Spinal cord stimulation in the treatment of chronic back and lower extremity pain syndromes. Nebr. Med. J.: 180–183.

Meglio, M. and Cioni, B. (1994) Spinal cord stimulation in low back and leg pain. Stereotact. Funct. Neurosurg., 62(1-4): 263–266.

Meglio, M., Cioni, B., and Rossi, G.F. (1989) Spinal cord stimulation in management of chronic pain: a 9-year experience. J. Neurosurg., 70: 519–524.

Meilman, P.W., Leibrock, L.G., and Leong, T.L. (1989) Outcome of implanted spinal cord stimulation in the treatment of chronic pain: arachnoiditis versus single nerve root injury and mononeuropathy. Clin. J. Pain, 5: 189–193.

Nielson, K.D., Adams, J.E., and Hosobuchi, Y. (1975) Experience with dorsal column stimulation for relief of chronic intractable pain: 1968–1973. Surg. Neurol., 4: 148–152.

North, R.B., Ewend, M.G., Lawon, M.T., and Piantadosi, S. (1991a) Spinal cord stimulation for chronic intractable pain: superiority of multichannel devices. Pain, 44: 119–130.

North R.B., Ewend M.G., Lawton M.T., Kidd D.H., and Piantadosi, S. (1991b). Failed back surgery syndrome: 5-year follow-up after spinal cord stimulator implantation. Neurosurgery, 28(5): 692–699.

North, R.B., Kidd, D.H., Zahurak, M., James, C., and Long, D.M. (1993) Spinal cord stimulation for chronic intractable pain: experience over two decades. Neurosurgery, 32: 384–395.

North, R.B., Kidd, D.H., Lee, M.S., and Piantodosi, S. (1994) A prospective, randomized study of spinal cord stimulation versus reoperation for failed back surgery syndrome: initial results. Stereotact. Funct. Neurosurg., 62(1-4): 267–272.

North, R.B., Kidd, D.H., and Piantadosi, S. (1995) Spinal cord stimulation versus reoperation for failed back surgery syndrome: a prospective, randomized study design. Acta Neurochir. Suppl., 64: 106–108.

North, R., Kidd, D., Olin, J., and Sieracki, J. (2002) Spinal cord stimulation electrode design: prospective, randomized, controlled trial comparing percutaneous and laminectomy electrodes – Part I: technical outcomes. Neurosurgery, 51: 381–390.

Rainov, N.G., Heidecke, V., and Burkert, W. (1996) Short test-period spinal cord stimulation for failed back surgery syndrome. Minim. Invasive Neurosurg., 39(2): 41–44. Jun.

Segal, R., Stacey, B.R., Rudy, T.E., Baser, S., and Markham, J. (1998) Spinal cord stimulation revisited. Neurol. Res., 20(5): 391–396.

Sharan, A., Cameron, T., and Barolat, G. (2002) Evolving patterns of spinal cord stimulation. Neuromodulation, 5: 167–179.

Turner, J.A., Loeser, J.D., and Bell, K.G. (1995) Spinal cord stimulation for chronic low back pain: a systematic literature synthesis. Neurosurgery, 37(6): 1088–1095.

Van De Kelft, E. and De La Porte, C. (1994) Long-term pain relief during spinal cord stimulation. The effect of patient selection. Qual. Life Res., 3(1): 21–27. Feb.

Villavicencio, A., Leveque, J.C., Rubin, L., Bulsara, K., and Gorecki, J. (2000) Laminectomy versus percutaneous electrode placement for spinal cord stimulation. Neurosurgery, 46: 399–406.

Wilkinson, H.A. (1991) *The Failed Back Syndrome: Etiology and Therapy*, 2nd ed., Harper and Row, Philadelphia.

Electrical Stimulation and the Relief of Pain
Pain Research and Clinical Management, Vol. 15
Edited by Brian A. Simpson

CHAPTER 7

Spinal cord stimulation for neuropathic pain

John C. Oakley*

Yellowstone Neurosurgical Associates, and Northern Rockies Pain and Palliative Rehabilitation Center, 2900 12th N, Billings, MT 59101, USA

Abstract

Spinal cord stimulation (SCS) has been demonstrated to be effective in the treatment of a variety of chronic pain diagnoses due to injury of the nervous system. This chapter presents a definition of neuropathic pain and describes an accepted algorithm for treatment. The assessment of the patient with neuropathic pain is described. The place occupied by SCS in the treatment of neuropathic pain syndromes is discussed, along with selection criteria for implementation of SCS. A description of stimulation technique is presented and the outcome from stimulation in the most common syndromes treated is discussed.

Keywords: Spinal cord stimulation; Neuropathic pain; neuropathy

1. Neuropathic pain

1.1. Neuropathic pain definitions

Neuropathic pain is defined in the lexicon of the International Association for the Study of Pain (IASP) as 'pain initiated or caused by a primary lesion or dysfunction in the nervous system' (Merskey and Bogduk, 1994). This definition avoids terms that imply a mechanism (e.g. deafferentation or neurogenic pain) or clinical features (dysaesthetic or causalgic) and focuses on abnormality within the nervous system, which may occur at any level. This definition is not without controversy (Max, 2002). The controversy exists because of the inclusion of the term 'dysfunction'. However, we now understand that many of the well-accepted features of neuropathic

pain may exist in some clearly non-neuropathic pain states. For example allodynia, lowered threshold and temporal summation, may be found in fibromyalgia, and in certain visceral pains. The broader definition of neuropathic pain including the term 'dysfunction' allows for more accurate assessment of mechanism for the treatment of various pain states, and allows for the realization that central plasticity of the spinal cord due to intense C-fibre input accounts for much of the commonality in pain description between differing pain syndromes (Woolf and Mannion, 1999; Woolf and Salter, 2000).

Nevertheless, in spite of diversity in aetiology and clinical findings, neuropathic pain syndromes have been generally accepted to have many common clinical characteristics. These characteristics are summarized in Table I. The most

---

*Correspondence to: Dr. John C. Oakley, Northern Rockies Pain and Palliative Rehabilitation Center, 2900 12th N, Billings, MT 59101, USA. Phone: +1-406-238-6650; Fax: +1-406-651-5514; E-mail: joshir@aol.com

TABLE I

Common clinical characteristics of neuropathic pain

A. Pain persists in the absence of ongoing or potential tissue damage.
B. Burning and/or electrical quality.
C. Delay in onset after the presenting injury.
D. There is a paroxysmal component described often as shooting/stabbing or electric shock-like.
E. The non-paroxysmal component is usually unremitting, and described as a continuous often aching presence.
F. Allodynia is present; ordinarily non-painful stimuli are perceived as painful.
G. Pain is felt in an area of sensory deficit.
H. There is a pronounced summation and painful after-reaction with repetitive stimuli.

TABLE II

Diagnoses which may result in neuropathic pain syndromes

Peripheral nervous system
  Sensory neuropathies
    Diabetes mellitus
    Proximal motor neuropathies (mononeuritis multiplex)
    Distal sensory neuropathies (polyneuropathy)
    Toxic neuropathies
    Vitamin deficiency (beri beri)
    Collagen vascular disease
    Lead poisoning
    Guillain–Barré syndrome
    Leprosy
    Ischaemic neuropathy
    Hereditary neuropathies
    Idiopathic neuropathy
  Peripheral nerve tumours (especially neurofibroma, cancer)
  Entrapment neuropathies
  Peripheral nerve injury (partial or complete transection; neuroma formation, including post-amputation stump pain)
  Brachial plexopathy
  Intercostal neuralgia
  Post-rhizotomy, post-ganglionectomy pain
  Post-herpetic neuralgia
  Post-nerve root injury pain (failed laminectomy or failed back or neck surgery syndrome)

Spinal cord
  Spinal cord injury pain
  Syringomyelia
  Brachial plexus avulsion
  Phantom or post amputation pain
  Postcordotomy pain

Central nervous system proximal to the spinal cord
  Cranial nerve neuralgias (trigeminal, glossopharyngeal, sphenopalatine, geniculate)
  Wallenberg syndrome
  Multiple sclerosis
  Syringobulbia
  Thalamic pain syndrome (Dejerine–Roussy syndrome)

Sympathetic nervous system
  CRPS types I, II

frequently used descriptive terms for neuropathic pain are those associated with burning, shooting, tingling and electric shock-like qualities. Neuropathic pain may have a predominantly paroxysmal component, e.g. trigeminal neuralgia, or often a constant background of persisting pain, e.g. diabetic neuropathy.

Neuropathic pain diagnoses may be organized according to the level of injury to the nervous system (Table II). In the peripheral nervous system, sensory neuropathies such as occur in diabetes mellitus may be amenable to spinal cord stimulation (SCS) for control of related pain. The outcome literature lacks any systematic approach to relief using SCS with the majority of these diagnoses. Peripheral nerve tumours may produce neuropathic pain, especially neurofibromas and cancer. Entrapment neuropathies may result in pain in the distribution of specific peripheral nerves such as carpal tunnel syndrome (median nerve), cubital tunnel syndrome (ulnar nerve), tarsal tunnel syndrome (tibial nerve) and the many varieties of entrapment of other peripheral nerves. The peripheral nervous system may also be affected by nerve injury with partial or complete transection, and with neuroma or neuroma-in-continuity formation. A number of other peripheral nerve problems may present with pain amenable to SCS. These include brachial plexopathy, intercostal neuralgia, post-rhizotomy, post-ganglionectomy pain, post-herpetic neuralgia (PHN) and the most common indication for stimulation: the failed back surgery syndrome (radicular pain following lumbar spine surgery; an analagous condition can also follow cervical spine surgery).

At the level of the spinal cord, a number of diagnoses are related to neuropathic pain. SCS has been used in most of these syndromes. With spinal cord injury pain for example, SCS has benefited patients with incomplete lesions and distal neuropathic pain, but has not been shown to be of help in the zonal pain at the level of the lesion. This is an area which may better be approached through the use of a dorsal root entry zone (DREZ) procedure. The outcome results with PHN using SCS have at best been mixed.

More central diagnoses include the cranial neuralgias such as trigeminal, glossopharyngeal, geniculate and sphenopalatine. A cerebrovascular accident may result in a Wallenberg syndrome and pain. Multiple sclerosis may produce trigeminal neuralgia and syringobulbia may result in pain. A more central cerebrovascular accident may result in a post-stroke, thalamic or Dejerine–Roussy syndrome. Various injuries may produce atypical facial pain, most often treated today with motor cortex stimulation, but Gasserian ganglion stimulation has been successfully used. Most of the entities associated with central nervous system injury or involvement are not generally demonstrated to be amenable to SCS.

Controversial diagnoses have included complex regional pain syndrome (CRPS) type I (formerly reflex sympathetic dystrophy), and CRPS type II (formerly causalgia). These have been associated with the concept of sympathetically maintained or sympathetically independent pain. These entities represent a neuropathic pain of a special variety and have their own unique treatment algorithm. SCS may be used effectively. This topic is covered elsewhere in this volume.

1.2. Mechanism of neuropathic pain

The mechanism of neuropathic pain generation has been the subject of intense research interest for many years. Because of the diverse presentation of neuropathic pain, more than one mechanism of action is likely. Observations in the treatment of neuropathic pain and ischaemic pain made

TABLE III

Observations in the treatment of neuropathic pain and ischaemic pain with SCS that have been consistently reported and must figure into any explanation of mechanism

Neuropathic pain
- Stimulation does not clinically give nociceptive pain relief.
- Relief of pain is not instantaneous but occurs gradually over 15–30 min, and may not maximize for several weeks.
- The reported relief of pain outlasts the period of stimulation.
- There is an increase in tactile stimulation thresholds in patients who have a disturbance of cutaneous sensibility (allodynia).
- SCS does not influence thresholds to noxious stimuli.
- There is inhibition of a component of the flexor reflex (R III) seen only in patients with pain relief, while the R II component is not affected.
- Somatotopographic coverage of the painful area by SCS produced paraesthesiae is necessary.

Ischaemic pain
- There is improved peripheral blood flow.
- There are clear autonomic effects.
- The most effective relief has been in vasospastic diseases such as Raynaud's disease.
- Stimulation has a pre-emptive effect on vasospasm.

during the treatment with SCS that have been consistently reported are presented in Table III.

It is known that injured axons develop alpha-adrenergic receptor-like activity. This may permit a chemical 'coupling' between sympathetic efferents and A-delta and C fibres. A-beta fibres mediate most hyperalgesia, which may explain sympathetically dependent pain. Injured axons are also mechanically sensitive, for example, the presence of a 'Tinel's' sign at a neuroma. Injured axons also become hyperactive with ischaemic or hypoxic injury, perhaps as seen with entrapment or when caught in poorly vascularized scar tissue. Dorsal root ganglia also become spontaneously active electrically after nerve injury. This may play a role in phantom pain and suggests there may be a role in pain mediation from the ventral root afferent fibres.

Wide dynamic range (WDR) cells, activated by thermal, mechanical and chemical stimuli, increase their receptive fields within the spinal cord after nerve injury. WDR cells change their threshold for activation becoming sensitized and respond to non-noxious stimulation (A-beta fibres) with high frequency discharge. It is speculated that this behaviour signals pain. Some of these WDR cells may degenerate and may represent an example of excitotoxicity.

Fields (1990) listed six specific mechanistic possibilities in the generation of neuropathic pain: spontaneous hyperactivity of deafferented spinal pain transmission neurons (e.g. brachial plexus avulsion); central neuronal plasticity due to intense C fibre input to the spinal cord; loss of afferent inhibition; ectopic impulse generation in damaged nociceptive primary afferents; ephaptic transmission and sympathetic activation or facilitation of primary afferents (e.g. CRPS I, II). Peripheral neuropathic pains show a strong correlation between the abnormal electrical behaviour of sensory axons after injury and symptoms seen in clinical pain syndromes. This degree of congruence encourages the hypothesis that pathophysiological changes in the peripheral nervous system are the principle causes of neuropathic and radiculopathic pain. However, dysfunction in the central nervous system has also been described to result in neuropathic pain. Tasker has described spontaneous and evoked pains and dysaesthesia appearing after injury to the spinal cord, brainstem, thalamus and cortex (Tasker, 1990). In such patients with central neuropathic pain it has been commonly accepted that there is some damage to at least a part of the spinothalamic system (Cassinari and Pagni, 1969; Boivie et al., 1989). Evidence has suggested that the initial injury to the nervous system may produce one mechanism of pain production which results in other pain producing mechanisms, resulting in a change of the pain over time. This evolution of pain over time may alter the way we necessarily must treat neuropathic pain over time.

Most difficult to comprehend are pain syndromes which result from deafferentation or from central nervous system injury. Not all patients with a given lesion develop pain, the onset of pain may be delayed after the causative event, and there is no involvement of nociceptors. This type of pain is somatotopically related to somatosensory function and may be evoked or spontaneous. When evoked it may take the form of allodynia and can occur in areas of partial somatosensory dysfunction. The spontaneous pain may be steady or intermittent usually in similar but not identical sites to somatosensory dysfunction.

As with all neuropathic pain states the intermittent spontaneous pain, which is rarely seen in the absence of a steady component, is characteristically described as lancinating, shooting, electric shock-like. When present, the intermittent spontaneous component of the pain is more intense than the steady or background component. The background is often described as burning or tingling. These responses are most likely generated centrally, possibly through denervation hypersensitivity, somatotopic reorganization, transmitter alteration, synaptic reorganization, loss of inhibition or the establishment of new connections.

Evoked pain as a component of central pain is usually in the form of hyperaesthesias, hyperpathia or allodynia and characterized by the usual descriptions. This aspect of neuropathic pain appears to be mediated through nociceptors, the input from which is abnormally processed centrally.

A commonly associated component of neuropathic pain disorders is sympathetic hyper function. Although not invariant, the presence of sympathetically mediated neuropathic pain may be a predictor of a good outcome from the use of SCS in its treatment (Rossi and Rabar, 1994). Kim and colleagues feel that the evoked and spontaneous intermittent elements of neuropathic pain respond to the same treatment strategies as nociceptive pain, and the steady background pain represents the more difficult aspect of neuropathic pain to treat successfully (Kim et al., 2001).

1.3. Assessment of the patient with neuropathic pain

In the application of SCS to neuropathic pain it is critical that the clinician gain insight into all the possible pain generators for each patient. In assessing each patient the presence of physiological, psychological and social factors contributing to the syndrome must be addressed. A set of goals should be developed and a treatment plan to meet these goals set forth. The primary goals of assessment include gaining insight into the pathophysiologic aetiology of the pain, the patient's response to the pain, the functional status of the patient, the presence of any co-morbid conditions such as medical or psychological conditions, the development of a treatment strategy appropriate for the patient and, if necessary, the development of a multidisciplinary evaluation and treatment plan. The pain manager in these cases needs to be a good neurologist, pharmacologist, psychologist, physiatrist and vocational counsellor or have them available.

1.3.1. Patient history

An important piece of information in developing a treatment programme includes assessment of the pain characteristics. The onset of the symptoms, sudden or gradual and the presence of the typical neuropathic characteristics such as numbness, tingling and weakness, or signs of nervous system dysfunction are recorded. Actions which provoke and which palliate the pain are assessed. The location of the pain and whether it has changed over time is determined. The quality of the pain is described, such as burning, aching, electric shock-like, sharp or dull and whether there are any other unusual or abnormal sensations present. A determination of the patient's functional status is made. Often a standardized form or forms such as the Roland–Morris current function scale, or Oswestry disability questionnaire will be helpful (Fairbank et al., 1980; Roland and Morris, 1983).

Co-morbid conditions are prevalent with neuropathic pain states. Such problems as sleep disturbance, depression, anxiety, post-traumatic stress disorder and legal issues all affect the ability to treat the neuropathic pain. The response to prior treatments can often give clues as to how the patient may respond to any proposed further

therapies such as SCS. Prior treatments may include medication. The type, dose, pain relief and any side effects should be recorded. The response to nerve blockade may be helpful in determining the anatomical site of the pain generator. What blocks were given? Who performed the procedures? What effect did they have?

A fundamental part of neuropathic pain management has been the use of physical activation. What physical or occupational strategies have been employed? What modalities were used? Was there an active exercise programme, manual therapies, myofascial release, craniosacral manipulation, massage or ultrasound/diathermy used? What functional outcomes were obtained?

1.3.2. Physical examination

The physical examination in neuropathic pain is directed toward confirming that indeed neuropathic pain is present. It is important to document the presence of nervous system injury correlating with the pain syndrome. The presence of dynamic allodynia, static allodynia, thermal allodynia and hyperalgesia within the painful area can confirm that the pain is indeed neuropathic. Myofascial examination, usually in proximal muscle groups, demonstrating decreased range of motion and painful trigger areas with referral of the pain into the painful region is common. Motor testing showing weakness, apraxia or neglect can verify the presence of a nervous system lesion.

1.3.3. Laboratory evaluation

Neuroradiologic testing, including magnetic resonance imaging (MRI), computed tomography (CT) and myelography, provide exquisite and detailed evaluation of the soft tissue components of nervous system anatomy. The difficulty that faces the clinician is that they are very sensitive but not very specific and careful correlation must be made between the history, physical examination and the radiographic findings. Unfortunately, these elegant studies do not provide any functional information regarding the structures imaged or their role in the generation of symptoms.

Assuming that an abnormal appearing structure is the source of pain can be erroneous. The presence of scarring around a nerve root does not guarantee that that nerve root is painful.

Electrophysiologic studies such as nerve conduction velocity (NCV) studies, and electromyography (EMG) can accurately measure how well a nerve is conducting an impulse and give accurate information regarding the presence of demyelination or axonal injury. However, these tests do not give much aid in the diagnosis or treatment of chronic pain. They can help to confirm that the nerves innervating the painful area are indeed injured. However, these studies measure predominantly large fibre function and are unable to assess small fibre function. Many neuropathies affect only small fibre nerve function and the NCV/EMG studies will often be normal.

Quantitative sensory testing (QST) has been reported to show changes in response to SCS and, in determining the presence of neuropathic pain, can be a useful diagnostic test (Alo and Chado, 2000). These techniques have traditionally been relegated to the research clinic due to the requirement for meticulous and time-consuming methods. These tests do measure both large and small fibre function by detecting the threshold for vibration (large fibre) and hot and cold thermal sensation (small fibres).

Unfortunately, in many neuropathic pain syndromes the results of diagnostic tests are normal. The absence of positive diagnostic testing does not imply that the patient's pain is psychogenic, or that the patient is a malingerer. The problem often lies with a lack of specificity in our testing. Numerous pathophysiologic processes are involved in producing neuropathic pain, most of which are not currently accessible through standard diagnostic testing.

1.3.4. Current treatment algorithm for neuropathic pain

The mainstay of treatment for neuropathic pain disorders is medical management. There are primarily three classes of drugs that are used to treat neuropathic pain. These include topical analgesics, adjuvant analgesics and opioid analgesics. The order of application of these drugs is determined by their demonstrated efficacy, tolerability and safety. All of the drugs mentioned have some literature support for their application. Fig. 1, represents a commonly accepted diagnostic algorithm for neuropathic pain and Fig. 2 presents an algorithm for treatment.

The point at which SCS is tried in the algorithm of treatment for neuropathic pain is somewhat dependent on the experience of the pain manager and the availability of the modality. Whether stimulation is offered early or as a treatment of last resort is somewhat dependent on the particular syndrome. Certainly in cases of CRPS, a neuropathic pain syndrome covered elsewhere in this volume, SCS is being shown to be effective early in the course of the process (Oakley and Weiner, 1999; Kemler et al., 2000). For the post lumbar spine surgery patient with persisting leg pain of a neuropathic origin, SCS is offered after medication, physical therapy and perhaps therapeutic blockade therapies have been unsuccessful but before repeat surgical intervention (North et al., 1994).

2. Spinal cord stimulation

2.1. History

Descriptions of the biological effects of electrical stimulation date far into antiquity, most likely first described by fishermen dealing with such creatures as the electric fish, *Torpedo mamorata*, *Malopterurus electricus*, and *Gymnotus electricus*. These species are known to have been abundant near the sites of ancient civilizations and fishermen noted their presence in the nets when experiencing a painful electric shock, often leaving them with a numb sensation. The first application of this effect was possibly reported by Scribonius Largus in 46 A.D. in his 'Compositiones Medicae', for the treatment of acute gouty attacks and headache.

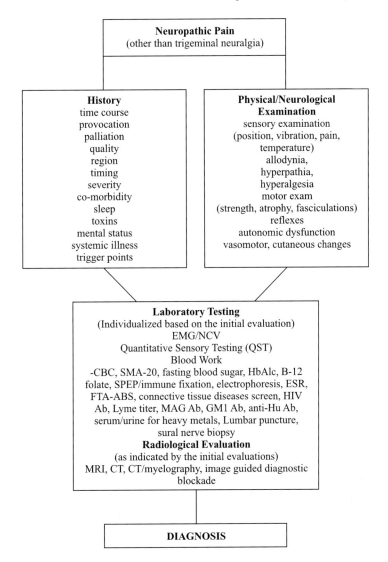

Fig. 1. Diagnostic algorithm for neuropathic pain.

He writes, "headache even if it is chronic and unbearable is taken away and remedied forever by a live torpedo placed on the spot which is in pain, until the pain ceases." (Kane and Taub, 1975).

With the publication of the 'gate control theory' of pain by Melzack and Wall in the 1960s, came the modern era of SCS (Melzack and Wall, 1965). Based on the argument that electrical stimulation of large diameter afferent fibres would close the gate to input from the smaller diameter and unmyelinated A-delta and C fibres mediating pain,

Shealy and co-workers reported pain relief in a patient with cancer related pain by the epidural application of spinal cord electrical stimulation (Shealy et al., 1967). With encouraging early results, albeit in an application for malignant origin pain no longer thought to be indicated, SCS began as a treatment modality for pain. Unfortunately, the initial belief was that SCS would be applicable to all pain types. Its broad application in the early 1970s almost resulted in its demise as a treatment modality due to poor

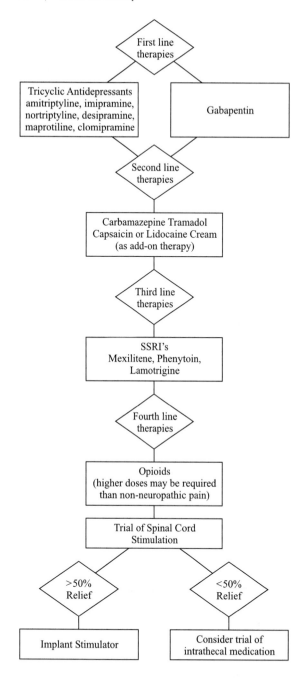

Fig. 2. Therapeutic algorithm for neuropathic pain.

outcomes. Careful observers began to note that SCS was most beneficial in patients with chronic pain of peripheral neurogenic origin, although some groups still claimed relief could be obtained in musculoskeletal pain. The primary indication

for the use of SCS became neuropathic pain due to peripheral nerve injury and almost exclusively in the USA for the treatment of the so-called failed back surgery syndrome. Syndromes with a predominantly neuropathic component were demonstrated to be relatively refractory to the usual medications including opioid medications in the customary dose ranges (Arner and Meyerson, 1988; Mao et al., 1995). In the currently accepted treatment algorithms, SCS often falls as a treatment of almost last resort when the pain has been designated drug-resistant. Unfortunately, even well selected patients may not experience significant pain relief. In general for failed back surgery syndromes, which offer the most literature data, the efficacy of SCS is about 60–70% (Meyerson, 1990; Simpson, 1994; Barolat, 1995). Currently the application of SCS encompasses not only neuropathic pain due to peripheral nerve or nerve root injury, but also selected primarily sympathetically mediated pain syndromes such as ischaemic pain due to peripheral vascular disease, angina pectoris, and CRPS type I and II (Mannheimer et al., 1988; Claeys and Horsch, 1993; Oakley and Weiner, 1999). Other applications of SCS have been tried, especially when other therapies have proven ineffective (Simpson, 1994; Barolat, 1995).

Spinal cord stimulation, like neuromodulation procedures in general, is a non-destructive, screenable and reversible treatment option. Since there are no long-term side effects that have been reported, SCS generally is preferable as a first step when other less invasive treatments have failed to produce acceptable control of the pain.

2.2. Selection of patients and outcomes of SCS

Special selection criteria apply to specific pain syndromes such as angina, peripheral vascular disease, CRPS and peripheral neuropathic pain. These criteria are generally the diagnostic criteria to establish the presence of the disease or syndrome (Gonzalez-Darder et al., 1991; Claeys and Horsch, 1993; De Jongste et al., 1994a).

TABLE IV
General inclusion and exclusion criteria for SCS intervention

General inclusion criteria
1. Appendicular pain following at least one previous spine surgery.
2. Pain of at least 6 months duration.
3. No chronic or recurring pain complaint above the level of the T10 dermatome (in failed back surgery syndrome).
4. Leg pain which radiates below the knee greater than back pain.
5. Informed consent.
6. Clearance after psychological evaluation by a Clinical Psychologist; the evaluation should include at least one objective, normalized psychological test felt to be helpful in making this determination, e.g. MMPI-II; evaluation of motivation for return to work, etc.

General exclusion criteria
1. Surgical procedure within the 6 months prior to screening trial.
2. Evidence of an active disruptive psychiatric disorder including dissociative disorder, major affective disorder with psychotic features, active drug or alcohol abuse, personality disorders significant enough to impact the perception of pain, compliance to intervention and/or ability to evaluate treatment outcome as determined by a qualified psychological or psychiatric consult.
3. Patients younger than 18 years of age.
4. Patients who have not received an adequate course of optimum non-surgical care.
5. Patients who have failed a previous SCS trial or system.

General inclusion and exclusion criteria have been developed and may be found in Table IV. For the majority of neurological surgeons, the primary indication for SCS will be a persisting radicular pain syndrome following primarily lumbar but also cervical spine surgery. When optimum medical management has failed to adequately restore function and relieve pain, it may be necessary to consider SCS to move the patient toward improved quality of life and functional ability.

The neurological surgeon may also be in a position to see a number of patients referred with central pain syndromes such as thalamic pain syndrome (post-cortical infarction pain syndrome) or a painful Wallenberg's syndrome (infarction of the posterior inferior cerebellar artery territory), or

post-spinal cord injury pain. Generally SCS has not been helpful in managing these diagnoses. SCS may be helpful in some cases of spinal cord injury pain when the lesion is incomplete, but in general does not relieve the end-zone pain.

Treatment outcomes have become an important part of justifying the application of newer and more expensive technologies. SCS is no exception. The specific outcome measures that are applied are as varied as the groups reporting results. Frequently success is determined by patients' self-reports of pain reduction. Other criteria such as decreased utilization of healthcare resources, improved function, return to work or closure of industrial insurance claims are reported as outcomes. Patient satisfaction is important, especially so to the treating physician, but it may not be a major concern for a third party insurance carrier.

Beginning in the early 1970s, numerous reports, predominantly case review studies, appeared in the literature. Significant changes in equipment were made throughout the 1970s, especially the introduction of multi-channel devices, and particularly the complication rates due to mechanical failure of the equipment changed for the better (North et al., 1991) There have appeared numerous reviews of these reports (Simpson, 1994; Barolat, 1995; Turner et al., 1995). To summarize what has become an extensive literature, the analysis of Turner et al. (1995) is helpful. In attempting to apply an evidence based literature review technique, they discovered that the predominantly case review nature of the literature did not lend itself to this type of scrutiny. However, it was felt that certain conclusions could be drawn, although further, more rigorous, randomized outcome approaches should be undertaken to verify these conclusions. A total of 39 studies met the review criteria. At the average follow-up of 16 months, 59% of the patients had 50% or greater pain relief. Complications occurred in 42% of patients but were considered to be minor. The lack of randomized trials prevented any conclusion as to the effectiveness of SCS relative to other forms of treatment, placebo or no treatment.

With developing pressure to produce randomized and prospective studies, preliminary results of a randomized study comparing SCS to repeat surgery for persisting leg pain following an initial spinal surgery was published after the Turner et al. (1995) article, by Richard North (North et al., 1994). Using the crossover from one treatment modality to the other after 6 months as the primary outcome measure, results for 27 patients showed a statistically significant advantage for SCS over repeat operation.

In a prospective, multicentre study combining 70 patients with at least 1 year follow-up, a variety of outcome measures including the average pain visual analogue scale, the McGill Pain Questionnaire, the Oswestry Disability Questionnaire, the Sickness Impact Profile and the Beck Depression Inventory were analyzed (Burchiel et al., 1996). Success of stimulation was considered achieved if 50% pain relief and patient satisfaction were reported. SCS was successful in managing the pain in 55% of the patients in whom 1-year follow-up was available. Statistically significant improvement was reported in all the outcome measures confirming that SCS can be an effective treatment modality for the management of chronic lower extremity pain.

Ohmeiss et al. (1996) reported a prospective study evaluating SCS in patients with intractable leg pain. An isometric lift task measured lower extremity function as an attempt to identify a measurable outcome parameter. This function was statistically significantly improved 6 weeks after the initiation of SCS. Other outcome measures such as the Sickness Impact Profile also significantly improved, confirming the results of other studies. Barolat and colleagues (1998), have reported a retrospective analysis of 102 patients evaluated by extensive questionnaire and telephone interview techniques from a disinterested third party. The average follow-up was 3.8 years. Twenty-one percent never experienced any pain relief. Of the remaining 80, 75% were still using their stimulator. In patients experiencing a reported 75% pain relief there was no reduction in relief over time. Patients experiencing only 50% reduction in their pain relief showed a dramatic reduction in their relief over the follow-up period. These authors felt that psychological screening contributed to a successful outcome.

Another method of analyzing the results of SCS is to evaluate results by specific syndrome. SCS has been applied in a number of pain syndromes. In the world literature, the most successful application of SCS is in the relief of intractable angina pectoris (Sanderson et al., 1992; De Jongste and Staal, 1993; Mannheimer et al., 1993; Anderson et al., 1994; De Jongste et al., 1994a,b,c; Sanderson et al., 1994). These patients have been selected as having refractory angina pectoris and not candidates for revascularization. Stimulation appears to improve cardiac function in these patients coincident with relieving pain. Success rates between 80 and 90% have been consistently reported. Electrodes are generally placed at the C_7–T_2 spinal level to the left of the midline with average stimulation parameters. Most notably in the European literature, peripheral vascular disease is the next most successful indication for SCS with relief of ischaemic pain in the extremity reaching 70–80% and limb salvage rates for extremities deemed appropriate for amputation are in the 60–70% range (Claeys and Horsch, 1993). CRPS type I and II is successfully treated at an 80–90% rate especially if the pain is sympathetically maintained. It is interesting that neuropathic pain in the extremity, such as is found in the patient with persisting radicular pain after spinal surgery, responds at a 60–70% rate. While representing the most common indication for SCS in the United States, it is the least successful in the long term. This may largely be due to the psychosocial problems associated with any pain management for the failed back surgery syndrome.

The most frequent use of SCS in the USA comes as a result of the prevalence of lumbar spinal surgery. There has grown a definable population of patients, estimated at 20–40% of those operated upon, who experience persistent or recurrent pain following intervention. SCS is indicated in patients who have failed to improve with optimum medical management. Optimum medical management of this problem includes such interventions as active physical rehabilitation. Generally a physical therapy directed programme is prescribed by a physical medicine and rehabilitation physician and carried out by a licensed physical therapist. This may consist of strengthening and flexibility exercises, aerobic conditioning and patient education to address lifting, posture, strengthening etc.; neuromuscular and modality therapy may be included in this programme but are not considered to alone constitute adequate therapy. Behavioural and psychological rehabilitation may also be a part of optimum management and consists of the application of pain control and stress management procedures including, but not limited to, relaxation therapy, guided imagery, cognitive restructuring, biofeedback, behavioural modification and group or individual education. Pharmacological management is probably the mainstay of optimum medical management and consists of the prescription of medication as required to control pain. This therapy may include narcotics, non-steroidal anti-inflammatory drugs, antidepressants, muscle relaxants and/or anticonvulsants as required by the patient's condition and deemed appropriate by the attending physician. In addition to standard pain management treatments, patients may seek, within various insurance systems, relief from acupuncturists, chiropractors and homeopaths.

It is generally after these treatments have failed that the interventionalist is asked to consider invasive pain treatments such as SCS. The implanter should be an integral part of a total pain management team, providing the necessary resources, experience and follow-up to ensure excellent patient management.

Some neuropathic pain conditions can be treated successfully with neurostimulation techniques other than SCS, for example peripheral nerve stimulation (Long, 1983). There has recently been an upsurge of interest in this application, particularly for CRPS (Hassenbusch et al., 1996)

and occipital neuralgia (Weiner and Reed, 1999) and in sacral and other nerve root stimulation for interstitial cystitis (Feler et al., 1999) and other neuropathic conditions (Alo et al., 1999). Whether SCS or a more peripheral stimulation modality may be more effective for a particular patient or condition is not yet established; for further discussion the reader is referred to Chapters 4, 5 and 8.

2.3. Technique

Certain requirements are necessary for SCS to be effective in relieving neuropathic pain. The stimulation produced paraesthesia must cover as large a percentage of the area of pain as possible and this effect must be maintained over time to obtain the best possible relief over time (Barolat, 1995). With SCS, the active electrode, the cathode or negative electrode, must be located near the level of the spinal cord dorsal columns that anatomically represents the level to be stimulated. If the pain is bilateral, a single electrode must be located on the physiologic midline of the spinal cord, or multiple electrode arrays may be used to allow the ability to access bilateral structures. If unilateral pain is present, the electrode is positioned to the side of the patient's pain (Barolat et al., 1993). With axial as well as appendicular pain multiple electrode arrays are useful to cover the axial portion of the pain with paraesthesia, as well as the painful extremity. How stimulation is applied to activate the desired paraesthesia pattern is nicely reviewed by Alo and Holsheimer (2002). Unfortunately, even the most elegant production of a paraesthesia pattern does not guarantee relief of pain. The paraesthesia may be nothing more than an epiphenomenon which is necessary for targeting the stimulation but not sufficient alone for relief.

2.3.1. Screening trial

While there is no literature proven method of screening for the efficacy of SCS, it is generally believed that a trial of 1 week or longer of externalized lead wires utilizing a temporary external transmitter can be effective in excluding from permanent implant up to 30% of patients screened. These patients are generally excluded due to lack of pain relief with the stimulation, or to uncomfortable stimulation effects. Table V presents criteria that must apply during a screening trial of 1 week or more for the patient to be eligible to go on to permanent receiver implant.

2.3.2. Equipment

The ability of SCS to modulate the nervous system is based on the delivery of electrical impulses to the spinal cord. This can be achieved by placing the

active part of the SCS lead, the electrode, on the spinal cord. This was historically the earliest approach utilizing a laminectomy and durotomy. However, within a short period of time, about 6 weeks to 6 months, the electrodes became ineffective due to fibrosis and occasionally due to spinal cord injury. Placing the lead wire in the epidural space solved this problem. In doing so, long term stimulation was possible without complication due to lead location. This also made the dorsal CSF space an important parameter in establishing stimulation amplitude and introduced stimulation variability with movement as a side effect.

Spinal cord stimulation electrodes are contained within lead wires. These are manufactured in numerous configurations and are available for implantation either percutaneously or via laminotomy (Fig. 3). The simplest form of lead contains two electrodes and allows bipolar stimulation. Lead wires progress in the number of electrodes from four to eight to sixteen contacts (the last being available in laminotomy paddle or plate leads only). Currently available leads are generally linear arrays of either one or two columns. A newer lead configuration deals with

TABLE V

SCS screening trial criteria

1. A minimum of 50% (optimum is at least 70%) pain reduction based on difference in VAS scores at pre-implant and post-lead implant, (anchors for the VAS are 'no pain' and 'worst possible pain').
2. The area of paraesthesia must be concordant with the area of pain.
3. Patient does not find the paraesthesia to be undesirable.
4. Functional improvement assessed by functional outcome evaluation as determined by each clinic, although some form of physical capacities evaluation is desirable.

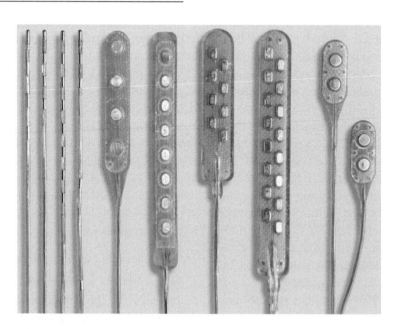

Fig. 3. Examples of existing SCS leads.

a transverse tripolar arrangement allowing programming across the spinal cord but must be used with a special transmitter.

Two types of power sources for producing stimulation at the electrode sites are currently manufactured (Fig. 4). The totally implantable pulse generators have a finite battery lifetime of 2–5 years on the average, depending on stimulation parameters, before they must be replaced by a surgical procedure, (Fig. 4b). An implantable pulse generator is programmed transcutaneously. The patient may control on, off, amplitude, and rate parameters with a handheld controller. The newest version of the implantable pulse generator (IPG) allows independent control of two, four contact, leads. Historically a radio frequency transmitter, which is worn externally, powers the first, and currently all other devices and broadcasts a signal to a subcutaneously implanted receiver connected to the lead wire (Fig. 4a). Radio frequency devices are programmed externally at the transmitter. Some devices allow the storage of multiple 'programs' of electrode positive and negative combinations which the patient may select at will (patient controlled stimulation) or which may be run in sequence independent of the patient (multiple stimulation mode) (Alo et al., 1998).

Electrical stimulation of the nervous system may excite or inhibit neuronal action. With SCS the active electrode that excites the desired paraesthesia response is the negative electrode or cathode (see Chapter 3). The cathode depolarizes neurons within its field and the neuron becomes more active. The positive electrode or anode inhibits the neurons in its field by hyperpolarization. Hence, various combinations of positive and negative electrodes are used to achieve the desired paraesthesia coverage. This forms the basis for programming the stimulation device. There are numerous ways to approach programming and to optimize paraesthesia coverage of the painful area (North, 1997). The success of SCS at relieving pain correlates with the percentage of the painful area covered by stimulation-induced paraesthesiae making these techniques important for any implanter.

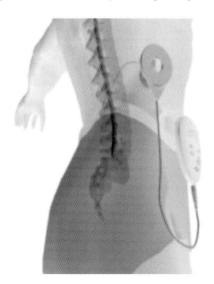

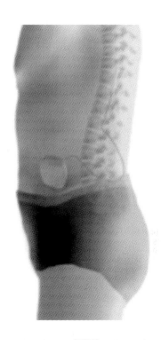

Fig. 4. There are two types of SCS systems. A: radiofrequency units with an external power source. B: completely implantable pulse generators. (A) Internal and external components; battery and controls outside. (B) Totally internal, power source internal; power controls external.

2.3.3. Lead implant techniques

Once a patient has been selected as a candidate for a trial of SCS, the implanting physician should be certain that the patient and the patient's support system, spouse, family, close relative or care giver, have been thoroughly educated concerning the intended procedure, its potential risks and expected outcomes. It should not be beyond the ability of the patient to understand the use of the intended system.

2.3.3.1. General technical concerns. Handling of lead wires requires special care so as not to break the lead insulation. The lead wires should not be kinked or bent or handled with sharp instruments. Rubber shod forceps or clamps or vascular type instruments such as Debakey style forceps should be used. Sutures should not be placed directly around the lead wires, silastic or hard plastic anchors and 2-0 braided suture or larger should be used to avoid cutting the insulation. Care should be taken to plan the length of lead necessary for subsequent permanent implantation. For example, a cervical lead wire with a proposed abdominal or buttock position of the receiver or transmitter will require a longer lead wire or extension wire than normal to avoid the lead being dislodged with flexion and extension movement. If an obstruction is encountered when moving the lead in the epidural space, do not force the lead. A guide wire technique may be tried, but it may be necessary to terminate the procedure and carefully evaluate the status of the spinal canal with regard to previously undetected stenosis or lesions.

2.3.3.2. Percutaneous leads. A general rule is to select a target for the active electrode, the negative electrode or cathode, based on the distribution of the patient's pain. If the predominant rhizopathy is in the S_1 root, the cathode will usually give appropriate paraesthesiae at the T11 or 12 vertebral levels. Always bear in mind that the anatomical midline of the spinal anatomy may not correlate with the physiologic midline for the purpose of producing paraesthesiae and some movement of the electrode position medio-laterally may be necessary to find the physiologic midline.

For percutaneous lead implantation, the operating room contains an operating table enabling fluoroscopic imaging. A C-arm image intensifier is used throughout the procedure to guide lead placement. If the implanter is right handed, the room is configured to allow the C-arm and video screen to be located on the patient's right side when the patient is prone (Fig. 5). The scrub table is placed to the operator's right side. These procedures are generally performed with monitored anaesthesia care under local anaesthesia. The anaesthesiologist is placed at the head of the table allowing enough room for the nurse or technician performing the screening trial.

Each manufacturer provides the necessary accessories with each lead that will allow either complete system implantation or placement of a tunnelled electrode for screening purposes (Fig. 6). These accessories include a modified Tuohy needle, a guide wire or lead blank, tunnelling instrumentation, anchors, insulation boots and hexagonal wrenches. For trial screening, disposable percutaneous extension wires are provided as well as the necessary external screening cable to allow testing.

The patient is placed prone on the operating table, prepped and draped from table to table. A chest-breast drape has a large fenestration that

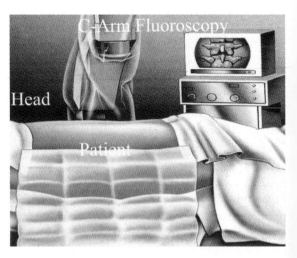

Fig. 5. Operating room configuration for a right handed implanter.

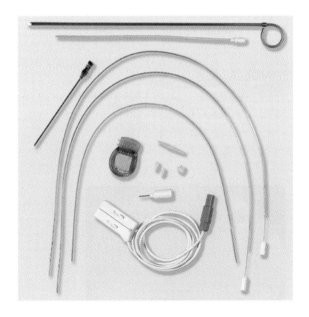

Fig. 6. Surgical accessories for implantation of SCS leads.

works particularly well for lead implantation. The vertebral interspace where the Tuohy needle will be placed in the epidural space is localized fluoroscopically. A 1–2 in. incision is made caudal from this point. Some clinics prefer to perform the needle placement first and confirm access to the epidural space and lead placement before making the incision (Fig. 7a). The Tuohy needle is inserted from a paraspinous approach at a 45° angle and directed toward the midline at the target level (Fig. 7b). This configuration allows insertion of the electrode more parallel to the epidural space. A loss of resistance technique or 'hanging drop' technique may be used to localize the epidural space. A positive contrast epidurogram may be performed if there is any question as to localization, but generally is not needed.

The electrode is then introduced through the Tuohy needle into the epidural space and 'steered' to the desired starting location using fluoroscopic guidance, as shown in Fig. 7c,d. The electrode is then connected to the screening cable. One end of the cable is passed over the ether screen to the implant assistant who connects it to the screening stimulator. Stimulation is then trialed. If a long

eight contact electrode is used, one method of intraoperative screening starts by stimulating the distal two electrodes the proximal two electrodes and two in the middle as anode–cathode bipoles. This establishes the upper middle and lower extent of the paraesthesiae. Adjustments as to electrode positions to locate the 'sweet spot' may then be made. Starting with the distal electrode negative and the proximal electrode positive and then reversing this sequence to determine the highest and lowest level of stimulation may screen four contact electrodes. The medio-lateral orientation will determine the medio-lateral position of the paraesthesiae in the extremity. Too far lateral will result in intercostal root stimulation and uncomfortable paraesthesiae. Perfectly midline stimulation may result in bilateral paraesthesiae and some interesting effects in the low back, or reaching the legs if stimulating the cervical spinal cord. Occasionally, a process called 'trawling' may ascertain the ideal location for the electrode. The electrode is placed higher than the expected stimulation level. The stimulator is adjusted to the perception threshold for paraesthesiae and slowly pulled caudally with the patient reporting the pattern of paraesthesia perception as the electrode is moved. The desired position is reached when the paraesthesiae 'paint over' the painful areas.

When the desired electrode location has been determined, the needle is removed and the lead is anchored to the fascia by using the anchors provided with the lead (Fig. 7e). If using a silastic anchor, one method of anchoring is to place a loop through the fascia and tie the suture. The stitch is then looped around the anchor and tied again. A single loop around the anchor and fascia may loosen. Anchoring should be done only to tissue not likely to necrose or absorb. Examples of tissue to not use would be muscle or fat. The lead is then attached to a disposable percutaneous extension and sealed with a silastic boot. A subcutaneous tunnel is then fashioned to the flank using tunnelling devices provided with the lead and the disposable lead is then brought through the tunnel

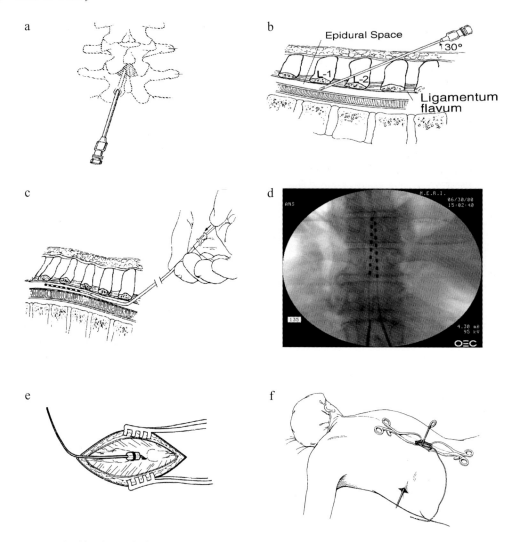

Fig. 7. Percutaneous lead implant technique. The procedure should take place under fluoroscopy.

and externalized (Fig. 7f). The back incision is then closed. The externalization stab wound is dressed by placing an antiseptic patch (for example, a BioPatch™, antimicrobial dressing, Johnson and Johnson Medical, Inc.) around the lead and a suitable overlying dressing. The patient is now ready to undergo a screening trial.

With the conclusion of a successful screening trial, the patient is returned to the operating room to implant the pulse generator or radio frequency receiver. The intended implant site determines the patient's position. Common sites are abdominal or upper outer buttocks for the pulse generator, and supracostal or upper outer quadrant of the buttocks for the radio frequency receiver to allow a more solid position for placing the external antenna. For abdominal or costal positions, the patient is positioned in the lateral decubitis position. For buttocks placement, the patient is prone. The prior implant site is prepped extending the prep to the proposed pocket site for the receiver or generator. After draping, the lead implant incision is opened and the disposable extension is cut and pulled out from under the drape by the circulator. The back incision and electrode are then packed with an antibiotic solution soaked sponge. Attention is turned to the pocket site. An 8–10 cm incision is made. Subcutaneous dissection is used to fashion the pocket, paying attention to haemostasis. The lead wire or extension wire is then tunnelled subcutaneously, connecting to the pocket. The lead or extension is connected to the receiver or pulse generator which is placed into the pocket being careful to coil any excess wire behind the unit. The wounds are closed with an interrupted inverted absorbable stitch and dressed.

Before discharge from the clinic, the patient and a significant other are instructed in the use of the device and if an implantable pulse generator has been used the device is programmed. The importance of this follow-up after the procedure cannot be overemphasized. Some clinics delay programming or activating the unit until the first post-operative visit when the patient may be more alert, and immediate post-operative effects have decreased. This initial session of education and initiation of stimulation should not be missed to begin a successful treatment plan using stimulation.

2.3.3.3. Laminotomy electrode implant. The general approach to the patient is similar to the percutaneous lead implant. One significant difference is the level of implant. The level of lead placement may have been determined by a percutaneous screening trial and the implanting neurosurgeon is asked to reproduce the paraesthesiae of the screening trial with a potentially more stable laminotomy lead. A percutaneous lead may have migrated twice necessitating the placement of a more stable electrode. Another candidate for the laminotomy implant is a patient whose predicted target is in the area of prior surgery which has obliterated the epidural space.

The operating room is set up identically to that for a percutaneously implanted lead. C-arm fluoroscopy is used to guide lead orientation. The patient is placed prone on the radiolucent operating table. It is often helpful to position a pillow or bolster under the patient's abdomen and have the patient lie prone, not on the arms or elbows. The patient is then prepped over the intended implant site, most commonly $T_{10,11}$ for the lower extremities, and, if the lead will be used as a screening lead, the prep is extended laterally to the table.

A midline incision is extended caudally from the implant level for 5–10 cm, after anaesthetizing with a long acting local anaesthetic such as bupivacaine. The deep fascia and paraspinous muscles are blocked with the local anaesthetic. When the block is established a subperiosteal dissection is performed using the electrocautery and a Cobb elevator or similar tool (Fig. 8a). After placing a self-retaining retractor in the wound, the inferior portion of the superior spinous process is resected exposing the ligamentum flavum (Fig. 8b). A window is made in the ligamentum flavum and enlarged using a 2 or 3 mm angled Kerrison rongeur. The dura is exposed and the opening widened by removing bone as necessary to allow placement of the lead. The lead is then introduced into the epidural space under fluoroscopic guidance to control for side-to-side orientation (Fig. 8c,d). The electrode may be sutured to the dura with a 4-0 braided stitch if there is excessive movement. The electrode is then intraoperatively screened for appropriate paraesthesia coverage as with the percutaneous lead. The position is adjusted as necessary. However, the ability to move the lead in a cephalic direction is limited, emphasizing the need for choosing the appropriate entry point or using a very large array electrode to allow electronic selection of the 'sweet spot'. With appropriate positioning, the wound is closed with an 'O' absorbable stitch through the muscle and a second layer apposing the muscle fascia. The lead or leads are then anchored to the fascia as described for percutaneous leads. The leads may then be tunnelled for a screening trial or connected to a pulse generator or radio frequency receiver. The position of the generator or receiver pocket and its creation may be chosen as with the percutaneous leads. Before proceeding to a laminotomy style implant a study such as MRI,

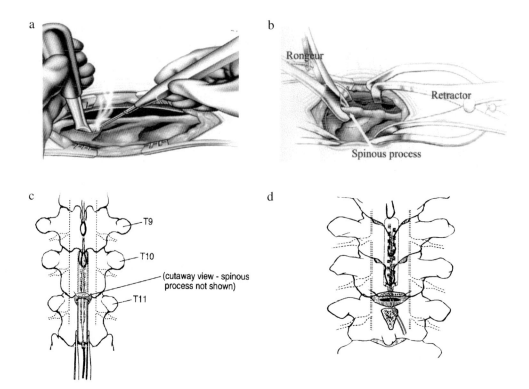

Fig. 8. Surgical lead implant technique.

or myelogram/CT should be performed to assess the diameter of the central canal and whether there exists a risk of spinal cord or cauda equina injury by placing a lead into the canal.

2.4. Complications

Complications are events whose incidence may be known but whose occurrence is unanticipated. These events imply an adverse outcome but do not suggest, in and of themselves, negligence. Complications will occur but every effort should be taken to eliminate preventable errors.

Complications during the placement and management of spinal cord stimulators fall in three categories:

(1) Surgical complications
(2) Device related complications
(3) Stimulation related complications

Overall complications occurred about 42% (20–75%) of the time in 13 case studies reviewed by Turner and colleagues (1995). The majority of these complications were considered to be minor and dealt with easily.

2.4.1. Surgical complications

The primary surgical related complication has been perioperative infection. This occurred in the review by Turner et al. (1995), surveying 31 studies in which complications were reported, 5% of the time (range 0–12%). Many clinics use antibiotic prophylaxis to avoid this complication. One method is to administer a cephalosporin intravenously 1-h before the procedure. Continuation of antibiotic coverage during the externalized screening trial is variable and there are no specific data to suggest a 'best' management technique. Biological complications other than infection occur about 9% (0–42%) of the time. These complications include spinal fluid leakage, haemorrhage and neurological injury. In the large prospective study of Burchiel and colleagues (1996) there were no infections either at lead implant or internalization. In 219 cases in this study there was one case each of cerebrospinal fluid leak, and reported muscle spasm. In their review of two decades of SCS experience, North's group (1993) reported no major morbidity defined as spinal cord injury, meningitis or life-threatening infection. The overall incidence of infection in this study was 5%.

2.4.2. Device related complications

In the analysis by Turner et al. (1995), stimulator complications occurred 30% of the time in 13 studies in which this could be determined. The electrodes were a problem 24% of the time. Most commonly this represented migration of the electrode(s), or movement, especially side to side, with a subsequent loss of paraesthesia coverage. The generator or receiver was a problem 2% of the time. In the Burchiel et al. (1996) study, 12 of 219 patients required surgical procedures for revision or replacement of at least one component of the system (5%). North and his colleagues (1993), in their survey of 20 years experience at the Johns Hopkins Hospital, defined electrode failure as a loss of stimulation paraesthesiae overlapping a patient's usual distribution of pain. A Kaplan–Meier survival curve was then generated demonstrating that multichannel devices were significantly more reliable than single channel laminectomy or percutaneous leads. A similar analysis for discontinuation of use for all reasons again demonstrated the superiority of newer multichannel devices.

2.4.3. Stimulation induced complications

Rarely, patients report that the stimulation paraesthesiae are uncomfortable, or increase the underlying pain. The exact incidence is difficult to ascertain from the literature. In the Burchiel et al. (1996) study, the incidence of these patient related complications was less than 3% (5 of 219 patients). One source of discomfort or lack of satisfaction with stimulation is posture-induced changes in paraesthesia intensity, as the spinal cord moves relative to the electrode contacts. Cameron and Alo (1998) investigated stimulation thresholds as a function of posture and found that in 20 patients the threshold for paraesthesia was lowest when lying; while in three patients thresholds were lowest when sitting for thoracic electrodes.

Efficacy reports for SCS in the management of chronic pain syndromes have consistently demonstrated that 50–60% of patients initially receiving more than 50% relief of pain are still using their stimulators at or after 1 year. It has been suggested that even after the 1-year period there remains a portion of the initially successfully treated population who return reporting a failure of stimulation to control their pain. In a review of 126 patients (74 female) followed for longer than 2 years in the author's clinic (24–168 months, average 37.8 months) reporting initially more than 50% pain relief, 26 (20%) were documented to have discontinued the use of stimulation or requested removal of the system. A retrospective analysis was conducted to determine the reasons why such patients with long-term relief ultimately fail therapy. Diagnoses at system implant included: myelographically proven arachnoiditis (61, 48%), radicular extremity pain (30, 24%), CRPS both types (8, 6%), spinal stenosis (7, 5%), peripheral neuropathy (6, 5%), peripheral vascular disease (5, 4%), other neuropathic pain (9, 7%). All patients were implanted with four contact percutaneous or paddle electrodes (Medtronic Quad™ or Resume™ style electrodes).

Three reasons for failure were determined:

(1) Progression of disease was determined in 12 patients (55% of failures). Seven patients were discovered to have new spine disease (32% of failures). Five patients presented with increased symptoms of peripheral neuropathy (23% of failures).
(2) Tolerance, defined as continued appropriate paraesthesiae with loss of relief. This was found in nine patients (41% of failures),

five with arachnoiditis and four others including two with post herpetic neuralgia.
(3) Pain at the pulse generator implant site occurred in one patient (4% of failures).

Four patients or 3% of the total enjoyed enough resolution of their pain that they no longer required stimulation (at 58, 60, 142, 57 months of stimulation), two with arachnoiditis, and two with radicular leg pain.

3. Specific neuropathic pain syndromes and SCS

SCS has been applied in a number of specific neuropathic pain syndromes. In addition to the major specific applications covered in this text, there are other infrequent reports of application in painful diabetic neuropathy, peripheral neuropathy of other origin, PHN and post amputation pain syndromes.

Post-herpetic neuralgia represents an application of SCS that has had a mixed history. However, Meglio and co-workers in 1989 demonstrated that in 10 patients with chronic PHN, six of the patients experienced 52.5% mean analgesia and underwent successful long-term implant (Meglio et al., 1989). A study using more contemporary stimulation techniques was reported by Harke and colleagues (2002). Twenty-eight patients with long-term (more than 2 years) PHN were prospectively evaluated and long-term pain relief was achieved in 82% (23 patients). Eight patients became completely pain free during the follow-up period. Four patients with acute PHN had improved pain immediately with SCS, but it is difficult to know if this was better than the natural history of the disease.

Diabetic peripheral neuropathy has always represented an enticing diagnostic entity for using SCS to relieve symptoms. Results of intervention have generally been disappointing. The literature has been predominantly sporadic cases reported as a part of more general case review studies of SCS (Kumar et al., 1998). The

results of individual cases have been no better than an estimated 40–50% relief of pain. One promising study from the Walton Centre, Liverpool, UK, describes 10 patients unresponsive to conventional treatment, six with type II diabetes with a mean duration of neuropathy 5 years. A standard thoracic epidural SCS target covering the pain distribution was used. A placebo external stimulator was used as well as the real external stimulator. Statistically significant relief of pain was seen in eight patients. Both background and peak neuropathic pain were statistically significantly relieved at 3, 6 and 14 months when compared to placebo. In addition exercise tolerance was measured and improved in this group of patients (Tesfaye et al., 1996). Further studies of this type are needed to validate SCS as a consideration in patients with pain due to diabetic peripheral neuropathy.

Post-amputation pain syndromes, which include phantom limb pain and post-amputation stump pain, have been treated with SCS. The IASP taxonomy defines phantom limb pain as pain referred to a surgically or traumatically removed limb or portion thereof (IASP subcommittee on taxonomy, 1986). Many forms of phantom pain actually exist involving structures such as a tooth, rectum, penis, scrotum, bladder, breast, nose and eye (Marbach, 1978; Pollman, 1981; Reisner, 1981; Sherman et al., 1984; Melzack, 1990; Kroner et al., 1991; Ovesen et al., 1991; Jensen and Rasmussen, 1994). Variations of phantom pain phenomena such as phantom angina and phantom sciatica have also been described (Mester et al., 1988; Kroner et al., 1991). Stump pain according to the same taxonomy is pain at the site of an extremity amputation. Phantom limb pain affects 0.5–5% of amputees severely (Sherman et al., 1984; Jensen and Rasmussen, 1994). Up to 97% of amputees may experience some phantom discomfort at some point following amputation (Ramheit, 1989). Stump pain obviously is present in the immediate post-amputation period but resolves within weeks. Persistent stump pain is reported to occur as infrequently as 5% of cases up to 71% of the time

(Loeser, 1990; Pohjolainen, 1991). Stump pain may have many aetiologies including neuroma formation, deafferentation pain or autonomic effects. Stump pain is not always a neuropathic phenomenon and may be related to skin changes, circulatory problems, infection and bone abnormalities (Jensen and Rasmussen, 1994).

The therapeutic use of SCS in the treatment of phantom pain is not extensively reported in the literature. Anecdotal reports appear usually as patients included in a larger retrospective review of stimulation for all types of chronic pain. Tasker and Dostrovsky (1989) reported that 56% of 16 personal patients responded favourably to dorsal column stimulation. Early reports of SCS in post-amputation pain syndromes suggested a similar response rate (Krainick et al., 1975; Richardson et al., 1980). Unfortunately, from the small reports that have been presented it is impossible to give a confident statement about when SCS should be used in these pain syndromes, or whether it is more effective in neuropathic stump pain or in the relief of a painful phantom. In the author's personal experience, in a small series of 15 patients, five with stump neuropathic pain and 10 with painful phantom, all of the stump pain patients experienced improvement of more than 50%. The mechanical sensitivity of the stump appeared to be relieved very quickly allowing the application of prosthesis, which before had been difficult. The phantom pain was less predictably relieved. Four out of the 10 patients reported they no longer experienced the phantom in an uncomfortable position although they could still experience the phantom. Most commonly relief was associated with some subjective experience of the stimulation paraesthesiae in the phantom. SCS is a modality which anecdotally may offer control of phantom limb and/or stump neuropathic pain but needs to be validated in a formal study setting.

In cases of general peripheral neuropathy of multiple origins, there exist even fewer reported cases. There has been an emerging interest in re-exploring the application of SCS in the treatment of painful peripheral neuropathy (Kumar et al.,

1996; Benbow and Macfarlane, 1999; Baheti, 2001). While being touted as a useful adjunct to the treatment of painful peripheral neuropathies, the actual supporting data are lacking. That is not to say it does not work, but merely to suggest further investigation is needed, as in all applications of SCS.

Acknowledgements

Figures 2, 3, 5 and 6 are reproduced courtesy of Advanced Neuromodulation Systems, Inc., Plano, Texas, and Fig. 7 by courtesy of Medtronic, Inc., Minneapolis, Minnesota and Advanced Neuromodulation Systems, Inc.

References

Alo, K.M. and Chado, H.N. (2000) Effect of spinal cord stimulation on sensory threshold functional measures. Neuromodulation, 3: 145–154.

Alo, K.M. and Holsheimer, J. (2002) New Trends in neuromodulation for the management of neuropathic pain. Neurosurgery, 50: 690–703.

Alo, K.M., Yland, M.J., Kramer, D.L., Charnov, J.H., and Redko, V. (1998) Computer assisted and patient interactive programming of dual octrode spinal cord stimulation in the treatment of chronic pain. Neuromodulation, 1: 30–45.

Alo, K.M., Yland, M.J., Redko, V., Feler, C., and Naumann, C. (1999) Lumbar and sacral nerve root stimulation (NRS) in the treatment of chronic pain. A novel anatomic approach and neurostimulation technique. Neuromodulation, 2: 23–31.

Anderson, C., Hole, P., and Oxhoj, H. (1994) Does pain relief with spinal cord stimulation for angina conceal myocardial infarction?. Br. Heart J., 71: 419–421.

Arner, S. and Meyerson, B.A. (1988) Lack of analgesic effect of opioids on neuropathic and idiopathic forms of pain. Pain, 33: 11–23.

Baheti, D.K. (2001) Neuropathic pain – recent trends in management. J. Indian Med. Assoc., 99: 692–697.

Barolat, G. (1995) Current state of spinal cord stimulation. Neurosurg. Quart., 5: 98–124.

Barolat, G., Massaro, F., He, J., Zeme, S., and Ketcik, B. (1993) Mapping of sensory responses to epidural stimulation of the intraspinal neural structures in man. J. Neurosurg., 78: 233–239.

Barolat, G., Ketcik, B., and He, J. (1998) Long-term outcome of spinal cord stimulation for chronic pain management. Neuromodulation, 1: 19–29.

Benbow, S.J. and Macfarlane, I.A. (1999) Painful diabetic neuropathy. Baillieres Best Pract. Res. Clin. Endocrinol. Metab., 13: 295–308.

Boivie, J., Leijon, G., and Johansson, I. (1989) Central post-stroke pain – a study of the mechanisms through analyses of the sensory abnormality. Pain, 37: 173–185.

Burchiel, K.J., Anderson, C.A., and Brown, F.D. (1996) Prospective, multicenter study of spinal cord stimulation for relief of chronic back and extremity pain. Spine, 21: 2786–2794.

Cameron, T. and Alo, K.M. (1998) Effects of posture on stimulation parameters in spinal cord stimulation. Neuromodulation, 1: 177–183.

Cassinari, V. and Pagni, C.A. (1969) Central Pain: A Neurological Survey. Harvard University Press, Boston.

Claeys, L., Horsch, S. (1993) Epidural spinal cord stimulation (ESCS) in chronic vascular pain. In: Kepplinger B, Pernak J.M., Ray A.L., Schmid H., (Eds.) *Pain – Clinical Aspects and Therapeutical Issues*, Part II. Edition Selva Verlag, Linz. pp. 45–51.

De Jongste, M. and Staal, M.J. (1993) Preliminary results of a randomized study on the clinical efficacy of spinal cord stimulation for refractory severe angina pectoris. Acta Neurochir. (suppl), 58: 161–164.

De Jongste, M.J.L., Haaksma, J., Hautvast, R.J.M., Hillege, H.L., Meyler, P.W.J., Staal, M.J., Sanderson, J.E., and Lie, K.I. (1994a) Effects of spinal cord stimulation on myocardial ischaemia during daily life in patients with severe coronary artery disease. Br. Heart J., 71: 413–418.

De Jongste, M.J.L., Hautvast, R.W.M., Hillege, H.L., and Lie, K.I. (1994b) Efficacy of spinal cord stimulation as adjuvant therapy for intractable angina pectoris: a prospective, randomized clinical study. J. Am. Coll. Cardiol., 23: 1592–1597.

De Jongste, M.J.L., Nagelkerke, D., Hooyschuur, C.M., Journee, H.L., Meyler, P.W.J., Staal, M.J., De Jonge, P., and Lie, K.I. (1994c) Stimulation characteristics, complications, and efficacy of spinal cord stimulation systems in patients with refractory angina: a prospective feasibility study. Pacing Clin. Electrophysiol., 17: 1751–1760.

Eliasson, T., Jern, S., Augustinsson, L.-E., and Mannheimer, C. (1994) Safety aspects of spinal cord stimulation in severe angina pectoris. Coronary Artery Dis., 5: 845–850.

Fairbank, J.C.T., Couper, J., Davies, J.B., O'Brien, J.P. (1980) The Oswestry low back pain disability questionnaire. Physiotherapy 66, 271-173.

Feler, C.A., Whitworth, L.A., Brookoff, D., and Powell, R. (1999) Recent advances: sacral nerve root stimulation using a retrograde method of lead insertion for the treatment of pelvic pain due to interstitial cystitis. Neuromodulation, 2: 211–216.

Fields, H.L. (1990) Introduction. In: H.L. Fields (Ed.), *Pain Syndromes in Neurology*. Butterworth Heinemann, Oxford.

Gonzalez-Darder, J.M., Canela, P., and Gonzalez-Martinez, V. (1991) High cervical spinal cord stimulation for unstable angina pectoris. Stereotact. Funct. Neurosurg., 56: 20–27.

Harke, H., Gretenkort, P., and Ladleif, H.U. (2002) Spinal cord stimulation in postherpetic neuralgia and in acute herpes zoster pain. Anesth. Analg., 94: 694–700.

Hassenbusch, S.J., Stanton-Hicks, M., Schoppa, D., Walsh, J.G., and Covington, E.C. (1996) Long-term results of peripheral nerve stimulation for reflex sympathetic dystrophy. J. Neurosurg., 84: 415–423.

International Association for the Study of Pain Subcommittee on Taxonomy. Classification of chronic pain. Description of chronic pain syndromes and definitions of pain terms. (1986) Pain Suppl. 3.

Jensen, T.S. and Rasmussen, P. (1994) Phantom pain and other phenomena after amputation. In: P.D. Wall, and R. Melzack (Eds.), *Textbook of Pain*, 3rd ed. (pp. 651–665). Churchill Livingstone, Edinburgh.

Kane, K. and Taub, A. (1975) A history of local electrical analgesia. Pain, 1: 125–138.

Kemler, M.A., Barendse, G.A., and van Kleef, M. (2000) Spinal cord stimulation in patients with chronic reflex sympathetic dystrophy. N. Engl. J. Med., 343: 618–624.

Kim, S.H., Tasker, R.R., and My, O. (2001) Spinal cord stimulation for nonspecific limb pain versus neuropathic pain and spontaneous versus evoked pain. Neurosurgery, 48: 1056–1065.

Kroener, K., Krebs, B., Skov, J., and Joergensen, H.S. (1989) Immediate and long-term phantom breast syndrome after mastectomy: incidence of clinical characteristics and relationship to pre-mastectomy breast pain. Pain, 36: 327–334.

Kumar, K., Toth, C., and Nath, R.K. (1996) Spinal cord stimulation for chronic pain in peripheral neuropathy. Surg. Neurol., 46: 363–369.

Kumar, K., Toth, C., Nath, R.K., and Laing, P. (1998) Epidural spinal cord stimulation for treatment of chronic pain – some predictors of success. A 15-year experience. Surg. Neurol., 50: 110–120.

Loeser, J.D. (1990) Pain after amputation: phantom limb and stump pain. In: J.J. Bonica (Ed.), *The Management of Pain*, 2nd ed. (pp. 255–256). Lea and Febiger, Philadelphia, PA.

Long, D.M. (1983) Stimulation of the peripheral nervous system for pain control. Clin. Neurosurg., 331: 323–343.

Mannheimer, C., Augustinsson, L.-E., Carlsson, C.-A., Manhem, K., and Wilhelmsson, C. (1988) Epidural spinal electrical stimulation in severe angina pectoris. Br. Heart J., 59: 56–61.

Mannheimer, C., Eliasson, T., Andersson, B., Bergh, C.-H., Augustinsson, L.-E., Emanuelsson, H., and Waagstein, F. (1993) Effects of spinal cord stimulation in angina pectoris induced by pacing and possible mechanisms of action. Br. Med. J., 307: 477–480.

Mao, J., Price, D.D., and Mayer, D.J. (1995) Experimental mononeuropathy reduces the antinociceptive effects of morphine: implications for common intracellular mechanisms involved in morphine tolerance and neuropathic pain. Pain, 61: 353–364.

Marbach, J.J. (1978) Phantom tooth pain. J. Endodont., 4: 362.

Max, M.B. (2002) Clarifying the definition of neuropathic pain. Pain, 96: 406–407.

Meglio, M., Cioni, B., Prezioso, A., and Talamonti, G. (1989) Spinal cord stimulation (SCS) in the treatment of post-herpetic pain. Acta Neurochir. Suppl. (Wien), 46: 65–66.

Melzack, R. and Wall, P.D. (1965) Pain mechanisms: a new theory. Science, 150: 971–979.

Merskey, H. and Bogduk, N. (Eds.) (1994) *Classification of Chronic Pain. Descriptions of Chronic Pain Syndromes and Definitions of Pain Terms.* 2nd ed. IASP Press, Seattle, WA.

Mester, S.W., Cintron, G.B., and Long, C. (1988) Phantom angina. Am. Heart J., 116: 1627–1628.

Meyerson, B.A. (1990) Electric stimulation of the spinal cord and brain. In: J.J. Bonica, J.D. Loeser, R.C. Chapman, and W.E. Fordyce, (Eds.), *The Management of Pain* (pp. 1862–1877). Lea and Febiger, Philadelphia.

North, R.B. (1997) Spinal cord stimulation. In: RB North, and R.M. Levy (Eds.), *Neurosurgical Management of Pain* (pp. 271–282). Springer-Verlag, New York.

North, R.B., Ewend, M.G., Lawton, M.T., and Piantadosi, S. (1991) Spinal cord stimulation for chronic, intractable pain: superiority of 'multi-channel' devices. Pain, 44: 119–130.

North, R.B., Kidd, D.H., Zahurak, M., James, C.S., and Long, D.M. (1993) Spinal cord stimulation for chronic intractable pain: two decades' experience. Neurosurgery, 32: 384–395.

North, R.E.B., Kidd, D.H., Lee, M.S., and Piantodosi, S. (1994) A prospective randomized study of spinal cord stimulation versus reoperation for failed back surgery syndrome: Initial results. Stereotact. Funct. Neurosurg., 62: 267–272.

Oakley, J.C. and Weiner, R.L. (1999) Spinal cord stimulation for complex Regional Pain Syndrome: a prospective study at two centers. Neuromodulation, 2: 47–50.

Ohmeiss, D.D., Rashbaum, R.F., and Bogdanffy, G.M. (1996) Prospective outcome evaluation of spinal cord stimulation in patients with intractable leg pain. Spine, 21: 1344–1351.

Ovesen, P, Kroener, K, Ornsholt, J, and Bach, K. (1991) Phantom-related phenomena after rectal amputation: prevalence and clinical characteristics. Pain, 44: 289–291.

Pohjolainen, T. (1991) A clinical evaluation of stumps in lower limb amputees. Prosthet. Orthot. Int., 15: 178–184.

Pollman, L. (1981) Phantom tooth phenomenon: painless and painful sensations. In: J. Siegfried, and M. Zimmermann (Eds.), *Phantom and Stump Pain* (pp. 77–80). Springer-Verlag, Berlin.

Reisner, H. (1981) Phantom tooth. In: J. Siegfried, and M. Zimmerman (Eds.), *Phantom and Stump Pain* (pp. 81–83). Springer-Verlag, Berlin.

Roland, M. and Morris, R. (1983) A study of the natural history of back pain. Part I. Development of a reliable and sensitive measure of disability in low back pain. Spine, 8: 141–144.

Rossi, U., Rabar, J. (1994) Spinal cord stimulation in the failed back syndrome: A reappraisal. Presented at the American Pain Society Meeting 11/10-13.

Sanderson, J.E., Brooksby, P., Waterhouse, D., Palmer, R.B.G., and Neubauer, K. (1992) Epidural spinal electrical stimulation for severe angina: a study of its effects on symptoms, exercise tolerance and degree of ischaemia. Eur. Heart J., 13: 628–633.

Sanderson, J.E., Ibrahim, B., Waterhouse, D., and Palmer, R.B.G. (1994) Spinal electrical stimulation for intractable angina-long-term clinical outcome and safety. Eur. Heart J., 15: 810–814.

Shealy, C.N., Taslitz, N., Mortimer, J.T., and Becker, D.P. (1967) Electrical inhibition of pain: experimental evaluation. Anesth. Analg., 46: 199–305.

Sherman, R.A., Sherman, C.J., and Parker, L. (1984) Chronic phantom and stump pain among American veterans: results of a survey. Pain, 18: 83–95.

Simpson, B.A. (1994) Spinal cord stimulation. Pain Rev., 1: 199–230.

Tasker, R.R. (1990) Pain resulting from central nervous system pathology (central pain). In: J.J. Bonica (Ed.), *The Management of Pain* (pp. 264–283). Lea and Febiger, Philadelphia.

Tasker, R.R. and Dostrovsky, J.O. (1989) Deafferentation and central pain. In: PD Wall, and R Melzack (Eds.), *Textbook of Pain*, 2nd ed. (pp. 154–180). Churchill Livingstone, Edinburgh.

Tesfaye, S., Watt, J., Benbow, S.J., Pang, K.A., Miles, J., and Macfarlane, I.A. (1996) Electrical spinal-cord stimulation for painful diabetic peripheral neuropathy. Lancet, 348: 1698–1701.

Turner, J.A., Loeser, J.D., and Bell, K.G. (1995) Spinal cord stimulation for chronic low back pain: a systematic synthesis. Neurosurgery, 37: 1088–1095.

Weiner, R.L. and Reed, K.L. (1999) Peripheral neurostimulation for control of intractable occipital neuralgia. Neuromodulation, 2: 217–221.

Woolf, C.J. and Mannion, R.J. (1999) Neuropathic pain, aetiology, symptoms, mechanisms and management. Lancet, 353: 1959–1964.

Woolf, C.J. and Salter, M.W. (2000) Neuronal plasticity: increasing the gain in pain. Science, 288: 1765–1768.

Electrical Stimulation and the Relief of Pain
Pain Research and Clinical Management, Vol. 15
Edited by Brian A. Simpson

CHAPTER 8

Spinal cord stimulation for complex regional pain syndromes

Daniel S. Bennett[a],* and Tracy L. Cameron[b]

[a]*Integrative Treatment Centers, 8406 Clay St.,*
Denver, CO 80031-3810, USA
[b]*Department of Biomedical Engineering, University of Texas, Southwestern Medical School,*
Dallas, TX 75390, USA

Abstract

Complex regional pain syndromes (CRPS) comprise a constellation of symptoms which together bridge neuropathic and vasculopathic pain syndromes. Diagnosis is based on the clinical history coupled with physical examination; no definitive diagnostic test is available. Increasing evidence of effectiveness of spinal cord stimulation in CRPS is being realized. Early recognition of this syndrome combined with multidisciplinary therapeutic aggressiveness should promote optimal functional recovery.

Keywords: Complex regional pain syndrome (CRPS); Reflex sympathetic dystrophy (RSD); Causalgia; Spinal cord stimulation; High frequency stimulation

1. Introduction

The complex regional pain syndromes (CRPS: Type I = reflex sympathetic dystrophy, RSD; Type II = causalgia) comprise a constellation of symptoms which together bridge neuropathic and vasculopathic pain syndromes, being characterized by both sensory and autonomic disturbances. It is important to keep in mind that we are discussing a syndrome (i.e. constellation of symptoms) defined by a phenotypic presentation. Since the first published descriptions of the syndrome over a century ago, definitive neurophysiologic pathways and mechanisms have remained elusive leading to considerable disparity between disciplines as to the appropriate treatment. Unfortunately, this has also led some to relegate this syndrome to nebulous psychodynamic origins rather than neurophysiologic ones, an attitude similar to that held towards depression at the turn of the 20th century. To date, no specific personality trait or psychological factor predisposing to the syndrome has been found (Lynch, 1992). Experimental animal evidence has emerged which suggests a hypothesis as to the formation of neuropathic circuits but a definitive model does not exist to adequately study the phenomena in CRPS. What may actually be occurring is a diverse phenotypic

*Correspondence to: Daniel S. Bennett, MD, Integrative Treatment Centers, 8406 Clay St., Denver, CO 80031-3810, USA. Phone:
+ 1-303-487-0932; Fax: + 1-303-487-0934; E-mail: dbennett@denverpain.com

representation of common neuropathic circuits, in which case treatment which negatively impacts the neuropathic circuit should prove effective in the treatment of the syndrome.

2. Background

The syndrome was first described in 1864 (Mitchell et al., 1864) in patients sustaining partial nerve injury and was labelled causalgia. As time progressed, various terms including algodystrophy, Sudeck's atrophy and post-traumatic vasomotor disorder were used. Evans coined the term RSD in 1946, describing his observations of sustained sympathetic responses and later trophic changes in the extremity (Evans, 1946). In 1994, the International Association for the Study of Pain (IASP) introduced the term CRPS as a more accurate description than RSD, subdividing this into Type I, previously RSD, and Type II, reserved for association with a known peripheral nerve injury (causalgia) owing to the paucity of evidence for a 'reflex' mechanism and with dystrophic changes occurring in only a subset of patients (Merskey and Bogduk, 1994). CRPS was further subdivided into sympathetically maintained pain (SMP), based upon cessation of pain with sympathetic fibre interruption and sympathetically independent pain (SIP). The two sub-types are thought to exist on a continuum; neither defines (includes or excludes a patient from) the syndrome. This newer classification also removed the concept of stages, recognizing that defined stages offer little help in treatment planning or in understanding probable neurophysiologic pathways responsible for the symptom complex.

3. Diagnosis of CRPS

A wide range of injuries can precipitate CRPS, from seemingly harmless injuries which do not even produce visible bruising to significantly traumatic injuries which require multiple surgeries;

historical detail of injury is therefore often of no help. The syndrome can develop suddenly in a patient who has undergone previous surgeries or trauma to an extremity, following an uncomplicated surgical course. It can also present without any significant trauma being reported. Immobilization (e.g. splinting or casting) can also produce the syndrome.

In addition to the poor correlation of historical findings, the syndrome presents along a phenotypic continuum with some patients expressing a fulminant form (rapidly progressing, multiple features and intense pain) or a latent form (some of the features with varied intensity of pain) often changing with time. As time progresses, CRPS can also spread to involve different extremities or other parts of the body. We simply do not understand the pathophysiology sufficiently to be able to explain the clinical progression.

Two factors contribute to the difficulty in obtaining consistency in diagnostic criteria: (1) the tendency of the clinical features of CRPS to change with time; and (2) the divergent range of clinical features associated with CRPS (Fig. 1; Schott, 1999). Galer and colleagues applied the IASP criteria to a group of patients and found little differentiation between those with diabetic neuropathy and CRPS (positive predictive value ranged from 40 to 60%). By using a checklist and scoring the positives (i.e. features present), the specificity increased to 0.95, with a predictive value of 0.91 for 11 out of 20 features present (Fig. 2; Galer et al., 1998). Because of the variability of symptoms, Harden proposed a further set of inclusion criteria to permit more uniform guidelines in clinical research (Fig. 3; Harden et al., 1999; Harden, 2000).

There is no definitive quantitative test or imaging technique available to diagnose CRPS. It is important to remember that the clinical tests advocated thus far measure the presence or absence of sympathetic dysfunction or the downstream effects of sympathetic dysfunction (i.e. thermography, triple-phase bone scan, resting sweat output). The presence or absence of these

Atrophy of skin with loss of wrinkles (glossiness of skin)
Allodynia
Detrusor and urinary sphincter dysfunction
Dupuytren's and other contractures
Excessive, absent or reduced sweating
Hair changes (excessive or reduced growth, and/or fineness instead of coarseness)
Inappropriate warmth or coldness
Involuntary movements: tremor, dystonia, spasms
Joint stiffness (acute or chronic arthritic changes)
Muscle wasting and/or weakness
Nails (ridged, curved, thin, brittle or clubbed)
Osteoporosis: spotty, localized or widespread
Pigmentation changes
Skin colour changes (cyanotic, erythematous, pale or blotchy)
Subcutaneous atrophy or thickening
Swelling

Modified from Schott (1999)

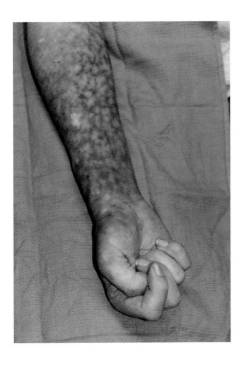 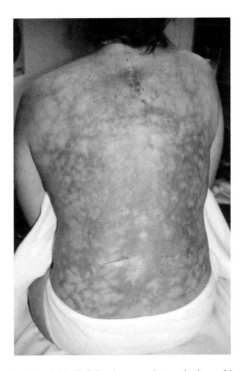

Fig. 1. (a) Clinical features of CRPS. (b) Clinical features in a patient who developed CRPS following carpal tunnel release. Note the significant trophic changes to nail beds, atrophy of muscles and vasomotor changes. (c) Centralized CRPS can involve regions of the body other than the extremities. Note the skin mottling, indicative of vasomotor instability and trophic changes to skin (shiny surface).

effects, however, does not define the syndrome. Laboratory evaluations (i.e. quantitative sudomotor axon reflex test, thermography) can be helpful in confirming the presence of SMP (Verdugo and Ochoa, 1993; Bruehl et al., 1996a,b; Gulevich et al., 1997; Sandroni et al., 1998). In the case of bone scintigraphy (triple-phase bone scan), there is a wide variability in changes making this test of low sensitivity and specificity (Lee and Weeks, 1995).

		No	Yes
Subject History			
1.	Burning Pain	___	___
2.	Skin sensitivity to touch (e.g. stroking of the skin, clothing, bedsheets)	___	___
3.	Skin sensitivity to cold	___	___
4.	Abnormal swelling	___	___
5.	Abnormal hair growth	___	___
6.	Abnormal nail growth	___	___
7.	Abnormal sweating	___	___
8.	Abnormal skin color changes	___	___
9.	Abnormal skin temperature changes	___	___
10.	Limited movement		
Physical Features (examination)			
11.	Mechanical allodynia (light touch, rubbing)	___	___
12.	Hyperalgesia to single pinprick	___	___
13.	Summation to multiple pinprick	___	___
14.	Cold allodynia	___	___
15.	Abnormal swelling	___	___
16.	Abnormal hair growth	___	___
17.	Abnormal skin color changes	___	___
18.	Abnormal skin temperature (> 1.0 C)	___	___
19.	Limited range of motion	___	___
20.	Motor neglect	___	___

From Galer, et al (1998)

Fig. 2. CRPS diagnostic checklist.

1. Continuing pain that is disproportionate to any inciting event.

2. Must report at least one symptom in each of the four following categories:

    a. **Sensory:** reports of hyperaesthesia
    b. **Vasomotor:** temperature asymmetry and/or skin color changes and/or sweating asymmetry.
    c. **Sudomotor:** edema and/or sweating changes and/or sweating asymmetry
    d. **Motor/Trophic:** decreased range of motion and/or motor dysfunction and/or trophic changes

3. Must display at least one sign in two or more of the following categories:

    a. **Sensory:** hyperalgesia and/or allodynia
    b. **Vasomotor:** temperature asymmetry and/or skin color changes and/or skin color asymmetry
    c. **Sudomotor:** edema and/or sweating changes and/or sweating asymmetry
    d. **Motor/Trophic:** decreased range of motion and/or motor dysfunction and/or trophic changes

From Harden (2000); Harden et al (1999).

Fig. 3. Experimental revision of diagnostic criteria for CRPS.

Sympathetic blockade has been advocated in both the diagnosis and treatment of CRPS. Sympathetic blockade may be useful in identifying SMP if one believes that only interruption of sympathetic fibres occurs when using standard regional techniques; it is more likely, however, that regional techniques produce a combined somatic and sympathetic blockade.

Some have proposed electro diagnostic studies as a way of narrowing the inclusion criteria for the diagnosis of CRPS. Traditional electromyography/ nerve conduction velocity (EMG/NCV) studies which measure large afferent and motor fibres are of no benefit in quantifying changes in small diameter myelinated afferents (A-delta) and unmyelinated afferent C fibres which are responsible for neuropathic signalling (Ochoa, 1994). Quantitative sensory testing (QST) has been advocated and preliminary data are encouraging, although normative data for CRPS are as yet insufficient to give the specificity required to be useful in narrowing the inclusion criteria (Lindblum, 1994; Tahmoush et al., 2000; Raj et al., 2001).

The diagnosis of CRPS is based on the clinical history coupled with strong indicators on physical examination. This 'bedside' approach was studied by Oerlemans and colleagues in patients who were classified as having CRPS with SMP; they concluded that this diagnostic approach correlated with objective evidence, i.e. laboratory measurements (Oerlemans et al., 1999).

4. Pathophysiology of CRPS

Although the pathophysiologic circuitry/pathways underlying CRPS have not been fully elucidated, evidence is accumulating for central pathway abnormalities, far removed from the affected extremity. The hypotheses used to explain CRPS (as well as neuropathic pain in general) are based on animal models which rely on somatic nerve injury or dorsal nerve root injury: (1) ligature of sciatic nerve (Bennett and Xie, 1988); (2) partial ligation of sciatic nerve (Seltzer et al., 1990); or (3) ligation of nerve root (Kim and Chung, 1992). In the purest sense, however, these really can only be extrapolated directly to CRPS II. Nevertheless, these models do provide a framework for our understanding of peripheral to central processes that are probably at play in producing the phenotypic constellation referred to as CRPS.

It is hypothesized that initial peripheral injury leads to inflammatory mediators (prostaglandins E2, D2 and F2, thromboxane B2, tumor necrosis factor, leukotrienes and interleukins) resulting in a production of free radicals. The presence of free radicals sensitizes C fibre and A-delta fibre ('silent') nociceptors leading to a change in the nociceptors to produce a predominant antidromic stimulus which facilitates peripheral swelling; histologic changes are similar to those found in diabetic neuropathy with superimposed changes reflective of a microangiopathy (Goris et al., 1987; Schmidt et al., 1994; Schmelz et al., 1996; Van der Laan et al., 1997a,b, 1998). Increased glutamate bombardment leads to an NMDA (*N*-methyl-D-aspartate) mediated increase in transduction of a perpetuating signal. The summation of the changes begins an afferent and efferent loop at the spinal segmental and suprasegmental levels which eventually leads to 'centralization' of pain (see also Chapter 5).

In an elegant study of human subjects' thermoregulatory responses, Wasner and co-workers found aberrant autonomic responses in patients with CRPS (Wasner et al., 2001). More specifically, in early presentations of CRPS, patients showed features consistent with inhibition of cutaneous vasoconstrictor neurons whereas in later presentations of CRPS they showed features consistent with peripheral hypersensitivity to norepinephrine. Schurmann and colleagues (2000) studied Doppler fluxmetry in patients with fractures of the radius. They found that in those who went on to develop CRPS, sympathetic vasoconstrictor responses were absent or diminished from the first day following injury. It is known that a key element in the diminution of nociceptive transmission is the firing of sympathetic vasoconstrictors. Schurmann also found that the autonomic disturbances displayed were not restricted to the painful extremity; they were more generalized. Riedl and colleagues (2001) found that stroke patients had similar autonomic dysfunction in the absence of pain, although the patterns were the same as those seen in CRPS. Therefore, CRPS patterns of autonomic dysfunction are probably a reflection of central pathway dysfunction rather than spinal segmental or suprasegmental dysfunction (Maleki et al., 2000). PET (positron emission tomography) scan data have shown decreases in thalamic activity in patients with post-traumatic neuropathic pain (Iadarola et al., 1995). Thimineur and colleagues (1998) studied 145 patients (including 26 normals and 69 with non-CRPS neuropathic pain) and found a high incidence of trigeminal hypoaesthesia in the CRPS I subgroup, including bilateral deficits and hemilateral sensory disturbances. They concluded that the abnormal pain, pressure and thermal perception noted in CRPS is evidence of central dysfunction in stimulus processing.

Gracely and colleagues (1992) postulated that central processing abnormalities coupled with peripheral sensitization and therefore abnormal input, are responsible for the sustained pain and distal changes observed in neuropathic pain syndromes. This is compatible with the various clinical observations noted in CRPS I and II. Functional magnetic resonance imaging (fMRI) has demonstrated widespread prefrontal hyperactivity, anterior cingulate gyrus activity and diminished activity in the contralateral thalamus (to the side of the body affected) occurring in CRPS I with SMP. The application of sympathetic blockade decreased the sensorimotor responses but had no effect on prefrontal regions of the brain (Apkarian et al., 2001).

Finally, the presence of myoclonic activity is probably the best physical indicator for a central mechanism to date and occurs in many cases of CRPS (Sandroni et al., 1998). Motor features are common in CRPS and may actually precede the occurrence of autonomic/sensory features (Schwartzman and Kerrigan, 1990; Veldman et al., 1993).

5. Treatment of CRPS

5.1. General review

Consensus groups have attempted to bridge the gap between quantitatively objectifiable testing, clinical treatment and the retrospective and prospective literature. Stanton-Hicks and colleagues

(2002) published their consensus statement that stressed the application of the 'conservative' over the 'invasive' therapy approach (Fig. 4).

The core basis of the approach in the treatment of CRPS has been physical/manual modalities, despite the lack of controlled clinical trials showing that these modalities change the course of CRPS. The rationale for the application of physical/manual therapeutic modalities is the prevention of contractures and the minimizing of muscular atrophy; these deleterious consequences of CRPS can add to functional impairment and disability. Physical therapy modalities, however, have not been shown to change the overall course of CRPS (Kingery, 1997).

Cognitive/behavioural therapies should be a core element in the treatment of CRPS, starting from the time of diagnosis. Although it has been postulated that psychological abnormalities are responsible for CRPS (Ochoa and Verdugo, 1995; Ochoa, 1999), data have not shown CRPS to be a consequence of psychological disturbance. Psychological problems can certainly be a *result* of chronic intractable pain which leads to depression, anxiety and other psychological sequelae (Lynch, 1992; Bruehl et al., 1996b; Gallagher, 1998a,b).

Systemic medication has shown significant variability in effectiveness in CRPS. Serotonin/norepinephrine reuptake blockers (Watson et al., 1982; Max et al., 1991), non-steroidal anti-inflammatory drugs (NSAIDS; Farah, 1993), steroids (Christensen et al., 1982; Oyen et al., 1993), opioids (Arner and Meyerson, 1988; Portenoy et al., 1990), alpha-adrenergic blocking agents (Davis et al., 1991; Byas-Smith et al., 1995), membrane stabilizers (Dejgard et al., 1988; Mellick and Mellick, 1995; Nicholson, 2000; Sandner-Kiesling et al., 2002) and NMDA antagonists (Kopf, 2000; Wallace et al., 2002) have all been advocated, with selective combination recommended (i.e. targeting multiple receptors to suppress abnormal nerve signalling). Certainly, in initial presentations, use of medications in combination for 'balanced' analgesia is appropriate to facilitate movement.

Sympathetic blockade has been advocated traditionally in the treatment of CRPS. Sympathetic (and/or somatic) blockade may be beneficial in quiescing early SMP thereby arresting the progression to permanent central changes in a subset of patients (theoretically by uncoupling peripheral nociceptor/efferent adrenergic stimulation). Data are lacking as to any positive long-term benefit with multiple and repeated sympathetic ganglion or neuroaxial blockades. Thus, unless significant diminution in pain and increased function are apparent over time, this approach is discouraged. Intravenous regional techniques (i.e. Bier blocks) show no evidence of any benefit, either in predictive value or in the modification of the course of CRPS (Cepeda et al., 2002). The question of whether the abolition of peripheral responses (i.e. weakness/dystonia) by placebo is causally predictive of secondary gain (with particular reference to worker's compensation) was discussed by Ochoa (1999). The problem with this argument, however, lies in the ill-defined nature of the placebo effect, which is ubiquitous throughout the population and affects any and all treatment modalities (Turner et al., 1994).

Given the impact of destructive lesions on the central nervous system, it does seem prudent that destructive modalities should be reserved as a 'last resort' in the treatment of any neuropathic process, particularly as evidence of peripheral–cord–brainstem interactions becomes more clearly defined. Tasker (1990) reviewed outcome data for sympathectomy for CRPS I and found that the long-term outcomes were poor.

5.2. *Electrical neuromodulation (spinal cord stimulation) and CRPS*

Spinal cord stimulation (SCS) had its beginning in the late 1960s with the application of electrical stimulation to the dorsal columns of a patient with neuropathic pain due to cancer (Shealy et al., 1967). Since that time stimulation has been used to treat a variety of pain syndromes, including CRPS.

5.2.1. Prospective studies

One of the main criticisms of the SCS literature in general arises from the possible role of placebo. Because a patient cannot be blinded to the therapy, few well-controlled studies have been attempted to determine the effects of placebo in SCS. In the present survey, no studies were identified that attempted to control for placebo and only one study was found that compared SCS with a control group (Table I).

In a prospective randomized trial, Kemler and co-workers (2000) examined the effects of SCS on a group of 24 patients diagnosed with RSD, selected from an initial cohort of 36 by trial stimulation and who had significant disability (of the initial group of 36, 10 required wheelchairs; eight required crutches and 13 required splints). Patients were included in this study if the disease was clinically restricted to one hand or foot, affected the entire hand or foot and had lasted for at least 6 months. They had also not shown a sustained response to psychological or medical therapies and had a mean pain intensity of at least 5 mm on a 10 mm visual analogue scale (VAS). The 24 patients were provided with SCS and physical therapy and the control group of 18 patients was provided with physical therapy alone. Outcome measures included pain measurements (VAS and McGill pain questionnaire) and quality of life measurements: the Nottingham Health Profile (NHP) and short version of the Sickness Impact Profile (SIP). Patients were assessed at 1, 3 and 6 months. Data were analyzed on an intention-to-treat basis. At 6 months, the results showed a significant improvement in the group ($N = 36$) assigned to receive SCS and physical therapy ($P < 0.0001$; mean reduction of pain intensity on VAS $= 2.4$ cm) compared to the group that received physical therapy alone (mean reduction 0.2 cm). The average reduction for the 24 actually treated with SCS was 3.6 cm. A significant improvement in the pain component of the NHP ($P = 0.02$) was also reported in the 24 patients who were treated with SCS. These positive results were

TABLE I

Articles for review were collected via Medline and Ovid search on all the available literature

Author	Patient diagnosis and intervention	Implanted patients (CRPS)	Mean follow-up (months)	Complications listed?	Outcome measures	Results
Kemler et al. (2000)	Pain due to CRPS I (RSD)	24	6	Y	2.3 mm reduction in VAS compared to control	VAS statistical significant improvement compared to control group $P<0.001$
Calvillo et al. (1998)	Upper extremity CRPS	31	36	Y	Changes in VAS scores, analgesic consumption	VAS statistically significant improvements ($P<0.0001$); 44.4% reduced narcotic use by 50%
Ebel et al. (2000)	CRPS I ($n=1$) and II ($n=1$), phantom limb	3 (2)	36	Y	Changes in VAS scores, analgesic consumption	100% success, >50% reduction in VAS, no analgesics required
Oakley and Weiner (1999)	CRPS	16	7.9	Y	Changes in VAS scores; overall benefit (four point scale)	80% success. (overall benefit); VAS statistically significant improvements ($P<0.05$)
Barolat et al. (1989)	RSD	15	14	Y	Benefit (four point scale; none, minimal, moderate, good)	73% success
Bennett et al. (1999)	CRPS I (RSD)	101	18.7/23.5	Y	Changes in VAS scores; overall satisfaction	70% quadripolar/91% octopolar success; VAS statistically significant to baseline ($P<0.0001$)
Broseta et al. (1982)	Causalgia	11	13	Y	Four categories: excellent, good, fair and poor	72% had excellent or good results
Devulder et al. (1990)	Phantom limb pain, failed back surgery (FBSS), polyneuropathy, causalgia	45 (6)	NA	Y	four point pain scale	83% had good pain relief, no narcotic analgesics
Hassenbusch et al. (1995)	Intractable low back and leg pain, RSD	42 (9)	25	Y	Changes in VDS scores and >50% reduction in pain (three point scale)	VDS statistical significance from baseline $P<0.001$; 67% patients had >50% pain relief
Kemler et al. (1999)	CRPS I (RSD)	18	32	Y	Changes in VAS scores and global perceived effect (GPE)	VAS statistical significant improvement from baseline $P<0.001$; 72% success GPE
Kumar et al. (1998)	FBSS, peripheral vascular disease, peripheral neuropathy, RSD	189 (13)	66	Y	Three point pain scale	100% had greater than 50% reduction in pain
Robaina et al. (1989a)	RSD	6	23	Y	Four point pain scale	100% had greater than 50% reduction in pain
Robaina et al. (1989b)	Raynauds syndrome, RSD	11 (8)	27	Y	Four point pain scale	87.5% had a greater that 50% reduction in pain
Sanchez-Ledesma et al. (1989)	Phantom limb pain, postherpetic neuralgia, RSD, causalgia, stump pain	36 (8/11)	66	Y	Four point pain scale	100% had greater that 50% long-term pain relief; 80% reduced narcotic use

Studies were included in the survey if they satisfied all the following criteria: patients were diagnosed as having CRPS; means, percentages, or statistics were available; the effectiveness of SCS was being studied; pain measurements such as the VAS were used as outcomes; and the number of patients studied was listed. Fifteen articles, involving 531 patients, were identified that met the inclusion criteria. These articles were subdivided into three groups that included prospective, randomized controlled or prospective controlled studies ($n=1$), prospective studies with no controls ($n=1$) and retrospective studies ($n=11$). The article in dark grey is a prospective, randomized, controlled study. Articles in light grey are prospective studies with no controls. The remaining articles are retrospective studies. (VAS: visual analogue scale; VDS: visual digital scale) demonstrated despite a significant surgical complication rate of 25%. Complications relating to unsatisfactory positioning of the electrode occurred in five patients. The correct position of the electrode was achieved in four patients after one additional procedure; however, one patient required three additional procedures to correct the electrode positioning. This study concluded that there is a beneficial effect of stimulation in this patient population. A criticism of Kemler's study has been that because all the patients that were selected had previously failed physical therapy, the control group was not given a true alternative therapy. Any permanent deficits secondary to structural surgeries in this patient population (that would preclude functional recovery) were not defined; such deficits would not be expected to respond to SCS. Kemler and his group did propose that better results would have been obtained if optimal leads (i.e. percutaneous vs. paddle, based on anatomy) had been employed at the outset and if multiple stimulation programmes had been available (as this has been shown retrospectively to be optimal). Nonetheless, Kemler's study did show that SCS produced improvement in a group of patients where nothing else was effective in reducing pain (39% 'much improved' in the global perceived effect with SCS and physical therapy vs. 6% with physical therapy alone); it is logical to predict that in a more favourable group of patients, results would indeed be better.

Calvillo's group (1998) examined 31 patients with CRPS affecting the upper extremity and found a significant ($P < 0.0001$) reduction in VAS scores with SCS compared to baseline. Ebel and colleagues (2000) examined the effects of SCS on deafferentiation pain syndromes due to peripheral nerve lesions. Three patients, diagnosed with phantom limb pain, causalgia and RSD, respectively, were treated with SCS and all three responded positively. The patient with causalgia had a 90% improvement in their VAS score while the patient with RSD had a 70% improvement. Another prospective study (Oakley and Weiner, 1999) reported on 19 patients. Sixteen were available at follow-up with 11 still using their devices; two patients were no longer in pain, one died (unrelated to the device) and two patients were unresponsive to the treatment. Eight of the 10 patients for whom follow up data were available and who were still using their stimulators obtained at least 50% pain relief. There was a significant change in the VAS score from pre-implant to post-implant ($P < 0.05$). Complications identified in these studies were minor and corrected without adverse effect on stimulation efficacy.

5.2.2. Retrospective studies

The majority of the published studies to date are retrospective (Table 1). The overall success rate for those patients diagnosed with causalgia (CRPS II) was 79% (23/29), while the overall success rate for those patients diagnosed with RSD (CRPS I) was 82% (148/180).

5.2.2.1 CRPS II. Causalgia (CRPS II) has been thought to be an indication for SCS for many years but few studies exist that examine the effectiveness of SCS specifically for this condition. Devulder and colleagues (1990) examined the effects of SCS on 45 patients with various chronic pain syndromes, six of whom were identified as having pain due to causalgia. Pain relief was assessed using a four point scale: (A) good pain relief, no need for medications; (B) good pain relief, need for nonnarcotic analgesics; (C) little pain relief, need for narcotic analgesics; and (D) no longer used the stimulator. At follow-up 83% of patients diagnosed with causalgia were considered successes with good pain relief without narcotic analgesics. Broseta's group (1982) reported on 11 patients with causalgia with an average follow-up of 13 months. They found that 64% of the patients reported a greater than 75% reduction in pain with only light analgesics required and that this same group was able to return to work. Finally Sanchez-Ledesma and colleagues (1989) reported on 11 patients diagnosed with causalgia and eight patients with RSD. At a mean follow-up of 5.5 years, all patients reported greater than 50% reduction in pain with stimulation; 90% of the causalgia (CRPS II) patients and 88% of the RSD (CRPS I) patients required no analgesics and were able to return to work and an active life.

5.2.2.2 CRPS I. The retrospective studies reflect a significantly positive experience with SCS in CRPS I. Kumar and colleagues (1998) reported on a 15-year experience of SCS for the treatment of chronic pain. A total of 235 patients were initially trialled with stimulation. Of these, 189 were considered successes and permanently implanted with internal pulse generator (IPG) or radio frequency (RF) systems; they were examined after a mean of 66 months. Of the 13 patients diagnosed as having RSD, all were found to have long-term satisfactory pain relief (mean 40 months). Barolat examined 18 patients with RSD. Three did not experience relief during the trial period; the remaining 15 patients underwent internalization with RF or IPG SCS systems. At a follow-up of 14 months, 11 patients (73%) were classified as successes. In Kemler's earlier retrospective study of 23 patients with RSD, of the 18 patients who were implanted with a SCS system, 13 (72%) responded favourably to stimulation, with a significant ($P < 0.001$) reduction in pain scores (VAS) compared to baseline (Kemler et al., 1999). Robaina's group reported in two papers (1989,a,b) their experience with SCS to treat RSD. Their first article described a retrospective examination of the clinical effectiveness of transcutaneous electrical nerve stimulation (TENS) and SCS for the treatment of RSD. Patients were followed for periods ranging from 10 to 36 months with a mean of 23 months. Of the six patients with RSD implanted with an SCS system, all reported a greater than 50% decrease pain. In their second paper they extended their study of the clinical effectiveness of SCS to eight patients with RSD and three with severe Raynaud's (vasospastic) disease of the upper limbs, followed for a mean of

27 months. Of the eight with RSD implanted with an SCS system, seven reported a greater than 50% decrease in pain. Hassenbusch et al. (1995) analyzed patients with intractable low back and leg pain treated with either SCS or spinal infusion. Patients included in this study had midline lower back pain and/or unilateral or bilateral leg pain. A multidisciplinary group involving anaesthesiology, neurosurgery, psychiatry, rehabilitation, nursing, orthopaedics and others as needed, assessed all patients. In nine patients implanted with stimulators, the leg pain was attributed to RSD. At the last follow-up, six of the nine were found to have greater than 50% pain relief.

We recently conducted a retrospective study to examine the current trends in the use of SCS to treat CRPS I (Bennett et al., 1999). This study was unique in that it not only examined the reduction of pain but also correlated this outcome with the type of stimulation hardware used. The goal of the study was to look for any similarities in those patients who were successfully treated with SCS and to compare the results of using single lead quadripolar systems with those using dual lead octapolar systems. We reviewed the data from 101 patients meeting the criteria for CRPS I as agreed in the IASP consensus statement (Merskey and Bogduk, 1994), with similar psychologic (psychometric testing) findings. Success was determined both by a reduction in the VAS score for pain and by patient satisfaction. Patients were divided into two groups: those that had single-lead quadripolar systems ($N = 30$) and those that had dual-lead octapolar systems ($N = 71$). There was a significant reduction in VAS pain intensity scores when compared to baseline for each group ($P < 0.0001$). The overall satisfaction of the group implanted with quadripolar leads was 70%, while the satisfaction of the group with dual-octapolar leads was 91%. Analysis of variance for improvement in pain score showed a significantly greater improvement (F-value 56.081, $P < 0.0001$) with dual-octapolar leads versus a single quadripolar lead. There was a mean pain improvement (Δ VAS) in the quadripolar group of 3.70 ± 0.79, while the mean pain improvement in the dual-octapolar group was 6.00 ± 1.59.

One major difference between the two groups was the ability to regain pain control after spontaneous lead movement. In the quadripolar group four patients (3.3%) required a surgical revision secondary to spontaneous lead migration, while in the dual-octapolar group no patients required surgical revision due to spontaneous lead migration. The larger number of electrodes available for programming in the dual-octapolar group provided an increased flexibility when rostral-caudal changes in lead placement occurred; patients who experienced spontaneous lead migration were able to recapture their pain coverage with reprogramming. An unexpected finding of the study was that, in addition to a larger number of available electrode combinations, the dual-octapolar group was also able to use higher frequencies (above 250 Hertz; Hz) to 'recapture' pain control; a subset of patients who had lost pain control in the presence of adequate paraesthesia coverage (15.5%) were able to regain control when their stimulation frequency was increased above 250 Hz (mean 455 Hz $\pm$ 104.5). A report by Alo et al. (1998a) supported this finding by demonstrating an increase in efficacy with the use of frequencies greater than 300 Hz.

In addition to the use of higher frequencies, the technology available to the dual-octapolar group enabled them to use multiple programmes. This was thought to be an important factor in the superior outcome in this group. We found that the overall reductions in VAS scores of the dual-octapolar group were comparable with data published by Alo in his prospective study of 80 patients treated with dual-octapolar systems, which included 22 with CRPS (Alo et al., 1998b, 1999). Of the dual-octapolar group in our study, 74.8% used multiple arrays to maximize paraesthesia coverage and 15.5% used frequencies above 250 Hz. Although both groups showed statistically significant improvements in pain scores and overall satisfaction compared to baseline, the dual-octapolar group consistently showed

greater improvements. With the use of frequencies greater than 250 Hz, patients were able to regain lost pain control. The percentage of patients that we found benefiting from higher frequencies is similar to that of patients who recently reported paraesthesia without pain relief (Barolat et al., 1998).

It is clear that the current literature suggests a significant benefit in the use of SCS to treat pain due to CRPS I and II when compared with other treatment modalities, with a low incidence of serious complications (Table II). However, it also demonstrates the relative lack of studies, in particular well-controlled studies, in this area. We were only able to find one study that compared SCS treatment to a control group and this study used a control group that was biased towards no improvement since they had previously failed all conservative therapy (Kemler et al., 2000). All other studies compared SCS outcomes with baseline measurements. The fact that any study

TABLE II

Table of the various complications identified in the studies detailed in Table I

Complication	Number of events	Total number of patients	Rate of occurrence (%)
Lead migration etc.	97	531	18.0
Infection	20	531	3.7
Epidural haemorrhage	0	531	0.0
Seroma	0	531	0.0
Haematoma	2	531	0.4
Paralysis	0	531	0.0
CSF leak	4	537	0.7
Undesirable stimulation	13	531	2.4
Intermittent stimulation	0	531	0.0
Pain over implant	5	531	1.0
Allergic reaction	1	531	0.2
Skin erosion	2	531	0.4
Lead breakage	17	531	3.2
Hardware malfunction	11	531	2.1
Loose connection	8	531	1.5
Battery failure	15	460	3.3
Other	9	531	1.7

This table examines the number of events, the total number of patients and the rate of occurrence.

showed improvement is extremely encouraging since SCS is routinely offered as a 'last chance' treatment after all more 'conservative' treatments have failed. In addition, most studies have reported results using stimulation systems with limited capabilities (few electrode contacts and limited output parameters). Recent studies are showing that for the CRPS population a more complex, technically advanced system may be required. Our recent observations and those of others have shown a positive advantage in using multiple electrode leads and high frequencies. Thus a more aggressive treatment strategy, which places neuromodulation therapies early on in the disease progression and the use of more advanced SCS systems, may prove to be more effective.

5.2.3. Physiology of spinal cord stimulation for neuropathic pain

A growing number of physiological studies examining the mechanisms of action of SCS is supporting the clinical data accruing from its use in the treatment of CRPS. Although the physiological mechanisms that are proposed are derived from studies in animals, it is clear that SCS affects the dorsal horn, segmental and suprasegmental regions of the spinal cord, as well as brainstem and higher cortical centres. To what extent neuromodulation affects each level is unclear; it is probable that no one neural structural level is responsible for the clinical effects documented in humans. Meyerson and Linderoth discuss these mechanisms fully in Chapter 11.

5.2.4. The place of SCS in the treatment of CRPS

The exact place for SCS in the treatment of CRPS remains controversial, in large part due to a lack of structured clinical studies comparing early intervention with SCS versus late intervention with SCS. Prospective studies detailing a comparison of electrode arrays and programming parameters between different types of system are needed. This is further complicated by the evolving criteria used to define study groups (Fig. 3) and stratification of study groups by given cognitive or behavioural subtype (i.e. one cannot compare individuals without considering how those individuals differ supratentorially). As discussed above, it is rational to treat patients who present with CRPS using a multimodal approach (Fig. 4). What has not been given competing credence in consensus statements is the place of neuromodulation therapies in CRPS. While other therapies have been proposed as 'more conservative' and therefore 'early' or 'initial' therapies, this rationale is not supported with favourable long term outcome data (i.e. a change in the course of the condition or significant long term diminution of pain). The conservative treatment algorithm is a 'We have always done it this way' approach, supported by anecdotal data and collections of case series. Thus, we propose a time oriented construct, which relies on the realization that timely reduction of pain should provide the best environment for functional recovery (Fig. 4). As the degree of pain and dysfunction is variable for any given patient, the exact timing of SCS in the treatment continuum is based on clinical judgement rather than on data.

5.2.5. Initial considerations: Who is an appropriate candidate for SCS in CRPS?

Patient selection is the key factor for a positive outcome in the application of SCS. Patients have to meet the clinical criteria for the diagnosis of CRPS, be able to understand how to use their stimulator (including being able to read appropriate handbooks/manuals), be motivated to have an active role in their management and be free of overwhelming and overriding psychological barriers such as psychosis or pathologic behaviour (e.g. obsessive compulsive disorder) and secondary gain. The selection of the appropriateness of the patient, therefore, should rely on a cohesive team of professionals each of whom has a key role during the selection process (Fig. 5).

The roles of the implant coordinator, nursing personnel and technical personnel (specialist nurse, neurophysiologist etc.) are invaluable. When patients are selected for implantation, they

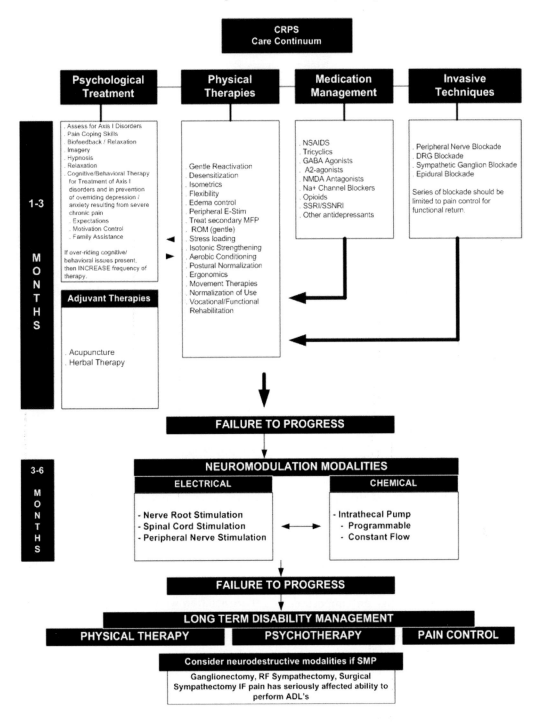

Fig. 4. CRPS Care continuum. CRPS treatment guidelines have been proposed via consensus (Stanton-Hicks et al., 2002) but without clear recommendations regarding the timing of implementations along the continuum, which should be considered a layered (in-parallel) multidisciplinary continuum with the goal being functional recovery with pain control. Data have shown that a 'golden window' exists from onset of injury to probability of returning to a functioning status. Thus, the above guideline is recommended. (SMP: sympathetically-maintained pain; ADLs: activities of daily living).

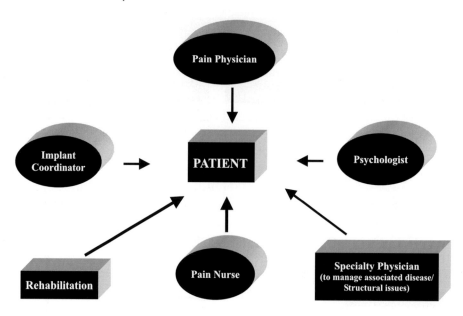

Fig. 5. Team approach. The team approach is crucial to the determination of the appropriate candidacy for neuromodulation techniques and the realization of optimal functional outcome.

are in essence marrying into your medical practice. Destructive behaviours can alienate staff from the patient and often present practical problems with programming and follow up care, which are crucial downstream in maximizing success. Just because a patient's medical classification predicts success with SCS it does not mean that one's practice is the place for them, or that they will respond in a meaningful way to the application of this therapy. It is usually the implant coordinator and/or pain nurse who provide crucial education and spend the most time with the potential stimulator candidate – listen to them.

The clinical psychologist is an important member of the implantation team who can assist the implanter in determining cognitive/behavioural suitability in preoperative preparation, as well as guiding the patient through their functional recovery. The psychologist can assist by identifying the presence of psychological conditions which require cognitive/behavioural management and of psychological conditions which need treatment prior to proceeding with SCS (e.g. severe extrinsic depression). Behavioural instruction, biofeedback, coping skills and strategies are examples of skills

these professionals bring to the table that greatly enhance the patient's readiness for and ultimate acceptance of, an implantable device. Cognitive/behavioural evaluation is best obtained over several visits to allow the medical psychologist time to profile the individual patient. However, the surgical selection of the patient should rest solely on the implanting physician.

5.2.6. SCS: Specifics related to CRPS

Surgical selection of the patient with CRPS begins with a complete review of the structural anatomy of the part of the spine to be accessed. Plain films in association with MRI (and/or CT) are strongly recommended to determine: (1) the width of the epidural space; (2) the distance from dura to cord; and (3) structural abnormalities (i.e. disc herniation, central canal stenosis, ligamentum flavum hypertrophy, spondylosis, spondylolisthesis etc.).

Technical considerations are discussed more fully in Chapter 12, but some points that are of particular relevance to CRPS will be highlighted here. Stimulation systems vary by: type of lead structure (percutaneous vs. 'paddle-type'); configuration (4-, 8-electrode or combinations thereof);

power source (internal vs. external); parameter limitations (pulse width, frequency, amplitude); programming modes (continuous, intermittent, dual-channel, multicycle, or patient controlled). In CRPS, the topography of the pain often changes with time. The more flexibility afforded in the programming of the implanted system (i.e. number of electrodes, range of pulse width, frequency and amplitude, dual channel capability) the more attractive the given system is for treating CRPS.

Law empirically determined that optimal electrode spacing comprised 3 mm electrode lengths, 4 mm apart; this provided optimal recruitment of deep fibres (Law, 1983) Electrode contacts with greater degrees of spacing are found to activate dorsal root fibres before recruitment of dorsal column fibres (Holsheimer et al., 1995). Indeed, consistent with Law's observations, Holsheimer's mathematical model predicts that narrowly spaced bipoles offer greater statistical superiority for capture of dorsal column neurons (Holsheimer, 1997; Holsheimer and Wesselink, 1997). Electrode configuration for paraesthesias in CRPS I and II should recruit dorsal column fibres preferentially as multiple dermatomes are involved; thus this type of electrode array is preferable. We recommend consideration of dual leads (or dual array paddle) with narrowly spaced bipoles to optimize both dorsal column fibre capture and programmability.

The amount of power required by the system is directly related to the number of electrodes that are active (i.e. cathodes), the amplitude, pulse width and frequency employed and the amount of time the patient utilizes the system. If more than 4 electrodes are needed, battery life of IPGs is greatly reduced which commits a patient to surgical replacements of the IPG at too frequent an interval to be practical or fiscally viable. In CRPS, when dual electrode arrays are employed the battery life of the currently available internal power systems is insufficient and thus radio-frequency controlled systems are preferable.

The frequency limitations of the system are also important to consider. In a recent multicentre data analysis, as discussed earlier, approximately 15% of patients with CRPS who lost pain control in the presence of paraesthesias regained pain control by increasing the frequency to >250 Hz (Bennett et al., 1999). Further, prospective, experience has shown a greater than 20% subset of patients with CRPS I will require frequencies exceeding 250 Hz (Bennett, unpublished data) many requiring 1025 Hz or greater to achieve 'recapture' of pain control. Cycling between high frequency and 'traditional' frequencies (with identical cathodes) also seems to provide a way of reducing exacerbations of pain in this population. Therefore, the utilization of a system with capabilities of higher frequency stimulation (without compromising available pulse width) should be given careful consideration.

The mode of programming must be considered. Simple continuous or intermittent stimulation is provided by all systems currently available. However, in a recent prospective 2-year study of patients with various pain syndromes, Alo and colleagues found that programmes that allowed multiple configurations of active electrodes and stimulation parameters to cycle automatically or to be chosen by the patient increased satisfaction from the previously reported 50–80% (Alo et al., 1998b, 1999). In addition, the ability to programme multiple configurations of guarded cathodes was found to recapture paraesthesia coverage without the need for multiple surgical lead revisions-an important cost consideration.

Finally, when implanting the IPG or the receiver–transducer of an RF system, care must be taken to avoid any area of the body affected by the CRPS as there is a real risk of exacerbating the condition.

5.2.7. Cost versus benefit of SCS in CRPS

Kemler and Furnee (2002) evaluated the economics of SCS for CRPS versus 'conventional' treatment and found that during the 1st year of therapy SCS was higher in cost than non-SCS therapy. They found, however, that in the lifetime analysis SCS was more effective than conventional therapy and was less expensive. These findings are similar to a recent comparison of conventional chronic pain therapies versus SCS in 104 patients with 'Failed Back Surgery Syndrome' (another complex symptom entity). Treatment costs with SCS were higher for the first 2.5 years and thereafter were approximately one-third lower. Additionally, 15% of the SCS treated group had returned to work (Kumar et al., 2002).

6. Conclusions

CRPS represents a challenge for the pain physician. Despite the syndrome being recognized for more than a century, phenotypic commonality is what ultimately defines inclusion. As the pathology of neural processes responsible for neuropathic pain is rapidly emerging, the application of therapies that interrupt or modulate these pathways is logical. SCS can modulate neuropathic pathways and thereby be effective in reducing the previously intractable pain and improving function and quality of life in patients suffering from CRPS.

References

Alo, K.M., Poli, P., Ghiara, M., Ciaramella, A., Varelli, G., Yland, M.J. (1998a) The treatment of refractory reflex sympathetic dystrophy with high frequency tripolar dual octrode spinal cord stimulation, a case report. Abstract from International Neuromodulation Society 4th International Congress, Lucerne, Switzerland.

Alo, K.M., Yland, M.J., Kramer, D.L., Charnov, J.H., and Redko, V. (1998b) Computer assisted and patient interactive programming of dual octrode electrode spinal cord stimulation in the treatment of chronic pain. Neuromodulation, 1: 30–45.

Alo, K.M., Yland, M.J., Charnov, J.H., and Redko, V. (1999) Multiple program spinal cord stimulation in the treatment of chronic pain: follow up of multiple program SCS. Neuromodulation, 2: 266–272.

Apkarian, A.V., Thomas, P.S., Krauss, Szeverenyi, N.M. (2001) Prefrontal cortical hyperactivity in sympathetically mediated chronic pain, Neurosci. Lett., 311: 193–197.

Arner, S. and Meyerson, B.A. (1988) Lack of analgesic effect of opioids on neuropathic and idiopathic forms of pain. Pain, 33: 11–23.

Barolat, G., Ketchik, B., and He, J. (1998) Long-term outcome of spinal cord stimulation for chronic pain management. Neuromodulation, 1: 19–29.

Barolat, G., Schwartzman, R., and Woo, R. (1989) Epidural spinal cord stimulation in the management of reflex sympathetic dystrophy. Stereotact. Funct. Neurosurg., 53: 29–39.

Bennett, G.J. and Xie, K. (1988) A peripheral mononeuropathy in rat that produces disorders of pain sensation like those seen in man. Pain, 33: 87–107.

Bennett, D.S., Alo, K.M., Oakley, J., and Feler, C. (1999) Spinal cord stimulation for complex regional pain syndrome [RSD]: a retrospective multicenter experience from 1995–1998 of 101 patients. Neuromodulation, 2: 202–210.

Broseta, J., Roldan, P., Gonzalez-Darder, J., Bordes, V., and Barcia-Salorio, J.L. (1982) Chronic epidural dorsal column stimulation in the treatment of causalgia pain. Appl. Neurophysiol., 45: 190–194.

Bruehl, S., Lubenow, T., Nath, H., and Ivankovich, O. (1996a) Validation of thermography in the diagnosis of reflex sympathetic dystrophy. Clin. J. Pain, 12(4): 316–325.

Bruehl, S., Husfeldt, B., Lubenow, T., Nathm, H., and Ivankovich, A. (1996b) Psychological differences between reflex sympathetic dystrophy and non-RSD chronic pain patients. Pain, 67: 107–114.

Byas-Smith, M.G., Max, M.B., Muir, J., and Kingman, A. (1995) Transdermal clonidine compared to placebo in painful diabetic neuropathy using a two-stage enriched enrollment design. Pain, 60: 267–274.

Calvillo, O., Racz, G., Didie, J., and Smith, K. (1998) Neuroaugmentation in the treatment of complex regional pain syndrome of the upper extremity. Acta Orthop. Belg., 64: 57–62.

Cepeda, M., Lau, J., and Carr, B. (2002) Defining the therapeutic role of local anesthetic blockade in complex regional pain syndrome: a narrative and systematic review. Clin. J. Pain, 18: 216–233.

Christensen, K., Jensen, E.M., and Noer, I. (1982) The reflex sympathetic dystrophy syndrome: response to treatment with systemic corticosteroids. Acta Chir. Scand., 148: 653–655.

Davis, K.D., Treede, R.D., Raja, S.N., Meyer, R.A., and Campbell, J.N. (1991) Topical application of clonidine relieves hyperalgesia in patients with sympathetically maintained pain. Pain, 47: 309–317.

Dejgard, A., Petersen, P., and Kastrup, J. (1988) Mexilitine for treatment of chronic painful diabetic neuropathy. Lancet, 1: 9–11.

Devulder, J., De Colvenaer, L., Rolly, G., Caemaert, J., Calliauw, L., and Martens, F. (1990) Spinal cord stimulation in chronic pain therapy. Clin. J. Pain., 6: 51–56.

Ebel, H., Balogh, A., and Klug, N. (2000) Augmentative treatment of chronic deafferentation pain syndromes after peripheral nerve lesions. Minim. Invasive Neurosurg., 43: 44–50.

Evans, J.A. (1946) Reflex sympathetic dystrophy. Surg. Gynecol. Obstet., 82: 36–43.

Farah, B.A. (1993) Ketorolax in reflex sympathetic dystrophy. Clin. Neuropharmacol., 16: 88–89.

Galer, B.S., Bruehl, S., and Harden, R.N. (1998) IASP diagnostic criteria for complex regional pain syndrome: a preliminary empirical validation study. Clin. J. Pain, 14: 48–54.

Gallagher, R.M. (1998a) Treating depression in patients with co-morbid pain: Part I. Dir. Psychiatry, 18: 81–97.

Gallagher, R.M. (1998b) Treating depression in patients with co-morbid pain: Part II. Dir. Psychiatry, 18: 149–171.

Goris, R.J.A., Dongen, L.M., and Winters, H.A. (1987) Are toxic oxygen radicals involved in the pathogenesis of reflex sympathetic dystrophy?. Free Radic. Res. Commun., 3: 13–18.

Gracely, R.H., Lynch, S.A., and Bennett, G.J. (1992) Painful neuropathy: altered central processing maintained dynamically by peripheral input. Pain, 51(2): 175–194.

Gulevich, S., Conwell, T., Lane, J., Lockwood, B., Schwettmann, R.S., Rosenberg, N., and Goldman, L.B. (1997) Stress infrared thermography is useful in the diagnosis of complex regional pain syndrome, type I (formerly reflex sympathetic dystrophy). Clin. J. Pain, 13(1): 50–59.

Harden, R.N. (2000) A clinical approach to complex regional pain syndrome. Clin. J. Pain, 16(2): S26–S32.

Harden, R.N., Bruehl, S., Galer, B.S., Saltz, S., Bertram, M., Backonja, M., Gayles, R., Rudin, N., Bhugra, M.K., Stanton-Hicks, M. (1999) Complex regional pain syndrome: are the IASP diagnostic criteria valid and sufficiently comprehensive? Pain, 83: 211–219.

Hassenbusch, S., Stanton-Hicks, M., and Covington, E.C. (1995) Spinal cord stimulation versus spinal infusion for low back and leg pain. Acta Neurochir., 64: 109–115.

Holsheimer, J. (1997) Effectiveness of spinal cord stimulation in the management of chronic pain: analysis of technical drawbacks and solutions. Neurosurgery 40(5): 990–996; discussions 996–999.

Holsheimer, J. and Wesselink, W.A. (1997) Optimum electrode geometry for spinal cord stimulation: the narrow bipole and tripole. Med. Biol. Eng. Comput., 35(5): 493–997.

Holsheimer, J., Struijk, J.J., and Tas, N.R. (1995) Effects of electrode geometry and combination on nerve fibre selectivity in spinal cord stimulation. Med. Biol. Eng. Comput., 33(5): 676–682.

Iadarola, M.J., Max, M.B., and Berman, K.F. (1995) Unilateral decrease in thalamic activity observed with positron emission tomography in patients with chronic neuropathic pain. Pain, 63: 55–64.

Kemler, M.A. and Furnee, C.A. (2002) Economic evaluation of spinal cord stimulation for chronic reflex sympathetic dystrophy. Neurology, 59(8): 1203–1209.

Kemler, M.A., Bardendse, G.A., Van Kleef, M., Van Den Wildenberg, A.J.M., and Weber, W.E.J. (1999) Electrical spinal cord stimulation in reflex sympathetic dystrophy: retrospective analysis of 23 patients. J. Neurosurg. (Spine. 1), 90: 79–83.

Kemler, M.A., Barendse, G.A., Van Kleef, M., De Vet, H.C., Rijks, C.P., Furnee, C.A., and van den Wildenberg, F.A. (2000) Spinal cord stimulation in patients with chronic reflex sympathetic dystrophy. NEJM, 343: 618–624.

Kim, S.H. and Chung, J.M. (1992) An experimental model for peripheral mononeuropathy produced by segmental spinal nerve ligation in the rat. Pain, 50(3): 355–363.

Kingery, W.S. (1997) A critical review of controlled clinical trials for peripheral neuropathic pain and complex regional pain syndromes. Pain, 73: 123–139.

Kopf, A. (2000) Novel drugs for neuropathic pain. Curr. Opin. Anaesthesiol., 13(5): 577–583.

Kumar, K., Toth, C., Nath, R., and Lang, P. (1998) Epidural spinal cord stimulation for treatment of chronic pain-some predictors of success: a 15 year experience. Surg. Neurol., 50: 110–120.

Kumar, K., Malik, S., and Demeria, D. (2002) Treatment of chronic pain with spinal cord stimulation versus alternative therapies: cost-effective analysis. Neurosurgery, 31(1): 106–116.

Law, J.D. (1983) Spinal stimulation: statistical superiority of monophasic stimulation of narrowly separated, longitudinal bipoles having rostral cathodes. Appl. Neurophysiol., 46: 129–137.

Lee, G.W. and Weeks, P.M. (1995) The role of bone scintigraphy in diagnosing reflex sympathetic dystrophy. J. Hand Surg., 20: 458–463.

Lindblum, U. (1994) Analysis of abnormal touch, pain and temperature sensation in patients. In: J. Boivie, P. Hansson, and U. Lindblom. (Eds.), *Touch, Temperature and Pain in Health and Disease: Mechanisms and Assessments* (pp. 63–84). IASP Press, Seattle.

Lynch, M.E. (1992) Psychological aspects of reflex sympathetic dystrophy: a review of the adult and paediatric literature. Pain, 49(3): 337–347.

Maleki, J., LeBel, A.A., Bennett, G.J., and Schwartzman, R.J. (2000) Patterns of spread in complex regional pain syndrome, type I (reflex sympathetic dystrophy). Pain, 88(3): 259–266.

Max, M.B., Kishore-Kumar, R., Schafer, S.C., Meister, B., Gracely, R.H., Smoller, B., and Dubner, R. (1991) Efficacy of desipramine in painful diabetic neuropathy: a placebo-controlled trial. Pain, 45: 69–73.

Mellick, G.A. and Mellick, L.B. (1995) Gabapentin in the management of reflex sympathetic dystrophy. J. Pain Sympt. Manage., 10: 265–266.

Merskey, H. and Bogduk, N. (Eds.) (1994) *Classification of Chronic Pain: Descriptions of Chronic Pain Syndromes and Definitions of Pain Terms,* 2nd edition, IASP Press, Seattle.

Mitchell, S.W., Morehouse, G.R., and Keen, W.W. (1864) *Gunshot Wounds and Other Injuries of Nerves*. Lippincott, Philadelphia.

Nicholson, B. (2000) Gabapentin use in neuropathic pain syndromes. Acta Neurol. Scand., 101(6): 359–371.

Oakley, J. and Weiner, R.L. (1999) Spinal cord stimulation for complex regional pain syndrome: A prospective study of 19 patients at 2 centers. Neuromodulation, 2: 47–50.

Ochoa, J.L. (1994) Pain mechanisms in neuropathy. Curr. Opin. Neurol., 7: 407–414.

Ochoa, J.L. (1999) Truths, errors, and lies around 'reflex sympathetic dystrophy' and 'complex regional pain syndrome'. J. Neurol., 246(10): 875–899.

Ochoa, J.L. and Verdugo, R.L. (1995) Reflex sympathetic dystrophy. A common clinical avenue for somatoform expression. Neurol. Clin., 13(2): 351–363.

Oerlemans, H.M., Oostendorp, R.A., de Boo, T., Perez, R.S., and Goris, R.J. (1999) Signs and symptoms in complex regional pain syndrome type I/reflex sympathetic dystrophy: judgement of the physician versus objective measurement. Clin. J. Pain., 15(3): 224–232.

Oyen, W.J., Arntz, I., Claessens, R.M., Van der Meer, J.W., Corstens, F.H., and Goris, R.J. (1993) Reflex sympathetic dystrophy of the hand: an excessive inflammatory response?. Pain, 55: 151–157.

Portenoy, R.K., Foley, K.M., and Inturrisi, C.E. (1990) The nature of opioid responsiveness and its implications for neuropathic pain: a new hypothesis derived from studies of opioid infusions. Pain, 43: 273–286.

Raj, P., Chado, H., Angst, M., Heavner, J., Dotson, R., Brandstater, M., Johnson, B., Parris, W., Finch, P., Shahani, B., Dhand, U., Mekhail, N., Daoud, E., Hendler, N., Somerville, J., Wallace, M., Panchal, S., Glusman, S., Jay, G., Palliyath, S., Longton, W., and Irving, G. (2001) Painless electrodiagnostic current perception threshold and pain tolerance threshold values in CRPS subjects and healthy controls: a multicenter study. Pain Pract., 1(1): 53–60.

Riedl, B., Beckmann, T., Neundorfer, B., Handwerker, H., and Birklein, F. (2001) Autonomic failure after stroke – is it indicative for pathophysiology of complex regional pain syndrome?. Acta Neurol. Scand., 103: 27–34.

Robaina, F.J., Rodrigez, J.L., de Vera, J.A., and Martin, M.A. (1989a) Transcutaneous electrical nerve stimulation and spinal cord stimulation for pain relief in reflex sympathetic dystrophy. Stereotact. Funct. Neurosurg., 52: 53–62.

Robaina, F.J., Dominguez, M.D., Diaz, M., Rodriguez, J.L., and de Vera, J.A. (1989b) Spinal cord stimulation for relief of chronic pain in vasospastic disorder of the upper limbs. Neurosurgery, 24: 63–67.

Sanchez-Ledesma, M.J., Garcia-March, G., Diaz-Cascajo, P., Gomez-Moreta, J., and Broseta, J. (1989) SCS in de-afferentation pain. Stereotact. Funct. Neurosurg., 53: 40–45.

Sandner-Kiesling, A., Seitlinger, G., Dorn, C., Koch, H., and Schwarz, G. (2002) Lamotrigine monotherapy for control of neuralgia after nerve section. Acta Anaesthesiol. Scand., 46(10): 1261–1264.

Sandroni, P., Low, P.A., Ferrer, T., Opfer-Gehrking, T.L., Willner, C.L., and Wilson, P.R. (1998) Complex regional pain syndrome I (CRPS I): prospective study and laboratory evaluation. Clin. J. Pain, 14: 282–289.

Schmelz, M., Schmidt, R., Forster, C., Handweker, H.O., Torebjork, H.E. (1996) Mechanoheat-insensitive chemonociceptors in human skin. In: Abstracts: 8th World Congress on Pain. IASP Press, Seattle, p. 12.

Schmidt, R.F., Schaible, H.G., Meßlinger, K., Heppelmann, B., Hanesch, U. Pawlak M. (1994) Silent and active nociceptors: Structure, functions, and clinical implications. In: G. Gebhart, G, et al. (Eds.), Proceedings of the 7th World Congress on Pain. IASP Press, Seattle, pp. 213–250.

Schott, G.D. (1999) Pain and the sympathetic nervous system. In: C.J. Mathias and R. Bannister (Eds.), *Autonomic Failure* 4th Ed. (pp. 520–526). Oxford University Press, Oxford.

Schurmann, M., Gradl, G., Zaspel, J., Kayser, M., Lohr, P., and Andress, H.J. (2000) Peripheral sympathetic function as a predictor of complex regional pain syndrome type I (CRPS I) in patients with radial fracture. Auton. Neurosci., 86: 127–234.

Schwartzman, R.J. and Kerrigan, J. (1990) The movement disorder of reflex sympathetic dystrophy. Neurology, 40: 57–61.

Seltzer, Z., Dubner, R., and Shire, Y. (1990) A novel behavioral model of neuropathic pain disorders produced in rats by partial sciatic nerve injury. Pain, 43(2): 205–218.

Shealy, S., Mortimer, J.T., and Reswick, J.B. (1967) Electrical inhibition of pain by stimulation of the dorsal columns. Anesthesia Analg., 46: 489–491.

Stanton-Hicks, M.D., Burton, A.W., Bruehl, S.P., Carr, D.B., Harden, R.N., Hassenbusch, S.J., Lubenow, T.R., Oakley, J.C., Racz, G.B., Raj, P., Rauck, R.L., Rezai, A.R. (2002) An updated interdisciplinary clinical pathway for CRPS: report of an expert panel. Pain Pract., 2(1): 1–16.

Tahmoush, A.J., Schwartzman, R.J., Hopp, J.L., and Grothusen, J.R. (2000) Quantitative sensory studies in complex regional pain syndrome type I/RSD. Clin. J. Pain., 16(4): 340–344.

Tasker, R. (1990) Reflex sympathetic dystrophy – neurosurgical approaches. In: W. Stanton-Hicks, W. Janig, and R. Boas (Eds.), *Reflex Sympathetic Dystrophy* (pp. 125–134). Kluwer Academic Publishers, Boston.

Thimineur, M., Sood, P., Kravitz, E., Gudin, J., and Kitaj, M. (1998) Central nervous system abnormalities in complex regional pain syndrome (CRPS): clinical and quantitative evidence of medullary dysfunction. Clin. J. Pain, 14: 256–267.

Turner, J., Deyo, R.A., Loeser, J.D., Von Korff, M., and Fordyce, W.E. (1994) The importance of placebo effects in pain treatment and research. JAMA, 271(20): 1609–1614.

Van der Laan, L., Kapitein, P.J.C., Oyen, W.J.G., Verhofstad, A.A., Hendriks, T., and Goris, R.J. (1997a)

A novel animal model to evaluate oxygen derived free radical damage in soft tissue. Free Rad. Res., 4: 363–372.

Van der Laan, L., Oyen, W.J.G., Verhofstad, A.A.J., Tan, E.C., ter Laak, H.J., Gabreels-Festen, A., Hendriks, T., and Goris, R.J. (1997b) Soft tissue repair capacity after oxygen derived free radical induced damage in one hindlimb of the rat. J. Surg. Res., 72: 60–69.

Van der Laan, L., ter Laak, H.J., Gabreels-Festen, A., Gabreels, F., and Goris, R.J.A. (1998) Complex regional pain syndrome type I (RSD): pathology of skeletal muscle and peripheral nerve. Neurology, 51: 20–25.

Veldman, P.H., Reynen, H.M., Arntz, I.E., and Goris, R.J. (1993) Signs and symptoms of reflex sympathetic dystrophy: prospective study of 829 patients. Lancet, 342: 1012–1016.

Verdugo, R.J. and Ochoa, J.L. (1993) Use and misuse of conventional electrodiagnostic, quantitative sensory testing, thermography and nerve blocks in the evaluation of painful neuropathic syndromes. Muscle Nerve, 16: 1056–1062.

Wallace, M.S., Rowbotham, M.C., and Katz, N.P. (2002) A randomized, double-blind, placebo-controlled trial of a glycine antagonist in neuropathic pain. Neurology, 59(11): 1694–1700.

Wasner, G., Schattschneider, K., Heckmann, K., Maier, C., and Baron, R. (2001) Vascular abnormalities in reflex sympathetic dystrophy (CRPS I): mechanisms and diagnostic value. Brain, 124: 587–599.

Watson, C.P., Evans, R.J., Reed, K., Merskey, H., Goldsmith, L., and Warsh, J. (1982) Amitriptyline vs. placebo in postherpetic neuralgia. Neurology, 32: 671–673.

Electrical Stimulation and the Relief of Pain
Pain Research and Clinical Management, Vol. 15
Edited by Brian A. Simpson

CHAPTER 9

Spinal cord stimulation in peripheral vascular disease

Geert H. Spincemaille*

Department of Neurosurgery, University Hospital Maastricht, P. Debyelaan 25,
6202 AZ Maastricht, The Netherlands

Abstract

Spinal cord stimulation (SCS) is used in atherosclerosis, particularly critical limb ischaemia (CLI), and in vasospastic conditions including Raynaud's, Buerger's and frostbite. CLI is the most common vascular indication for SCS. Much less information is available on vasospastic disease; only small series are published, indicating good results in selected cases. The primary goal of SCS in all these indications is pain relief and if possible limb saving. Expertise in microcirculatory diagnostic workup including transcutaneous oxygen tension measurement ($TcpO_2$), laser Doppler and/or capillary microscopy is required. Trial stimulation, which is almost an out-patient procedure, is an accepted procedure to further select the responders to SCS. It should be used in all patients who fulfil the inclusion criteria for the different vascular indications. The evaluation of trial stimulation must be based on both pain reduction and a change in the microcirculation. The results of SCS in CLI indicate that in a patient group selected according to microcirculatory criteria a positive response may be expected in 75–80% of the patients treated. Patients with CLI have negative characteristics regarding survival (mean age 71 years, mortality 50% within 5 years) and have multi-organ disease (cardiac, pulmonary, diabetes). Patients with primary Raynaud's phenomenon/disease are generally younger and otherwise healthy; the success rate seems to be around 50% but there are no prospective randomised studies available. Even less data are available on Buerger's disease and frostbite but SCS may also have a role in these conditions. SCS is usually used as a last resort. Lack of information on the possibilities of SCS is responsible for non-referral of eligible patients. Evaluation of patients implanted with SCS demands long-term follow-up for assessment of pain relief, use of medication, quality of life, microcirculatory changes and technical assessment of the hardware implanted.

Keywords: Critical limb ischaemia; Ischaemic pain; Microcirculation; Limb salvage; Vasospastic disease; Raynaud's; Buerger's; Frostbite; Spinal cord stimulation

1. Atherosclerosis and critical limb ischaemia

1.1. Introduction

The second European consensus document on chronic critical leg ischaemia defines critical limb ischaemia (CLI) in non-diabetic patients as the presence of rest pain or tissue necrosis (ulceration or gangrene; Fig. 1) with an ankle systolic pressure of 50 mmHg or less, or a toe pressure of 30 mmHg or less (European Working Group, 1992). Normal oxidative processes of cells need an oxygen supply. When blood flow to a tissue drops below the level needed for normal metabolic function, anaerobic

---

*Correspondence to: Dr. G.H. Spincemaille, Department of Neurosurgery, University Hospital Maastricht, P. Debyelaan 25, 6202 AZ Maastricht, The Netherlands. Phone: + 31-43-3874041; Fax: + 31-43-3876038; E-mail: gspi@snch.azm.nl or gspi@village.uunet.be

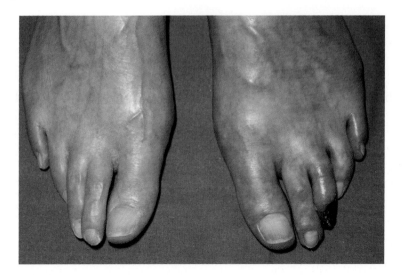

Fig. 1. The typical appearance of ischaemic changes in the feet secondary to proximal arterial atherosclerotic obstruction. The left third toe is already gangrenous. The pain which is present at rest can be extremely severe and is greatly exacerbated by exercise.

metabolism temporarily tries to compensate. This phenomenon is known as ischaemia. It becomes critical when blood flow drops to a level where cell survival is in danger. Cell death results in tissue necrosis. The best known symptom in the early stages of ischaemia is intermittent pain (vascular claudication).

CLI as defined is equivalent to Fontaine stages III and IV plus the blood pressure criteria. None of the criteria of the European consensus has been evaluated for its prognostic value in predicting outcome of the threatened limb. Thompson and Jacobs both found in their series that 50% of the patients classified as severely ischaemic fulfilled the criteria of the consensus document. The other 50% had an ankle systolic pressure greater than 50 mmHg and an outcome similar to those with an ankle systolic pressure less than 50 mmHg (Jacobs et al., 1988; Thompson et al., 1993). It is, however, agreed that patients with ulcers greater than 3 cm^2 in area have a much lower limb salvage rate (Broseta et al., 1986; Tallis et al., 1992). Wolfe and Wyatt (1997) presented an overview of the different definitions of CLI. Their suggestion to look for high- and low-risk patients is a step in the right direction. However, they do not mention the microcirculatory measurements. Carter and Bunt

and Holloway, proposed modified haemodynamic definitions for critical and subcritical ischaemia, which include measurements of pressures and indices of microcirculation (Bunt and Holloway, 1996; Carter, 1997).

The debate which might lead to a better classification of patients with CLI belongs to the vascular surgeons. An important part of the discussion will certainly be the value of microcirculatory measurements. There are different ways to assess blood flow and there is no consensus on the best prognostic indicator. This means that further studies are needed to find out which method has the best prognostic value and can discriminate responders (limb salvage) from non-responders. Ubbink suggests that a combination of toe blood pressure and transcutaneous oxygen tension (TcpO$_2$), using cut-off values of 38 mmHg for toe blood pressure and 35 mmHg for TcpO$_2$ in the supine position, has a better prognostic value (Ubbink et al., 2000). Gersbach uses the difference between sitting and supine TcpO$_2$ as a better predictor of outcome (Gersbach et al., 1997). Fiume reported that pain relief was obtained only in patients who showed an improved TcpO$_2$ during trial stimulation (Fiume et al., 1989), an observation also made by Jacobs

(Jacobs et al., 1988). Petrakis suggested that a trial period of two weeks should be considered before final implantation, because those who show a significant increase in $TcpO_2$ in that period have a better outcome (Petrakis and Sciacca, 1999).

The criteria of the second European consensus document concern patients with 'chronic' CLI. This means a constant pain persisting for, at least, more than 2 weeks as used in the Dutch trial (Klomp et al., 1999–see Section 1.5). In another study, by Kumar et al. (1997), only those patients treated conservatively for 6 months were included; this represents a different population (Kumar et al., 1997). With regard to limb survival of patients with CLI, it is obvious that the first two to three months after the diagnosis of CLI are very important because a large number of patients undergo amputation within this period.

Recently, in a consensus document on the definition of CLI, some recommendations have been proposed both for the definition and for the trials on CLI. It is clear from this document that there is no real consensus on inclusion criteria and investigation of patients at risk of an amputation within months of diagnosis of CLI (Chronic CLI, 2000).

1.2. Chronic pain

Ischaemic pain, the main symptom in CLI, is probably a combination of nociceptive and neuropathic pain. The simple clinical evidence that ischaemic pain is, at least partly, nociceptive is the positive effect of opiate drugs. Since the gate theory of Melzack and Wall (1965; and see also Noordenbos, 1959) inspired the introduction of spinal cord stimulation (SCS) (Shealy et al., 1967) it has become clear that SCS is effective against neuropathic, rather than nociceptive, pain. This theory was later expanded to include the involvement of supraspinal centres in the inhibition of hyperactivity in the dorsal horn of the spinal cord (Melzack, 1999). One may consider that, particularly in the presence of skin lesions, the peripheral nerves and their endings may degenerate following

ischaemia, and therefore ischaemic pain may be partially due to neuropathy. Moreover, a large number of patients with CLI also have diabetes; peripheral neuropathy is a common feature of diabetes. The effect of SCS on ischaemic pain is explained better if a combination of nociceptive and neuropathic pain is accepted as the underlying pathology (Linderoth et al., 1991). Evidence for the effect of SCS on pain due to diabetic neuropathy comes mainly from a single publication (Tesfaye et al., 1996). The relative contribution of various possible factors to the analgesic effect of SCS in PVD, such as antinociception, modulation of neuropathic pain, a primary anti-ischaemic effect, a secondary anti-ischaemic effect (secondary to pain relief), is still not fully understood (Franzetti et al., 1989; Petrakis and Sciacca, 2000) (see also Chapter 11).

1.3. Effects of SCS on ischaemia

Cook was the first to notice (in the early 1970s) that, in patients with a neurological disorder such as the spinal cord lesions or multiple sclerosis, SCS resulted in autonomic changes with warming of the cold lower extremities. He assumed that a regional increase in blood flow might be the underlying mechanism. Three years later he published a small study of nine patients with varying degrees of limb ischaemia persisting after failure of sympathectomy or bypass procedures. He observed a striking degree of pain relief, and although infarcted tissue was not restored, wound-healing was promoted after SCS. He concluded: "*It is indeed probable that persistent spinal cord stimulation will avert the need for amputation in some patients. It certainly can be considered as another alternative before progression to amputation after failure of all other known therapeutic modalities*" (Cook et al., 1976). Dooley observed the same phenomenon of increased peripheral blood flow in patients with SCS for central nervous system disorders such as multiple sclerosis, olivopontocerebellar atrophy, amyotrophic lateral sclerosis and Friedreich's ataxia (Dooley, 1977). To elucidate the phenomenon he used transcutaneous electrical nerve stimulation (TENS) in a patient with a cervical radiculitis. Electrodes were placed over the right side of the cervical spine. A one-channel impedance plethysmograph was connected to the right finger. Electrostimulation for $2\frac{1}{2}$ minutes resulted in a fall in impedance that was interpreted as being equivalent to a 154% increase in blood flow to the finger. He concluded: "*Electrostimulation over the posterior spinal roots and the spinal cord, although not new, has not been used extensively for the treatment of patients with arterial disease. Electrostimulation of the nervous system is not designed to replace standard therapeutic measures of treatment of patients with vascular disease, but to supplement them*" (Dooley and Kasprak, 1976).

Ghajar and Miles (1998) found that with SCS there was an increase in capillary blood flow and skin temperature in the lower extremities if the stimulating electrode was placed below the vertebral level T10, preferably at T12.

Tallis suggested three possible mechanisms whereby SCS could influence blood flow: (1.) Conventional pain relief might reverse the sympathetic vasoconstriction that occurs in response to pain. The observation that adequate pain relief correlates with improved capillary flow would be in accordance with this. (2.) SCS induces an electrical sympathetic paralysis (with or without concomitant stimulation of cholinergic vasodilators). (3.) The antidromic stimulation of dorsal root afferents causing sustained vasodilatation has been demonstrated both in man and in animals (Tallis et al., 1992). For a detailed discussion of mechanisms, the reader is referred to Chapter 11.

1.4. Case reports and cohort studies

In the second half of the 1980s and the beginning of the 1990s, epidural SCS was seen as an alternative treatment for patients with peripheral arterial occlusive disease no longer eligible for vascular reconstruction. SCS relieved the pain resulting in improved mobilisation which in turn enhanced blood flow, leading to ulcer healing (Groth, 1985; Broggi et al., 1987; Bracale et al., 1989; Meglio et al., 1989; Kasprzak and Raithel, 1994; Rickman et al., 1994).

Inclusion criteria were frequently loosely defined and many reports contained highly inhomogeneous groups of patients (arteriosclerosis, vasospastic disease and others) at different stages of the disease. The target population was composed of patients with severe limb ischaemia. The belief that an amputation could be avoided in at least in 40–50% of the patients motivated an increasing number of physicians to use the technique. The positive sentiment towards the therapy was further driven by the publication of Augustinsson, who stated that, indeed, almost all patients (90%) conservatively treated underwent amputation, but with SCS this was only 34% (Augustinsson et al., 1985). Some reports mentioned a near normalisation of the blood flow in larger vessels proven by a normalisation of Doppler ankle pressure or even Doppler waves. This was further emphasised by data revealing a significant increase in microcirculatory parameters (Jacobs et al., 1990). Vascular surgeons produced a consensus document, the main goal of which was to harmonise the patient population undergoing treatment. Macrocirculatory criteria were added to the classical Fontaine grading (Second European Consensus Document on Critical Limb Ischaemia, 1992). If SCS could avoid limb amputation in a substantial proportion of the patients with CLI, this would be a major therapeutic advance. The mortality rate of patients with CLI was already 45–75% within 5 years (Dormandy and Thomas, 1988; Bertele et al., 1999).

Apart from the clinical criteria described in the European Consensus Document, there was no consensus on the measurement of blood flow. In a leading article Jacobs and Jörning stated: "*Systolic ankle/arm pressure measurements at rest and after treadmill exercise are generally accepted as the best non-invasive method to document arterial obstruction of lower extremities . . . . It should be emphasised, however, that in patients with Fontaine stage III and IV not only is the macrocirculation inadequate but, especially in patients with ulcerations and gangrene, the microcirculation is also threatened. Tissue oxygen pressure measurement, laser Doppler flowmetry and isotope clearance techniques can be performed to study cutaneous blood flow. Intravital skin capillary microscopy is a direct and non-invasive method of studying the morphological pattern of skin microcirculation and allows the measurement of red blood cell velocity in the skin capillaries, which specifically reflects nutritional blood flow"* (Jacobs and Jörning, 1998).

1.5. Randomised studies on CLI and SCS

The first randomised study was performed in Belgium, on 38 patients with ischaemic rest pain, and concluded that there was no statistically significant difference regarding amputation. SCS did, however, give pain relief, increase the ability to walk and improved the quality of life (Suy et al., 1994).

Jivegard reported a randomised trial on the effect of SCS in 51 patients with inoperable severe lower limb ischaemia. The difference in amputation-free survival at 18 months between the SCS group and the control group was 17% in favour of SCS (62% vs. 45%; Jivegard et al., 1995).

Claeys and Horsch (1996) conducted a randomised study on 86 patients. Forty-five patients received a spinal cord stimulator and 41 had optimal medical treatment. Limb survival at 1 year follow up was 68% for patients treated with SCS and 65% for optimal medical treatment.

The Dutch randomised study recruited 120 patients and was published in 1999. Forty (67%) of 60 patients in the SCS group and 41 (68%) of 60 patients in the 'standard treatment' group were alive at the end of the study. There were 25 major amputations in the SCS group and 29 in the control group ($P = 0.47$). Limb survival after 2 years was 60% in the SCS group and 46% in the conservatively treated patients. The hazard ratio for survival at 2 years without major amputation in the

SCS group, compared with the standard group, was 0.96 (95% confidence limits $= 0.61–1.51$) (Klomp et al., 1995, 1999; Ubbink et al., 1999a).

These studies therefore did not generally confirm an overall limb saving effect of SCS.

1.6. Rationale for a different selection procedure

Microcirculatory investigation seems the target for better selection as it focuses on the distal blood flow and nutritional distribution. Experimental data suggest that SCS may have a beneficial effect upon the microcirculation in certain patients and that $TcpO_2$ might be able to distinguish responders from non-responders. Galley and colleagues (1992) found a significant increase in $TcpO_2$ (13.5–24 mmHg, $P < 0.001$) following 9 ± 4 days of SCS. The $TcpO_2$ (sitting) changed from 24.4 ± 22 (before stimulation) to 50.4 ± 18 (after stimulation). The gradient between sitting and supine $TcpO_2$ ($\Delta TcpO_2$) increased from 22.4 ± 22 (prestimulation) to 41.4 ± 18 (poststimulation). Horsch and Claeys (1994) reported on 177 patients in Fontaine stages III ($n = 114$) and IV ($n = 63$). A SCS system was implanted in 139 patients who had excellent pain relief after trial stimulation. The mean supine $TcpO_2$ was 24 mmHg in stage III and 16 mmHg in stage IV patients. During treatment, $TcpO_2$ increased to 48 and 37 mmHg respectively. Gersbach started with a trial period of SCS for one week irrespective of the initial microcirculatory data. The baseline-supine $TcpO_2$ was 19.5 ± 15 mmHg and baseline-sitting $TcpO_2$ was 42 ± 15 mmHg ($\Delta TcpO_2 = 23$ mmHg). Retrospective analysis of the different tests revealed that the supine–sitting $TcpO_2$ gradient was the strongest predictor of limb salvage. If the gradient was greater than 15 mmHg, the limb salvage rate was as high as 88%. All patients with a sitting $TcpO_2$ less than 20 mmHg underwent amputation of the ischaemic limb (Gersbach et al., 1997). Kumar treated patients only if they had undergone a 6-month period of conservative therapy for pain relief. Excellent ($>75\%$) pain relief and a substantial increase in $TcpO_2$ after trial stimulation showed a significant positive correlation with long-term success. Patients with a TcpO$_2$ of less than 10 mmHg following stimulation tended to undergo an amputation within the first 3 months. Improvement in pain control combined with an increase in TcpO$_2$ greater than 10 mmHg was a significant early predictor of long-term success. The best results were seen in patients with severe claudication and rest pain without trophic changes in the foot (Kumar et al., 1997).

Claeys and Horsch (1996) compared SCS with optimal medical treatment. Patients started with one week of prostaglandinE$_1$ treatment (PGE$_1$), after which they were randomised between SCS + PGE$_1$ and PGE$_1$ alone. The initial mean value of TcpO$_2$ was 10 mmHg (SCS group) versus 11 mmHg. At 12 months the TcpO$_2$ was 21 mmHg versus 11.4, respectively ($P < 0.0001$). The outcome in patients with an initial TcpO$_2$ less than 10 mmHg was significantly worse than for those with a TcpO$_2$ greater than 10 mmHg. Ubbink categorised patients according the status of their baseline skin microcirculation as 'good' (TcpO$_2$ above 30 mmHg), 'intermediate' (TcpO$_2$ between 10 and 30 mmHg) and 'poor' (TcpO$_2$ below 10 mmHg). Patients with a poor skin perfusion had a high amputation rate of 80% for SCS and 71% for standard treatment. Patients with a good microcirculation had a good outcome irrespective of the treatment given. The amputation rate in patients with an intermediate TcpO$_2$ value and treated with SCS was half that in the standard group (24 vs. 48%) (Ubbink et al., 1999a; Fig. 2). This categorisation had a predictive value regarding limb salvage (Ubbink et al., 1999b).

1.7. Algorithm design

Based on this rationale, patients with a baseline TcpO$_2$ (supine and sitting) below 10 or above 30 mmHg (Claeys and Horsch, 1996; Ubbink et al., 1999a,b) or a ΔTcpO$_2$ below 15 mmHg (Galley et al., 1992; Gersbach et al., 1997) are not candidates for SCS. Patients with a TcpO$_2$ between 10 and 30 mmHg or with a ΔTcpO$_2$

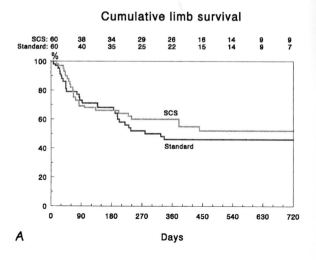

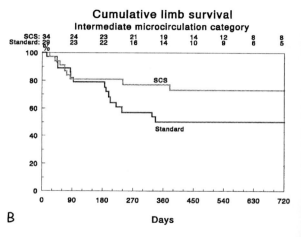

Fig. 2. (A) Overall cumulative limb survival (Kaplan–Meier) of patients receiving standard treatment and those receiving additional SCS. The numbers indicate the patients at risk at the different follow-up times. (B) Cumulative limb survival (Kaplan–Meier) of patients in the intermediate microcirculatory category (From Ubbink et al., 1999a).

above 15 mmHg are eligible and can proceed to a period of trial stimulation. At the end of that period pain relief and changes in TcpO$_2$ are recorded. If pain relief is below 50%, adjustment of medication is allowed to enhance the pain relief. If pain relief is above 50% and the change in TcpO$_2$ more than 15 mmHg full implantation is considered. If no positive response is obtained, SCS is not indicated and symptomatic treatment is

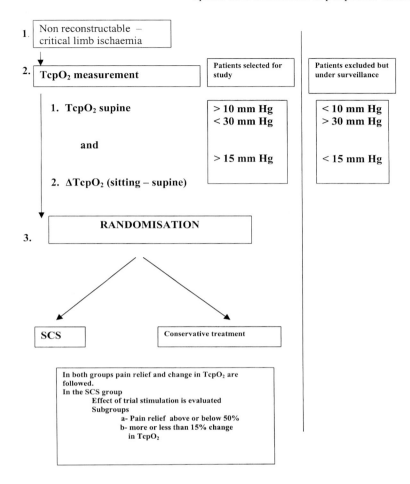

Fig. 3. Algorithm for patient selection for SCS in CLI.

given, consisting of analgesics, vasoactive drugs and adequate care of foot ulcers (Fig. 3).

1.8. Remaining problems

1.8.1. Pain reduction

Pain reduction after trial stimulation was repeatedly suggested to correlate with limb salvage (Horsch and Claeys, 1994; Kumar et al., 1997). In the Dutch randomised study, trial stimulation was not performed; a retrospective analysis examined the limb salvage at 6 months and 1 year in all patients who had good or excellent pain relief, with or without SCS, scored at 1-month follow-up.

The results in both treatment groups were comparable. Patients with a bad response with regard to pain relief had significantly lower limb salvage rates in both treatment groups, suggesting that pain relief was related to limb salvage, irrespective of how the pain relief was obtained. One of the effects of pain relief is certainly an enhanced mobility, which may be responsible for a secondary improvement in blood flow (Klomp et al., 1999).

1.8.2. Hypertension

Jivegard concluded from his results that hypertension was a prognostic factor in relation to limb survival (Jivegard et al., 1995). This has not been confirmed by others and as such remains questionable.

2. Primary and secondary Raynaud's phenomena

2.1. Primary Raynaud's phenomenon and Raynaud's disease

Raynaud's phenomenon is characterised by transient attacks of pallor, cyanosis and numbness of the fingers and sometimes palms followed by vasodilatation which results in swelling. It is usually precipitated by cold, but can also be precipitated by emotion in susceptible individuals. The lower extremities are less commonly affected. Most cases are benign and are not seen by a physician. As many as 15% of healthy adolescents may be affected. This phenomenon is different from the normal peripheral vasoconstriction that occurs on exposure to cold. Diagnosis is based on the bilateral occurrence of characteristic changes in the presence of normal distal pulses, the absence of trophic skin lesions and the absence of any causative underlying disease. Although symptoms are usually benign, severe and chronic cases can cause considerable pain and even, in the later stages, ulcerative skin lesions (Raynaud's disease).

2.2. Secondary Raynaud's phenomenon

The main conditions in which secondary Raynaud's phenomenon is seen are connective tissue disorders such as scleroderma, vasculitic and hyperviscosity syndromes, vascular occlusive disease and thoracic outlet syndrome. It can also be drug induced.

2.3. Pathophysiology

The paleness of the skin is caused by vasospasm. The subsequent cyanosis is due to a reduced blood flow and stasis in skin capillaries and veins. The last phase is a vasodilatation resulting in redness and swelling of the fingers. In Raynaud's disease vasospasm occurs within the arteriovenous shunt system of the skin. In secondary Raynaud's phenomenon vasoconstriction occurs in small arterioles, shunts, capillaries and, to some extent, in veins in the presence of diffuse vessel wall thickening. The mechanism in primary Raynaud's may be an increased sympathetic nervous system outflow or an altered sympathetic–parasympathetic balance and/or a generalised or specific hyperreactivity of the vascular smooth muscle wall. In secondary Raynaud's, decreased ability for vasodilatation, immunologically mediated vasculitis, thrombosis and haemorheological factors all play a role.

2.4. Diagnosis

Diagnosis relies mainly on the clinical history, but physical examination is important, combined with blood and urine analysis (sedimentation rate, full blood count, creatinine, cryoglobulins, antinuclear antibody, proteinuria, casts). If secondary Raynaud's is suspected, a more extensive laboratory analysis is necessary. Examination of the microcirculation by capillaroscopy and laser Doppler velocimetry may be helpful. Postocclusive reactive hyperaemia plays a role in the follow up of patients, but is too insensitive to classify patients according to the severity of the disease.

2.5. Therapy

Multiple therapies are used to treat primary Raynaud's ranging from simple explanation and reassurance, avoiding cold or medication causing vasoconstriction, through the use of vasodilators, thrombocytic aggregation inhibitors, physiotherapy and TENS, to invasive measures (stellate ganglion block, sympathectomy). In secondary Raynaud's the above can be used depending on the underlying disease with, in addition, non-steroidal anti-inflammatory drugs (NSAID), immunosuppressive drugs and plasmaphoresis. SCS is not widely used although there are several reports indicating a beneficial effect (see Section 2.6).

2.6. Review of the literature

The largest series of patients with Raynaud's treated with SCS was published by Raso. He treated 40 patients of whom 45% had excellent results and 30% a good to moderate outcome (Raso, 1989). Robaina had excellent results in 10 of 11 of the patients treated (Robaina et al., 1989). Further reports indicate an excellent effect of SCS on secondary Raynaud's phenomenon (Francaviglia et al., 1994; Kahaleh, 1995). Neuheuser described microcirculatory changes in severe Raynaud's phenomenon after SCS (Neuhauser et al., 2001).

3. Thromboangiitis obliterans (Buerger's disease)

Buerger's disease is a segmental inflammatory vasculitis that involves the small and medium-sized arteries, and veins and nerves. It is causally related to tobacco use. The diagnosis is usually made on the basis of the presence of distal arterial disease in individuals who smoke and in whom other potentially causative conditions have been excluded. The most effective treatment for Buerger's disease is cessation of smoking. Without strict adherence to tobacco avoidance, disease progression is likely and may lead to amputation. Methods to control the ischaemic pain include medication, sympathectomy, and surgical revascularization. The effect of sympathectomy is unpredictable, and the chances of a successful revascularization procedure are small because distal target vessels are often extensively diseased. Very little has been published on the effects of SCS in Buerger's disease but it does appear to be effective in controlling the pain and may improve the vascular parameters (Claeys et al., 1997; Swigris et al., 1999; Chierichetti et al., 2002).

4. Frostbite

The effects of frostbite after freezing of the extremities probably result from a standstill of the circulation for a varying period of time. If this circulatory arrest lasts for hours it may result in metabolic and structural changes in tissues and arteries. Cauchy described a new classification of frostbite based on clinical factors and on bone scans (previously validated). Four degrees of severity were defined: first degree, leading to recovery; second degree, leading to soft tissue amputation; third degree, leading to bone amputation, and fourth degree, leading to large amputation with systemic effects (Cauchy et al., 2001).

Experimental data suggest that second order sensory neurons—wide dynamic range (WDR) and high threshold (HT) neurons—show an enhanced response to cold and heat stimuli after a mild freeze injury (Khasabov et al., 2001). It is likely that they contribute to thermal hyperalgesia. The effect of SCS is primarily related to the vascular response. A search of the literature revealed no treatment data. Su and colleagues put it in the following way: "*The literature is full of various treatment protocols that allegedly are beneficial despite addressing different mechanisms. Mills described 10 different categories of medication, each addressing one of four possible mechanisms, used in the clinical treatment of frostbite injury over a 30-year period. Analysing this information is even more confusing when one realizes that there is little uniformity in animal models employed to generate these data. This is further complicated by the lack of clinical correlation with the most common experimental model—liquid nitrogen rapid freezing. Traditionally, observation and delayed amputation have been employed to manage frostbite. More recently, triple-phase bone scans have been used to distinguish between tissue that is irreversibly destined for necrosis and tissue that is at-risk for necrosis, but potentially salvageable. Early operation can be used to provide at-risk tissue with a new blood supply and preserve both function and length in the upper extremity*" (Su et al., 2000).

It is proposed that SCS would enhance recuperation, reduce pain and might result in a more peripheral level of amputation. The real effect and efficacy of SCS in frostbite is not proven; more data are required (Arregui et al., 1989). The use of trial stimulation is advocated as an adjunct to conservative treatment, during the period of observation.

5. Conclusion

As far as pain relief is concerned, SCS significantly reduces ischaemic pain and the need for pain-relieving medication. The mechanism may be complex and is not fully understood. There is a clear anti-ischaemic effect. In CLI, SCS is not, however, proven to be superior to best medical treatment in terms of limb salvage, under the selection criteria as used in the available randomised studies. As indicated, a further refining of the selection procedure seems to be the only way to target the possible responders for this therapy. If the updated selection criteria are used, we may expect to prove the effectiveness of SCS therapy in a smaller population than the one indicated by the European consensus document.. The recent European PVD Outcome Study (EPOS) gives further evidence of the importance of the microcirculatory measurements; limb salvage in a *selected group* of patients can reach 80–85% at 1 year (Amann et al., in press). The selection criterion of a sitting $TcpO_2 > 20$ mmHg seems to be the most important prognostic factor, perhaps even making trial stimulation redundant.

With regard to vasospastic diseases, anecdotal evidence is compelling but there is too little information to give clear evidence of long term success. A prospective randomised trial in patients with severe vasospastic disease is badly needed. A combined multinational effort may be the best option.

References

Amann, W., Berg, P., Gersbach, P., Gamain, J., Raphael, J.H., Ubbink, D. (2003 in press). Spinal cord stimulation in the treatment of non reconstructable, stable critical limb ischaemia. Results of European peripheral vascular disease outcome study. Eur. J. Vasc. Endovasc. Surg.

Augustinsson, L.E., Carlsson, A., Holm, J., and Jivegard, L. (1985) Epidural electrical stimulation in severe limb ischemia. Evidences of pain relief, increased blood flow and a possible limb-saving effect. Ann. Surg., 202: 104–111.

Bertele, V., Roncaglioni, M.C., Pangrazzi, J., Terzian, E., and Tognoni, E.G. (1999) Clinical outcome and its predictors in 1560 patients with critical leg ischaemia. Eur. J. Vas. Endovasc. Surg. 18: 401–410.

Bracale, G.C., Selvetella, L., and Mirabile, F. (1989) Our experience with spinal cord stimulation (SCS) in peripheral vascular disease. Pace, 12: 695–697.

Broggi, G., Servello, D., Franzini, A., Giorgi, C., Luccarelli, M., Ruberti, U., Cugnasca, M., Odero, A., Tealdi, D., and Denale, A. (1987) Spinal cord stimulation for the treatment of peripheral vascular disease. Appl. Neurophysiol., 50: 439–441.

Broseta, J., Barbera, J., de Vera, J.A., Barcia-Salorio, J.L., March, G., Gonzalez-Darder, J., Robaina, F., and Joanes, V. (1986) Spinal cord stimulation in peripheral arterial disease. A cooperative study. J. Neurosurg., 64: 71–80.

Bunt, T.J. and Holloway, G.A. (1996) TcpO₂ as an accurate predictor of therapy in limb salvage. Ann. Vasc. Surg., 10: 224.

Carter, S.A. (1997) The challenge and importance of defining critical limb ischemia. Vasc. Med., 2: 126–131.

Chronic critical limb ischaemia. (2000) In: Management of peripheral arterial disease (PAD). Transatlantic Inter-Society Consensus (TASC). Section D. Eur. J. Vasc. Endovasc. Surg. 19, Suppl A: S144–S243.

Claeys, L. and Horsch, S. (1996) Transcutaneous oxygen pressure as predictive parameter for ulcer healing in endstage vascular patients treated with spinal cord stimulation. Int. Angiology, 15: 344–349.

Cook, A.W., Oygar, A., Baggenstos, P., Pacheco, S., and Kleriga, E. (1976) Vascular disease of extremities: electrical stimulation of spinal cord and posterior roots. N.Y. State J. Med., 76: 366–378.

Dooley, D.M. (1977) Demyelinating, degenerative and vascular disease. Neurosurgery, 1: 220–224.

Dooley, D. and Kasprak, M. (1976) Modifications of blood flow to the extremities by electrical stimulation of the nervous system. South. Med. J., 69: 1309–1311.

Dormandy, J.A. and Thomas, P.R.S. (1988) What is the natural history of a critical ischaemic patient with and without his leg?. In: R.M. Greenhalgh, C.W. Jamieson, and A.N. Nicolaides, (Eds.), *Limb Salvage and Amputation for Vascular Disease* (pp. 11–26). Saunders, Philadelphia.

European Working Group on critical leg ischemia (1992) Second European consensus document on chronic critical leg ischemia. Eur. J. Vasc. Surg. 6, (Suppl A): 1–32.

Fiume, D., Palombi, M., Sciassa, V., and Tamorri, M. (1989) Spinal cord stimulation (SCS) in peripheral ischemic pain. Pace Clin. Electrophysiol., 12: 698–704.

Franzetti, I., De Nale, A., Bossi, A., Greco, M., Morricone, L., Ruggerini, M., Meazza, D., Sciolla, A., Caviezel, F., Oriani, G. (1989) Epidural spinal electrostimulatory system [ESES] in the management of diabetic foot and peripheral arteriopathies. Pacing Clin. Electrophysiol., 12: 705–708.

Galley, D., Rettori, R., Boccalon, H., Medvedowsky, A., Lefebvre, J.M., Sellier, F., Chauvreau, C., Serise, J.M., and Pieronne, A. (1992) La stimulation électrique médullaire dans les artériopathies des membres inférieurs: une étude multicentrique chez 244 patients. J. Mal. Vasc., 17: 208–213.

Gersbach, P., Hasdemir, M.G., Stevens, R.D., Nachbur, B., and Mahler, F. (1997) Discriminative microcirculatory screening in patients with refractory limb ischaemia for dorsal column stimulation. Eur. J. Vasc. Endovasc. Surg., 13: 464–471.

Ghajar, A.W. and Miles, J.B. (1998) The differential effect of the level of spinal cord stimulation on patients with advanced peripheral vascular disease in the lower limbs. Br. J. Neurosurg., 12: 402–408.

Groth, K.E. (1985) Spinal cord stimulation for the treatment of peripheral vascular disease-European Multi-center Study. In: Fields (Ed.), *Advances in Pain Research and Therapy.* Vol. 9. (pp. 861–870). New York, Raven Press.

Horsch, S. and Claeys, L. (1994) Epidural spinal cord stimulation in the treatment of severe peripheral arterial occlusive disease. Ann. Vasc. Surg., 8: 468–474.

Jacobs, M.J.H.M. and Jörning, P.J.G. (1998) Is epidural spinal cord stimulation indicated in patients with severe lower limb ischaemia?. Eur. J. Vasc. Surg., 2: 207–208.

Jacobs, M.J.H.M., Jörning, P.J.G., Joshi, S.R., Kitselaar, P.J.E.H.M., Slaaf, D.W., and Reneman, R.S. (1988) Epidural spinal cord stimulation improves microvascular blood flow in severe limb ischemia. Ann. Surg., 207: 129–133.

Jacobs, M.J., Jörning, P.J.G., Beckers, R.C.Y., Ubbink, D.T., van Kleef, M., Slaaf, D.W., and Reneman, R.S. (1990) Foot salvage and improvement of microvascular blood flow as a result of epidural spinal cord electrical stimulation. J. Vasc. Surg., 12: 354–360.

Jivegard, L.E., Augustinsson, L.E., Holm, J., Risberg, B., and Ortenwall, P. (1995) Effects of spinal cord stimulation (SCS) in patients with inoperable severe lower limb ischaemia: a prospective randomised controlled study. Eur. J. Vasc. Endovasc. Surg., 9: 421–425.

Kasprzak, O. and Raithel, D. (1994) Can spinal cord stimulation reduce the amputation rate in patients with critical limb ischemia. In: S. Horsch, and L. Claeys (Eds.), *Spinal Cord Stimulation. An Innovative Method in the Treatment of PVD* (pp. 165–169). Steinkopff, Darmstadt.

Klomp, H.M., Spincemaille, G.H., Steyerberg, E.W., Berger, M.Y., Habbema, J.D.F., and van Urk, H. (1995) Design issues of a randomised controlled clinical trial on spinal cord stimulation in critical limb ischemia. Eur. J. Vasc. Endovasc. Surg., 10: 478–485.

Klomp, H.M., Spincemaille, G.H., Steyerberg, E.W., Habbema, J.D., and van Urk, H. (1999) Efficacy of spinal cord stimulation in critical limb ischemia. Lancet, 353: 1040–1044.

Kumar, K., Toth, C., Nath, R.K., Verma, A.K., and Burgess, J.J. (1997) Improvement of limb circulation in peripheral vascular disease using epidural spinal cord stimulation: a prospective study. J. Neurosurg., 86: 662–669.

Linderoth, B., Fedorcsak, I., and Meyerson, B.A. (1991) Peripheral vasodilatation after spinal cord stimulation: animal studies of putative effector mechanisms. Neurosurgery, 28: 187–195.

Meglio, M., Cioni, B., and Rossi, G.F. (1989) Spinal cord stimulation in management of chronic pain. A 9-year experience. J. Neurosurg., 70: 519–524.

Melzack, R. (1999) From the gate to the neuromatrix. Pain, Suppl 6: S121–S126.

Melzack, R. and Wall, P.D. (1965) Pain mechanisms: a new theory. Science, 150: 971–979.

Noordenbos, W. (1959) *Pain. Problems Pertaining to the Transmission of Nerve Impulses which give rise to Pain*, Elsevier, Amsterdam.

Petrakis, I.E. and Sciacca, V. (1999) Epidural spinal cord stimulation in diabetic critical lower limb ischemia. J. Diabetes Complications, 13: 293–299.

Petrakis, I.E. and Sciacca, V. (2000) Does autonomic neuropathy influence spinal cord stimulation therapy success in diabetic patients with critical lower limb ischemia?. Surg. Neurol., 53: 182–188.

Rickman, S., Wuebbels, B.H., and Holloway, G.A. (1994) Spinal cord stimulation for relief of ischemic pain in end-stage arterial occlusive disease. J. Vasc. Nurs., 12: 14–20.

Second European consensus document on chronic critical leg ischemia. (1992) European working group on critical leg ischemia. Eur. J. Vasc. Surg. (Suppl A): 1–32.

Shealy, C.N., Mortimer, J.T., and Reswick, J.B. (1967) Electrical inhibition in pain by stimulation of the dorsal columns: Preliminary clinical report. Anesth. Analg., 46: 489–491.

Suy, R., Gybels, J., Van Damme, H., van Maele, R., and Delaporte, C. (1994) Spinal cord stimulation for ischemic rest pain. The Belgian randomised study. In: S. Horsch, and L. Claeys (Eds.), *Spinal Cord Stimulation: An Innovative Method in the Treatment of PVD* (pp. 197–202). Steinkoph-Verlag, Darmstadt.

Tallis, R., Jacobs, M., and Miles, J. (1992) Spinal cord stimulation in peripheral vascular disease (Editorial). Br. J. Neurosurg., 6: 101–105.

Tesfaye, S., Watt, J., Benbow, S.J., Pang, K.A., Miles, J., and MacFarlane, I.A. (1996) Electrical spinal cord stimulation for painful diabetic neuropathy. Lancet, 348: 1698–1701.

Thompson, M.M., Sayers, R.D., Varty, K., Reid, A., London, N.J.M., and Bell, P.R.F. (1993) Chronic critical leg ischaemia must be redefined. Eur. J. Vasc. Surg., 7: 420–426.

Ubbink, D.T., Spincemaille, G.H., Prins, M.H., Reneman, R.S., and Jacobs, M.J. (1999a) Microcirculatory investigations to determine the effect of spinal cord stimulation for critical leg ischemia: the Dutch multicenter randomized controlled trial. J. Vasc. Surg., 30: 236–244.

Ubbink, D.T., Spincemaille, G.H., Reneman, R.S., and Jacobs, M.J. (1999b) Prediction of imminent amputation in patients with non-reconstructible leg ischemia by means of microcirculatory investigations. J. Vasc. Surg., 30: 114–121.

Ubbink, D.T.h., Tulevski, I.I., de Graaff, J.C., Legemate, D.A., and Jacobs, M.J.H.M. (2000) Optimisation of the non-invasive assessment of critical limb ischaemia requiring invasive treatment. Eur. J. Vasc. Endovasc. Surg., 19: 131–137.

Wolfe, J.H.N., Wyatt, M.G. (1997) Critical and subcritical ischaemia. Eur. J. Vasc. Endovasc. Surg., 37: 578–582.

Raynaud's

Francaviglia, N., Silvestro, C., Maiello, M., Bragazzi, R., and Bernucci, C. (1994) Spinal cord stimulation for the treatment of progressive systemic sclerosis and Raynaud's syndrome. Br. J. Neurosurg., 8: 567–571.

Kahaleh, M.B. (1995) Raynaud's phenomenon and the vascular disease in scleroderma. Curr. Opin. Rheumatol., 7: 529–534.

Neuhauser, B., Perkmann, R., Klingler, P.J., Giacomuzzi, S., Kofler, A., and Fraedrich, G. (2001) Clinical and objective data on spinal cord stimulation for the treatment of severe Raynaud's phenomenon. Am. J. Surg., 67: 1096–1097.

Raso, A.M. (1989) Results of electrostimulation of the spinal cord in Raynaud's disease and syndrome. J. Mal. Vasc., 14: 52–54.

Robaina, F.J., Dominguez, M., Diaz, M., Rodriguez, J.L., and de Vera, J.A. (1989) Spinal cord stimulation for relief of chronic pain in vasospastic disorders of the upper limbs. Neurosurgery, 24: 63–67

Buerger's disease

Chierichetti, F., Mambrini, S., Bagliani, A., and Odero, A. (2002) Treatment of Buerger's disease with electrical spinal cord stimulation – review of three cases. Angiology, 53: 341–347.

Claeys, L.G.Y., Ktenidis, K., and Horsch, S. (1997) Effects of spinal cord stimulation on ischemic pain in patients with Buerger's disease. Pain Diag., 7: 138–141.

Swigris, J.J., Olin, J.W., and Mekhail, N.A. (1999) Implantable spinal cord stimulator to treat the ischemic manifestations of thromboangiitis obliterans (Buerger's disease). J. Vasc. Surg., 29: 928–935

Frostbite

Arregui, R., Morandeira, J.R., Martinez, G., Gomez, A., and Calatayud, V. (1989) Epidural neurostimulation in the treatment of frostbite. Pacing Clin. Electrophysiol., 12: 713–717.

Cauchy, E., Chetaille, E., Marchand, V., and Marsigny, B. (2001) Retrospective study of 70 cases of severe frostbite lesions: a proposed new classification scheme. Wilderness Environ. Med., 12: 248–255.

Khasabov, S.G., Cain, D.M., Thong, D., Mantyh, P.W., and Simone, D.A.J. (2001) Enhanced responses of spinal dorsal horn neurons to heat and cold stimuli following mild freeze injury to the skin. Neurophysiology, 86: 986–996.

Su, C.W., Lohman, R., and Gottlieb, L.J. (2000) Frostbite of the upper extremity. Hand Clin., 16: 235–247.

Electrical Stimulation and the Relief of Pain
Pain Research and Clinical Management, Vol. 15
Edited by Brian A. Simpson

CHAPTER 10

Neuromodulation for refractory angina pectoris

Tore Eliasson,[a],* Mike J.L. DeJongste,[b] and Clas Mannheimer[a]

[a]*Department of Internal Medicine, Multidisciplinary Pain Centre,*
Sahlgrenska University Hospital/Ostra, S-41685, Göteborg, Sweden
[b]*Department of Cardiology, Groningen University Hospital, Hanzeplein 1,*
PO Box 30 001, 9700 RB, Groningen, The Netherlands

Abstract

In this chapter we focus on neuromodulation therapies for patients suffering from the sequels of chronic ischaemic cardiac pain, refractory to standard therapies – refractory angina pectoris. For these patients new and promising therapies, e.g. neuromodulation, provide challenging perspectives for both patients and clinicians.

It is the purpose of this chapter to discuss the efficacy, safety, drawbacks and potential mechanisms of neuromodulation for patients with chronic refractory angina pectoris. By definition the angina pectoris of these patients is severe and chronic, results from coronary artery disease and reversible myocardial ischaemia, and standard pharmacological and surgical therapies have failed and are exhausted.

Keywords: Chronic refractory angina pectoris; Neuromodulation; Myocardial ischaemia

1. Ischaemic heart disease

1.1. Coronary artery disease and angina pectoris

The clinical presentation of a transient chest discomfort caused by physical strain was described for the first time in 1772 by William Heberden, (Heberden, 1772) though he did not recognise the symptom as a sign of cardiac distress. He originally named his observation 'pectoris dolor', the term which his son later changed to 'angina pectoris'. The famous physician Dr. William Heberden accurately described these patients as follows: "*There is a disorder of the breast ... while they are walking, and more particularly when they walk soon after eating, with a painful and most disagreeable sensation ... the moment they stand still all this uneasiness vanishes ... the os sternii is usually pointed to as the seat of this malady ... and sometimes there is with it a pain about the middle of the left arm*". To date, this description has been redefined by the American Heart Association as "*... a clinical syndrome characterized by discomfort in the chest, jaw, shoulder, back, or arm, typically aggravated by exertion or emotional stress*" (Gibbons et al., 1999).

The pathophysiological mechanism leading to angina pectoris is reversible myocardial ischaemia, a concept which was postulated more than 150 years later (Keefer and Resnik, 1928). Angina

---

*Correspondence to: Dr. Tore Eliasson, Present address: Department of Internal Medicine, Multidisciplinary Pain Centre, Sahlgrenska University Hospital/Ostra, S-41685, Göteborg, Sweden. Phone: +46313435063; Fax: +46313435933; E-mail: tore.eliasson@hjl.gu.se

pectoris was then recognised to be caused by an imbalance between the demand and the supply of oxygen to the heart. The decrease in supply is usually the consequence of either vessel obstruction or vasospasm, which subsequently reduces the local blood flow to the cardiac muscle. The increase in oxygen demand of the muscle, which may trigger anginal attacks, results from events such as physical activity, redistribution of the blood flow after meals and cold, or mental stress (Deanfield et al., 1984; Kim et al., 2003).

To date, coronary artery disease still accounts for the highest incidence of disease and is the major cause of death in the Western world. The morbidity, usually manifested as symptomatic angina pectoris and heart failure, also remains high, albeit that pharmacotherapeutical and surgical treatment strategies have significantly improved the quality of life and increased life expectancy of patients suffering from ischaemic heart disease.

A specific problem concerns patients suffering from angina pectoris with normal coronary angiographies, usually, and somewhat inadequately, referred to as cardiac (not to be confused with 'metabolic') Syndrome X, also referred to as 'microvascular angina', or 'small vessel disease'. These patients have typical exercise-triggered angina with ST segment depression on exercise ECG or other objective signs of myocardial ischaemia. They generally fail to respond to conventional anti-anginal therapy and therefore constitute a therapeutic problem. The cause of this specific type of exercise-induced chest pain has not been properly elucidated. Some of the causes suggested are endothelial dysfunction, abnormal distribution and function of adenosine receptors and estrogen deficiency (Panza, 2002). Syndrome X is more common in women than in men and the prognosis is excellent, with the exception of a subgroup that may develop dilated cardiomyopathy.

1.2. Pathophysiology of ischaemic heart disease

The heart is dependent on almost complete oxidation of nutrients to obtain energy and may only tolerate an oxygen debt within narrow limits and for a short period of time. Given the availability of sufficient nutrients, measurement of the oxygen consumption is therefore a good way to assess the heart's metabolism. The heart's basic flow is between 60 and 90 ml/min/100 g of tissue, but this flow may be increased four- or fivefold in healthy individuals – the so-called flow reserve (Maseri, 1995). Increases in heart rate, blood pressure and contractility increase the oxygen demand (Braunwald, 2002). The product of heart rate and blood pressure, the so-called double product or rate-pressure product, is proportionally related to myocardial oxygen consumption MVO_2. Coronary atherosclerosis, coronary vasospasm or a combination of these two conditions leads to a reduction in blood flow and subsequently to a decrease in oxygen supply. Irrespective of the initiating factors, during the so-called ischaemic cascade, the increase in oxygen demand of the myocardium induces changes in the coronary flow.

1.3. Conventional therapies for chronic ischaemic heart disease

Many theories of the pathogenesis of atherosclerosis have been proposed and are incorporated in the well-known model of the 'response to injury hypothesis', published by Ross and Glomset (1976). In fact, their theory of the induction of atherogenesis was a synthesis of Virchow's observations, which dated back to 1852, on the role of endothelial damage through inflammation and Rokitansky's finding of the incorporation of fibrin and platelets into atherosclerotic plaques. To tackle the progression in the narrowing of coronary arteries resulting from atherosclerosis, different strategies may be explored. The basic effect desired from anti-anginal therapy is a reduction of local ischaemia, either by increasing the oxygen supply (increased flow) or by reducing the demand (decrease in oxygen consumption). In brief, pharmacotherapeutical control of ischaemic heart disease is directed (1) to prevent clotting (i.e. of thrombocytes) in the coronary artery (antiplatelet agents, coumarins), (2) to decrease the cardiac oxygen demand (β-blockers and some calcium-blocking agents), (3) to increase the supply (nitrates and some calcium-blocking agents), or (4) to improve endothelial function (statins, ACE: angiotensin converting enzyme – inhibitors, NO: nitric oxide – donators). The interventional approach (i.e. restoring the vessel diameter through decreasing or bypassing the stenosis), is directed towards the improvement of blood flow in the coronary artery. The invasive methods, routinely used in the treatment of coronary artery disease when drug therapy fails to produce an adequate effect, are percutaneous transluminal coronary angioplasty (PTCA) and coronary artery bypass grafting (CABG). To emphasize the frequent use of stents and atherectomies, the term PTCA is often replaced with percutaneous transluminal intervention (PTI). In general, surgical procedures performed on patients with significant stenosis (above all, patients with three-vessel disease, i.e. significant stenoses in all three primary coronary vessels and main stem stenosis) results in increased survival and decreased cardiac morbidity.

2. Refractory angina pectoris

Pharmacotherapeutical and surgical treatment strategies have significantly improved the quality of life, in conjunction with an increased life expectancy, for patients suffering from ischaemic heart disease (Zanger et al., 2000). Notwithstanding these anti-anginal therapeutic merits, which usually supply appropriate symptom relief in the majority of patients, in an increasing number of patients with ischaemic heart disease the major goal, i.e. the control of angina pectoris (Parmley, 1997), is not met. Within the treatment of angina pectoris pain alleviation is fundamental, not only to reduce symptoms, but also because pain *per se* may aggravate myocardial ischaemia through an increase in both segmental and general sympathetic activity. It is therefore necessary to break

this vicious circle for these patients, in whom it results in severe disabling anginal complaints, which may occur during minimal exercise or even at rest. The patients are subsequently suffering from angina pectoris that is refractory to standard therapies.

The term 'chronic refractory angina pectoris' has been designated for patients with severe chest pain, resulting from coronary artery disease that is uncontrollable by both anti-anginal medication (aspirins, β-blocking agents, calcium-channel blockers, long-acting nitrates etc.) and revascularization procedures (PTI: percutaneous transluminal intervention and CABG: coronary artery bypass grafting; Eliasson et al., 1996; Jessurun et al., 1997a). Therefore, the European Study Group on the Treatment of Refractory Angina Pectoris has recently redefined this disorder as: "*A chronic condition characterized by the presence of angina, caused by coronary insufficiency in the presence of coronary artery disease, which cannot be adequately controlled by a combination of medical therapy, angioplasty, and coronary artery bypass surgery. The presence of reversible myocardial ischemia should be clinically established to be the cause of symptoms*" (Mannheimer et al., 2002). Patients suffering from this condition are usually characterized by a long history of coronary artery disease, previously treated with multiple CABG and PTI procedures, they are relatively young (mean age 63 years), predominantly male, have a slightly reduced left ventricular ejection fraction, and an elevated fibrinogen (Schoebel et al., 1997; TenVaarwerk et al., 1999). With regard to the latter the increased fibrinogen is most likely to be an epi-phenomenon, related to chronic inflammation induced by coronary artery disease (De Jongste and TerHorst, 2001).

Patients suffering from chronic refractory angina pectoris resistant to conventional therapies are classified as survivors of their coronary artery disease. It is estimated that in the US and in Europe about 100,000 patients fulfil this condition (Mukherjee et al., 1999). As coronary artery disease continues to worsen, they often require numerous admissions to control pain and experience a very poor quality of life. In addition, as a result of an acute worsening of their coronary artery disease, these patients often need hospital admission (Murray et al., 1999). Therefore, the search for and evaluation of adjunct therapies has to be encouraged in order to identify novel strategies that are able to reduce anginal complaints and subsequently improve the quality of life, without adversely influencing the prognosis of these severely disabled patients. However, several of these therapies have problems including a relatively short period of effectiveness, high costs, intolerable side effects, increased mortality and morbidity (Reynolds, 1974; Olausson et al., 1997; Clarke and Schofield, 1999).

3. Adjunct therapies

The first category of adjuvant therapies includes the administering of medication, either systemically like amiodarone (Singh, 1983), chelation (Kidd, 1998), opioids (Mouallem et al., 2000), and (intermittent) urokinase (Schoebel et al., 1997), or locally applied, such as thoracic epidural anaesthesia (TEDA) (Blomberg, 1994).

Second are therapies aiming at the restoration of functioning of the entire body or of the organ, by means of a rehabilitation programme (Wannamethee et al., 2000), Enhanced External Counter Pulsation: EECP (Urano et al., 2001), or an up-regulation of vascular endothelial growth factors, inducing gene-therapy i.e. angiogenesis. (Freedman and Isner, 2001). The latter adjuvant therapy is highly experimental and the (theoretical) risks of, for example, induction or growth of malignancies have not yet been established.

The third way to obtain an additional anti-anginal effect is provided by modulation of the nervous system. Neuromodulation and intermittent ablation has been performed for many years and may be executed by vagal stimulation (Zamotrinsky et al., 1997), by creating a temporary sympathetic block through injections with local anaesthetics into the stellate ganglion (Chester et al., 2000), through stimulation of the stellate ganglion (Braunwald, 2002), or through stimulation of the spinal cord or peripheral nerves, i.e. 'neuromodulation'. Neuromodulation is usually applied either by spinal cord stimulation (SCS), or by transcutaneous electrical nerve stimulation (TENS). Among all the available adjunct therapies, modulation of the nervous system through either TENS or SCS is considered as one of the more effective and safe adjuvant treatments for patients with angina pectoris resistant to conventional strategies (Mulcahy et al., 1994; Fallen, 1999). Relief of angina pectoris is most beneficial with SCS applied in the epidural space at levels T1–T2 inducing paresthesias covering the precordial chest (Jessurun et al., 1996, DeJongste, 2000). In a report from a European Society of Cardiology Joint Study Group on Refractory Angina Pectoris, SCS and TENS were therefore recommended as the treatment of choice for these patients (Mannheimer et al., 2002).

The final category consists of destructive therapies such as transmyocardial (Kraatz et al., 2001) and percutaneous 'revascularization' with laser beams (Clarke and Schofield, 2001), and denervation of the stellate ganglion (Wiener and Cox, 1966), or of the extrinsic cardiac nervous system. The latter can be applied through transthoracic (Palumbo and Lulu, 1966) or endoscopic sympathectomy (Wettervik et al., 1995; Khogali et al., 1999).

Taking all the available adjuvant therapies into account, heart transplantation cannot seriously be considered as an alternative for these patients.

4. Ischaemic heart disease: pain pathways

Following myocardial ischaemia, sensory nerve endings are activated in the adventitia of coronary arteries, in the subepicardial tissue, and in the myocardium. These receptors appear to be sensitive to chemical stimuli (Foreman et al., 1999). At local sites, a reduction in pH, as well as potassium ions, lactate, bradykinin and adenosine may activate nerves. The heart's pain afferents, together with sympathetic nerve branches, run to the upper four thoracic paravertebral sympathetic ganglia. Pain fibres continue uninterrupted through the ganglia to the upper thoracic, dorsal spinal roots to reach the segments in the spinal cord. The pain fibres are identical to somatosensory fibres in appearance and electrical conduction capacity. It has been shown that stimulation of the upper thoracic interspinal ligaments gives rise to pain that is indistinguishable from angina pectoris in terms of its quality and extension (Braunwald, 1992). Clinically, the pain manifests itself as a diffuse, poorly localised pain without any relationship to the cardiac cycle. During transient myocardial ischaemic periods afferent cardiac fibres are recruited in sympathetic and vagal nerves. Following ischaemic episodes the subsequently activated fibres activate sympathetic afferent fibres that enter the T1–T6 spinal cord segments. Stimulation of these afferent fibres in acute animal experiments excites spinal neurons that are found primarily in the dorsal horn of upper thoracic segments (Foreman, 1999). Sympathetic afferents from the heart convey noxious and mechanical information via the dorsal roots primarily to the upper thoracic segments.

Both centrally projecting as well as non-projecting neurons respond to noxious stimuli applied to the heart. These same neurons receive nociceptive somatic inputs from the upper chest and arm. It has also been shown that neurostimulation applied at the chest generates impulse transmission via somatic afferents to the upper spinal cord, inducing neuronal activity in the spinothalamic tract (STT; DeJongste et al., 1998; Foreman, 1999). This convergence of visceral and somatic input onto a common pool of STT cells provides a mechanism to explain pain referral to somatic structures in angina pectoris.

Pain from the heart is perceived as referred pain, as is pain from other visceral organs. The localisation corresponds to the dermatomes supplied by the upper four thoracic spinal roots.

Several observations have been made of the effects on the inner organs in the human body of cutaneous electrical stimulation. TENS of the abdominal wall may, for example, cause bladder inhibition and give rise to gastrointestinal hyperactivity. Cook and colleagues were the first to report that epidural electrical stimulation may increase blood flow in the lower extremities in patients with peripheral arterial circulatory insufficiency (Cook et al., 1976).

There is thus considerable support in the literature for the assumption that autonomic functions may be influenced by electrical stimulation. These effects require visceral reflex mechanisms that are controlled from higher centres.

5. History of neuromodulation for angina pectoris

Though the application of electricity as an alternative therapy against pain dates back to ancient history, a scientific background was not provided until 1965. The scientific base for the mechanism of action of electrical neuromodulatory therapies, such as SCS and TENS, in the treatment of various pain conditions is offered by the model of the 'gate control', proposed by Melzack and Wall (1965). Although the details of the theory have been the subject of intense debate and criticism, it has been extraordinarily important for the continued research into spinal segmentally modulated mechanisms. Shortly after the gate control therapy was proposed, the general principles of segmental pain inhibition came to be used as the basis for the development of electrical nerve stimulation as pain treatment.

The TENS method is a therapy that has been established and is reported to improve angina symptoms (Mannheimer et al., 1985), and, specifically when compared to other adjunct therapies, it is worthy of consideration (Meyler et al., 1994). By the late 1970s, TENS was already in use in Gothenburg, Sweden, to treat this group of patients. TENS was shown to have an anti-anginal effect secondary to a decrease in myocardial ischaemia and not reversible by the opiate antagonist naloxone (Mannheimer et al., 1982, 1985, 1989; Emanuelsson et al., 1987). However, it is hampered by practical problems. The patient's electrodes sometimes fall off, which causes some discomfort. In 10–15% of patients, the electrodes also induces skin reaction, the so-called ortho-ergic response, which is related to the high resistance of the skin complicating the use of this device (Strobos et al., 2001). However, in general this reaction affects, above all, patients in whom long-term, continuous stimulation is desirable. Compared with spinal cord stimulation, TENS must thus be considered an impractical method for long-term treatment. To date it is mainly used to test the effect of afferent stimulation/electrical stimulation in angina pectoris, to assess the patient's compliance in order to find suitable candidates for spinal cord stimulation, and for research purposes. TENS may also serve as a valuable auxiliary option in the treatment of unstable angina (Börjesson et al., 1997).

SCS has been used since the end of the 1960s, initially to treat neurogenic pain. Since 1976, several reports have been published on the beneficial effects of spinal cord stimulation in advanced peripheral arterial circulatory insufficiency (Chapter 9). The treatment appears to induce local peripheral perfusion, which in turn gives rise to improved healing of ischaemic ulcers. Following the beneficial effects of TENS for chronic refractory angina pectoris and SCS for peripheral vascular disease (PVD) the step towards SCS for chronic refractory angina pectoris was an easy move to make.

SCS has been used to treat refractory angina pectoris in Sweden since 1985. The first report on the anti-anginal effect of SCS in patients with chronic refractory angina pectoris was published by Murphy and Giles from Western Australia, in 1987 (Murphy and Giles, 1987). They observed a reduction in both the frequency and severity of anginal attacks in conjunction with a reduction in sublingual intake of glyceryl trinitrate. In contrast with the favourable results, the therapy initially

met with great scepticism (Mannheimer et al., 1988). Subsequently, however, many authors have advocated neuromodulation and especially SCS as an effective approach for patients chronically disabled by their anginal pain (Mannheimer et al., 1982, 1985, 1986, 1988, 1989, 1991, 1993a,b; Mannheimer, 1984; Emanuelsson et al., 1987; De Landsheere et al., 1992; Sanderson et al., 1992, 1994, 1996; DeJongste and Staal, 1993; Eliasson et al., 1993a, 1994, 1996, 1998; DeJongste et al., 1994a,b,c; Eliasson, 1994, 2000; Mannheimer and Eliasson, 1995; Hautvast et al., 1996, 1997, 1998a,b; Norrsell et al., 1997, 1998; Greco et al., 1999). To date, in selected patients, in view of the long-term beneficial effect (DeJongste et al., 1994b,c; Sanderson et al., 1994; Bagger et al., 1998), SCS may even be considered as an alternative to bypass surgery (Mannheimer et al., 1998). However, in view of the partially understood mechanism of action, it is important to demonstrate the safety of SCS in patients suffering from refractory angina pectoris. Therefore, in the past few years research has been performed to determine whether the observed analgesic effect of SCS is accompanied by an anti-ischaemic effect.

6. Anti-anginal and anti-ischaemic effects of neuromodulation

Both observational and randomised studies on SCS have demonstrated beneficial effects, expressed in a reduction in anginal complaints and use of short acting nitrates, and perceived quality of life, in conjunction with an improvement in exercise capacity (Mannheimer et al., 1982, 1985, 1986, 1988, 1989, 1991, 1993a,b; Mannheimer, 1984; Emanuelsson et al., 1987; De Landsheere et al., 1992; Sanderson et al., 1992, 1994, 1996; DeJongste and Staal, 1993; Eliasson et al., 1993a, 1994, 1996, 1998; DeJongste et al., 1994a,b,c; Eliasson, 1994, 2000; Mannheimer and Eliasson, 1995; Hautvast et al., 1996, 1997, 1998a,b; Norrsell et al., 1997, 1998; Greco et al., 1999). In approximately 80% of patients the beneficial effects of SCS last for at least 1 year and in nearly 60% of these patients improvement in exercise capacity and quality of life has been reported for up to 5 years (Bagger et al., 1998; TenVaarwerk et al., 1999; Ekre et al., 2002).

The anti-anginal effect of SCS is paralleled by a reduction in myocardial ischaemia. In many publications from different independent centres, the anti-ischaemic effect of neuromodulation has been demonstrated by making use of different tools to study the ECG, such as exercise stress testing (Mannheimer et al., 1988; Eliasson et al., 1993b; DeJongste et al., 1994b,c; Hautvast et al., 1998b) and ambulatory ECG monitoring (Sanderson et al., 1992; DeJongste et al., 1994b; Eliasson et al., 1994; Hautvast et al., 1998a; Jessurun et al., 1999; Di Pede et al., 2001). Both open and randomized studies have demonstrated that the reduction in anginal pain during SCS enables the patient to prolong the exercise without aggravating myocardial ischaemia. Furthermore, one study showed an increased tolerance to atrial pacing and delayed onset of anginal complaints during SCS accompanied by a decrease in myocardial ischaemia and reduced myocardial oxygen consumption on a comparable pacing rate (Mannheimer et al., 1993a). All patients ultimately experienced angina pectoris. Chauhan and colleagues (1994) demonstrated an increase in coronary flow velocity, using Doppler flow catheters during neuromodulation. The rise in the anginal threshold is probably caused by a reduction of myocardial ischaemia caused by a decrease in myocardial oxygen consumption and, possibly, redistribution of coronary blood flow from myocardial regions with a normal perfusion in favour of regions with impaired myocardial perfusion (Mannheimer et al., 1993a; Hautvast et al., 1996; Mobilia et al., 1998).

In contrast to the favourable influence of SCS on anginal complaints, many concerns remain with regard to the potential risk of an increase in myocardial ischaemia with serious ensuing sequelae, if SCS is indeed depriving the patient of the anginal 'warning' signal. Because SCS elevates the anginal threshold and patients are subsequently reporting a reduction, and not a complete elimination of anginal attacks during SCS, this concern is obviously not rational. In addition, since SCS appears to employ an anti-ischaemic effect, without increasing mortality (Mannheimer et al., 1998; TenVaarwerk et al., 1999; Ekre et al., 2002) and without concealing the anginal warning signal during an acute myocardial infarction (Andersen et al., 1994; Sanderson et al., 1994; Jessurun et al., 1997b; Gonzalez-Darder et al., 1998; Greco et al., 1999; Murray et al., 1999), neuromodulation is considered as a safe therapy for patients invalided by their refractory angina. The fear of a potential increase in myocardial events does not seem to be justified (DeJongste et al., 1994a; Eliasson et al., 1996). Rather than abolishing anginal pain, SCS enhances the anginal threshold. As a consequence patients report an increase in exercise capacity and a reduction in the severity, without a complete elimination, of anginal symptoms with intact pain perception during acute myocardial infarction (Andersen et al., 1994; Eliasson et al., 1996; Jessurun et al., 1997b). This is consistent with the absence of an adverse effect on mortality as demonstrated in prospective and retrospective studies on SCS for refractory angina pectoris. In addition, SCS was not able to suppress the conduction of cardiac pain signals to the cerebrum during cardiac distress (Hautvast et al., 1997).

With regard to safety, another important issue is the long-term effect of afferent stimulation with respect to side effects and complications. In a retrospective follow-up of 517 patients, no negative effects with regard to mortality were observed (TenVaarwerk et al., 1999). In a prospective randomised study, spinal cord stimulation was compared with bypass surgery in patients who only experienced symptomatic effects from bypass surgery (Mannheimer et al., 1998). After 6 months, there was no difference between spinal cord stimulation and bypass with regard to symptom relief. There was a lower mortality and cerebrovascular morbidity in the spinal cord stimulation group. A follow-up investigation after 2 years showed SCS to be superior to bypass surgery from a cost-effectiveness perspective (Andrell et al., 2002), and the 5-year follow-up showed no differences in mortality between the groups (Ekre et al., 2002). Compared with the pre-surgery situation, good symptom relief and improved quality of life were maintained after 5 years without any significant difference between the groups. SCS may thus be a possible alternative to coronary surgery for certain groups of patients in whom only a symptomatic effect of bypass surgery can be expected.

7. Neuromodulation and arrhythmias

Although systematic studies are lacking, SCS does not appear to influence heart rate variability (DeJongste et al., 1994b; Hautvast et al., 1998a; Norrsell et al., 2000; Di Pede et al., 2001) or have an arrhythmogenic effect (Eliasson et al., 1996). As has been previously described, patients with refractory angina pectoris generally have a long history of anginal complaints and may be considered survivors of coronary artery disease. They may therefore be at lower risk of developing arrhythmias. On the other hand, if SCS reduces myocardial ischaemia, this may potentially decrease the risk of rhythm disturbances. At the cardiac level SCS is thought to stabilize intra-cardiac neuronal function during ischaemia, and subsequently may potentially have a beneficial effect on the occurrence of reperfusion arrhythmias and autonomically induced sudden cardiac death (Foreman et al., 2000; Kingma et al., 2001; Armour et al., 2002; Tanaka et al., 2003). TENS and SCS do not appear to give rise to an increase in arrhythmias (DeJongste et al., 1994b).

8. Neuromodulation and myocardial function

No significant influence of SCS on left ventricular function has been observed in longitudinal studies (Hautvast et al., 1993). One study reported on the acute effects of SCS on left ventricular function, which was impaired by the infusion of adenosine. The investigators observed an improvement in ventricular function during SCS (Kujacic et al., 1993).

9. Mechanisms of action of neuromodulation

In 1965, Melzack and Wall published the 'gate-control theory' (Melzack and Wall, 1965). The model was based on the theory that stimulation of myelinated relatively fast conducting A fibres modulated the processing of pain in the non-myelinated slower conducting C fibres in the dorsal horn.

Initially, the anti-ischaemic effect of SCS was ascribed to modulation of the autonomic nervous system, more specifically, to the sympathetic branch. However, clinical data do not support this hypothesis, since no change in heart rate variability, or in (nor)-epinephrine metabolism has been found during spinal cord stimulation (DeJongste et al., 1994b; Norrsell et al., 1997; Hautvast et al., 1998b).

The rise in the anginal threshold, causing the delayed onset of angina, may be related to deferring the moment of critical balance between myocardial oxygen supply and demand. Whether the suggested redistribution in coronary blood flow takes place through recruitment of collaterals (Jessurun et al., 1998) or that other mechanisms are involved such as angiogenesis (Egginton and Hudlicka, 2000) or preconditioning (Marber et al., 1993) is a matter of further research.

The increased anginal threshold was emphasized by a study in which patients with refractory angina and SCS were randomized to control or stressed by right atrial pacing to their ischaemic threshold (Mannheimer et al., 1993a). During SCS the anginal threshold was higher, secondary to an anti-ischaemic effect, albeit that all patients ultimately reported angina. In a letter to the editor it was claimed that the results could be alternatively explained by preconditioning (Marber et al., 1993). Preconditioning and collateral recruitment are likely to play an important role in determining the ischaemic threshold in patients with refractory angina pectoris. To protect the heart, SCS apparently activates efferent and afferent neural projections to and from the heart. These projections may activate intrinsic cardiac neural processes that release various endogenous neuromediators and neuromodulators (i.e. norepinephrine, endorphins, neurokinins etc.). In one study, SCS turned a net uptake of beta-endorphin at rest to a release during cardiac stress in the heart (Eliasson et al., 1998). Caffrey and colleagues have found that naloxone enhances the myocardial performance and coronary blood flow in a dose-dependent manner in the dog, mediated by a direct effect on μ-opiate receptors, indicating that endogenous opioids have locally mediated, direct effects on the heart (Caffrey et al., 1985). Furthermore, the results indicated local myocardial turnover of leu-enkephalin, beta-endorphin and calcitonin-gene-related peptide. In addition, it was implied that SCS may induce myocardial release of beta-endorphin that could explain the beneficial effects in myocardial ischaemia. The net effect of this SCS-induced release of neurochemicals is likely to stabilize the heart during myocardial ischaemia.

In contradiction to ischaemic preconditioning data, from clinical experience it appears that the benefits of SCS on cardiac function are maintained for years. This may be related to an ability of the nervous system, under SCS control, to release the appropriate endogenous neurochemicals where and when they are needed and at levels that are sufficiently low to minimize the potential for receptor downregulation.

The prevalent opinion on the mechanism behind the pain-alleviating effect of TENS and SCS is that the electrical stimulation activates the body's own defence system against pain at the segmental level, but probably also via a system involving the brain stem which brings about pain alleviation.

The most common objection to afferent treatment methods, such as spinal cord stimulation, is the hypothesis that stimulation would only block the pain signal without affecting myocardial ischaemia and thus involve a risk to the patient. Several studies carried out at various centres show that when the heart is stressed during stimulation to comparable load the myocardial ischaemia is reduced, compared with a control situation without stimulation. However, when the patient is provoked to myocardial ischaemia during stimulation treatment (often at a higher load) the anginal pain returns. This indicates that the patient is not deprived of the warning signal that the pain constitutes. This applies regardless of the stress method used (bicycle test, pharmacological provocation or atrial pacing; Eliasson et al., 1996). Furthermore, Chandler and co-workers have shown that electrical stimulation of the spinal cord inhibits the conduction of nociceptive signals in the spinothalamic tract (Chandler et al., 1993), and additionally causes alterations in cerebral blood flow (Hautvast et al., 1997).

Theoretically, there are three possible explanations for the reduction in myocardial ischaemia by electrical stimulation of afferent neurons: increased coronary flow, reduced oxygen demand in the heart and, finally, a direct pain-inhibiting effect with a reduction in oxygen consumption in the myocardium as a secondary phenomenon. The positive effects obtained in peripheral arteriosclerotic disease in the legs, in the form of pain alleviation and healing of ischaemic ulcers, appear to be due to a redistribution of the blood flow. However, available data support the notion of an increase in microvascular flow.

There are studies indicating that afferent stimulation gives rise to a reduction in oxygen consumption in the myocardium under stress (Mannheimer et al., 1993a; Braunwald, 2002). Spinal cord stimulation has an anti-anginal and anti-ischaemic effect that appears to be secondary to reduced oxygen consumption rather than increased coronary flow. When the patients' heart rate was increased through atrial pacing to the myocardial ischaemia limit, anginal pain occurred. This indicates that the patient was not deprived of a warning signal. There is a linear relationship between the oxygen need of the myocardium and the coronary flow. This means that any measure influencing oxygen consumption also affects the coronary flow. Thus, if spinal cord stimulation reduces the consumption it will also reduce the coronary flow, as in the study referred to above.

With regard to the third alternative, it has been shown that anginal pain induces an increase in sympathetic activity. This gives rise to constriction of local arterioles. It has also been shown that anginal pain and increased sympathetic activity may give rise to life-threatening arrhythmias, particularly in the presence of ischaemia or infarction. Pain alleviation in itself may thus give rise to a segmental and general reduction in sympathetic activity and reduce myocardial ischaemia. In angina pectoris, the pain-alleviating effect normally occurs within 1–2 min and the pain relief is usually complete.

Although some experimental data indicate that SCS inhibits impulse transmission within the spinothalamic tract (Linderoth and Foreman, 1999), most clinical observations support the notion that SCS alters the myocardial oxygen-supply ratio. In this regard, SCS improves myocardial lactate production perhaps because of reducing cardiac myocyte metabolism and thus oxygen demand. It is also proposed that SCS redistributes myocardial blood flow to regions of ischaemia (Hautvast et al., 1996; Jessurun et al., 1998; Mobilia et al., 1998). In a clinical setting, the anti-anginal effects of SCS far outlast the duration of stimulation. Whether the suppressor effect of SCS on the intrinsic cardiac nervous system, or other cardiac and spinal cord mechanisms, are involved has to be addressed further.

Intracardiac neurons (ICN) are considered as the final common integrator of the nervous system in the heart (Armour, 1999). In recent experimental studies it was shown that SCS modulates, in a consistent pattern, the firing rate of these intrinsic cardiac neurons (Foreman et al., 2000;

Armour et al., 2002). SCS was effective in reducing intrinsic cardiac neuronal activity, whether it was applied before, during or following the onset of a 2-min coronary artery occlusion. This SCS-induced suppression of ICN activity persisted after cessation of SCS implying that the neural suppressing effects of SCS are long-lived and supports the clinical studies that indicate a similar cardio-protective benefit even after SCS is discontinued. In a follow-up study, SCS continued to suppress the activity generated by the ICN, even when coronary arteries were occluded for periods up to 15 min (Armour et al., 2002). In either case, transsection of the subclavian ansae eliminated the suppressor effects of SCS on ICN activity, indicating that the responses were due primarily to the influence of spinal cord neurons acting via the sympathetic nervous system. In summary, it appears that SCS may influence the function of the final common neural pathway of the heart, the intrinsic cardiac nervous system, in the presence of a severe ischaemic challenge.

In addition to the effect of SCS on spinal cord neurons and the ICN, in higher brain centres both angina pectoris and neuromodulation have been found to affect areas involved in cardiovascular control (Rosen et al., 1994). In addition to these putative actions at different levels in the central nervous system (CNS), a variety of neurotransmitters and vasoactive compounds, such as adenosine and endorphins, are thought to link shifts in the activity in CNS centres to control the cardiovascular state.

Finally, in the canine model the anti-anginal effects of SCS did not appear to be dependent upon redistribution of coronary blood flow alterations in cardiac work. In another recent study regional cardiac blood flow distribution evoked by transient occlusion of the left anterior descending coronary artery (LAD) in dogs was unaffected by SCS (Kingma et al., 2001). Moreover, left ventricular pressure–volume loops evoked by transient LAD occlusion were likewise unaffected. SCS by itself was ineffective in changing ventricular myocardial blood flow patterns or left ventricular pressure–volume loops. It should be pointed out that these studies were conducted in an animal model with a normal heart. Nevertheless, from these animal studies one might conclude that the anti-anginal effects of SCS do not reflect modulation of the cardiac supply/demand balance but rather involve other neuro-humoral mechanisms which protect the heart from some of the deleterious consequences attending myocardial ischaemia and the resultant angina.

10. Implantation techniques for neuromodulation and stimulation

Under local anaesthesia, an incision is made in the thoracic part of the back at the thoracic (T) 5–8 level and a four-pole electrode is inserted in the epidural space via a guiding device. The tip of the electrode is guided into the epidural space under fluoroscopy, usually to the level of the T1 and T2 vertebrae. The implantation procedure of SCS, a reversible non-destructive therapy, has been described in detail elsewhere (DeJongste et al., 1994b; Eliasson et al., 1996). The key to the success of SCS is an accurate placement of the stimulating electrode in the dorsal epidural space. During the pre-operative stimulation, the patient feels paraesthesiae in the chest. It is important to adjust the position of the electrode so that the paraesthesiae in the chest cover the area of the patient's anginal pain, even if the angina pectoris is atypically localised. This is the only way to verify that the area of the spinal cord that innervates the heart is being stimulated. A common reason for an inadequate effect is incorrect electrode position, i.e. the paraesthesiae in the chest do not cover the area of the anginal pain. With correct electrode positioning the anginal pain should disappear completely after 20–120 s of high-intensity stimulation, provided that the chest pain is angina pectoris caused by myocardial ischaemia.

When adequate paraesthesiae have been achieved, an electrical wire is tunnelled subcutaneously to the left upper abdomen where it is connected to a subcutaneous pulse generator about the size of a pacemaker. This means that this is a completely closed system and the patient can move around freely without any practical restrictions to daily life activities. With older systems the stimulator is turned on and off with the aid of an external magnet that activates two preset stimulation amplitudes, a stronger one to be used during and before an expected attack, and a weaker strength to be used as 'maintenance therapy' (stimulation for at least 1–2 h, 3–4 times a day). Instead of an external magnet, state-of-the-art stimulators have an external programming unit that allows the patient to turn the stimulator on and off with a push button and to increase and reduce the strength of the stimulation.

11. Indications, patient selection, and clinical experience

Since 1985, about 800 patients have been treated with spinal cord stimulation for angina at the Multidisciplinary Pain Centre in Gothenburg. Globally, approximately 2500 cardiac patients have received this treatment. The indications are severe angina, despite optimum drug and surgical therapy, in patients with coronary disease, and angina pectoris in patients with normal coronary angiographies, so-called Syndrome X. Side effects and complications are rare, compared with other medical and surgical treatment modes. The implantation requires only a minor surgical intervention as described above and is reversible. In the Gothenburg series superficial post-operative wound infections have occurred in approximately 1.5% of patients but no epidural infections have been observed.

Before implantation it is important to ensure that the patients have full intellectual capacity as a fairly high degree of compliance is required for the patient to manage the stimulator in a home setting. It is also very important to ensure that the patient's chest pain really is related to current reversible myocardial ischaemia, as chest pain of other origin usually responds less well to this therapy. An objective check should therefore be made by means of conventional examination methods, such as standard exercise test, heart scintigraphy, stress ECG and 24–48-h ECG recording (Holter technique). If current reversible myocardial ischaemia cannot be confirmed it is doubtful whether the patients should be implanted, even though severe coronary disease may be present. This is particularly important when psychological, psychosocial or other functional factors may be suspected to play a prominent role in the patient's disease picture.

Patients with severe coronary disease constitute a clinical and therapeutic problem. Therefore, long-term follow-up is important. In Sweden, a standardized programme for these patients has been developed, focussing on the above problems. It is also important to determine the patient's cerebral status. Most patients have undergone one or several bypass operations and have thus been connected to a heart–lung machine. This involves a certain degree of cerebral microembolisation with a consequent risk of hypoxic brain damage. A syndrome of diffuse cerebral damage with intellectual and cognitive dysfunction is not infrequently seen in these patients (Zamvar et al., 2002). It also has negative effects on the pain defence system, with increased pain perception and development of pain behaviour, which may be part of the reason why these patients respond inadequately to conventional therapy. CT scanning, or neuropsychiatric assessment by a psychiatrist with experience of pain patients is sometimes required. It is particularly important to identify the possible presence of a somatoform pain syndrome or other major psychosocial pain determinants. Should this be the case, somatically focussed therapeutic measures should not be initiated until the patient has been rehabilitated from his/her pain syndrome.

After implantation, patients should be hospitalized for at least 24 h in an ordinary medical ward. Personal patient instruction with written information should then be initiated. The use and handling of the stimulator should be demonstrated thoroughly several times. The patient should provoke him/herself several times to mild anginal pain and use the stimulator to relieve the symptoms. Close relations and family members should preferably also be instructed.

The stimulator is set using an external programming unit in the same way as with a modern artificial cardiac pacemaker. Amplitude, pulse width, frequency and electrode polarity may be altered so that adequate paraesthesiae in the chest are achieved. It is important to ensure that the stimulation really reaches the segments of the spinal cord that innervate the heart. This is done by setting the stimulator so that the paraesthesiae cover the area of the angina pectoris. If the patient's pain is atypically localized, the paraesthesiae must consequently cover this area (for example, the right hand). With older systems, the patient can activate the stimulator via a magnet to obtain a weak or strong current (see above). The small, portable, external programming device that accompanies modern systems allows the patient to gradually increase or reduce the strength of the current himself. In acute attacks or expected angina, the patient should use high-intensity stimulation, i.e. use a pulse amplitude that is tolerable for 30–120 s. So-called maintenance treatment is recommended for 1–2 h 3–4 times per day at a low, comfortable current level. There are other clinics that recommend continuous treatment.

After implantation, the patient's previous anti-anginal medication should be kept unchanged. In selected cases, long-acting nitrates and/or calcium antagonists may slowly be discontinued if the patient experiences adverse reactions. The use of beta-blockers should be maintained, if possible. The patients should be carefully followed up in an outpatient setting; among other things, to ensure that they are capable of handling the stimulator and that adequate paraesthesiae are present. During the first 12 months, we see the patients 4–6 times, as the epidural position of the electrode sometimes changes. When the patients are stable with regard to paraesthesiae, stimulator handling, etc. we usually see them once a year. The patient is always given the possibility to contact a nurse and be given an extra appointment with short notice at the clinic.

About 80% of patients experience good long-term effect of the treatment in the form of reduced attack frequency, increased physical activity and improved quality of life (Eliasson et al., 1996; DeJongste, 2000). These results can be compared to the long-term effects of SCS in chronic neurogenic pain (about 50%) or pronounced peripheral arterial circulatory insufficiency (60–70%). In patients who respond inadequately to treatment, psychological factors may be involved. It may also be uncertain whether the pain can be related to ongoing myocardial ischaemia. Furthermore, it has been observed that patients who are very active physically adapt themselves to a higher stress level after implantation, which results in a return to more or less the previous attack frequency after about 6 months.

The placebo effect is probably of considerable importance for the positive effects. However, this tends to decrease with time and is considered to be negligible after 2–3 months. Reduced myocardial ischaemia during stimulation, as well as the fact that the clinical effects last for several years, indicate that other mechanisms in addition to the placebo effect are of importance for the positive result (Bagger et al., 1998; TenVaarwerk et al., 1999). This is also supported by the fact that battery failure may lead to a deterioration in the patient's condition, in the form of increased angina frequency and impaired physical capacity, albeit without a rebound in myocardial ischaemia (Jessurun et al., 1999).

12. Conclusions

Spinal cord stimulation is an effective and safe therapy for patients with therapeutically refractory angina. It is patient-controlled and reversible with a low complication rate. Furthermore, symptoms from acute coronary events are not concealed. SCS does not affect morbidity and mortality adversely. SCS induces the release of neuromediators, neuromodulators and vasoactive substances at the heart and in the CNS. The mechanisms of action are complex and take place at multiple levels. Furthermore, the underlying mechanism appears to be related to a normalization of sensitized pain in conjunction with a reduction in myocardial ischaemia.

References

Andersen, C., Hole, P., and Oxhøj, H. (1994) Does pain relief with spinal cord stimulation conceal myocardial infarction? Br. Heart J., 71: 419–421.

Andrell, P., Ekre, O., Eliasson, T., Blomstrand, C., Börjesson, M., Nilsson, M. and Mannheimer, C. (2003) Cost-effectiveness of spinal cord stimulation vs coronary artery bypass grafting in patients with severe angina pectoris – long-term results from the ESBY study. Cardiology, 99: 20–24.

Armour, J.A. (1999) Myocardial ischaemia and the cardiac nervous system. Cardiovasc. Res., 41: 41–54.

Armour, J.A., Linderoth, B., Arora, R.C., DeJongste, M.J., Ardell, J.L., Kingma, J.G., Jr., Hill, M., and Foreman, R.D. (2002) Long-term modulation of the intrinsic cardiac nervous system by spinal cord neurons in normal and ischaemic hearts. Auton. Neurosci., 95: 71–79.

Bagger, J.P., Jensen, B.S., and Johannsen, G. (1998) Long-term outcome of spinal cord electrical stimulation in patients with refractory chest pain. Clin. Cardiol., 21: 286–288.

Blomberg, S.G. (1994) Long-term home self-treatment with high thoracic epidural anesthesia in patients with severe coronary artery disease. Anesth. Analg., 79: 413–421.

Braunwald, E. (1992) Heart Disease – A Textbook of Cardiovascular Medicine, WB Saunders, Philadelphia.

Braunwald, E. (2002) Personal reflections on effort to reduce ischemic myocardial damage. Cardiovasc. Res., 56: 332–338.

Börjesson, M., Eriksson, P., Dellborg, M., Eliasson, T., and Mannheimer, C. (1997) Transcutaneous nerve stimulation in unstable angina pectoris. Coronary Artery Disease, 8: 543–550.

Caffrey, J., Gaugl, J., and Jones, C. (1985) Local endogenous opiate activity in dog myocardium. Am. J. Physiol., 248: H382–H388.

Chandler, M.J., Brennan, T.J., Garrison, D.W., Kim, K.S., Schwartz, P.J., and Foreman, R.D. (1993) A mechanism of cardiac pain suppression by spinal cord stimulation: implications for patients with angina pectoris. Eur. Heart J., 14: 96–105.

Chauhan, A., Mullins, P., Thuraisingham, S., Taylor, G., Petch, M., and Schofield, P. (1994) Effect of transcutaneous electrical nerve stimulation on coronary blood flow. Circulation, 89: 694–702.

Chester, M., Hammond, C., and Leach, A. (2000) Long-term benefits of stellate ganglion block in severe chronic refractory angina. Pain, 87: 103–105.

Clarke, S.C. and Schofield, P.M. (1999) Myocardial laser revascularization. Eur. Heart J., 20: 1213–1214.

Clarke, S.C. and Schofield, P.M. (2001) Laser revascularization in the management of coronary artery disease. Hosp. Med., 62: 8–13.

Cook, A., Oygar, A., Baggenstos, P., Pacheco, S., and Kleriga, E. (1976) Vascular disease of the extremities. Electrical stimulation of spinal cord and posterior roots. NY State J. Med., 76: 366–368.

Deanfield, J.E., Shea, M., Kensett, M., Horlock, P., Wilson, R.A., de Landsheere, C.M., and Selwyn, A.P. (1984) Silent myocardial ischaemia due to mental stress. Lancet, 2: 1001–1005.

DeJongste, M.J. (2000) Spinal cord stimulation for ischemic heart disease. Neurol. Res., 22: 293–298.

DeJongste, M. and Staal, M. (1993) Preliminary results of a randomised study on the clinical efficacy of spinal cord stimulation for refractory severe angina pectoris. Acta Neurochir. Suppl., 58: 161–164.

De Jongste, M.J. and TerHorst, G.J. (2001) *The Nervous System and the Heart*, Human Press Inc., Totowa, NY.

DeJongste, M., Nagelkerke, D., and Hooyschuur, C. (1994a) Stimulation characteristics, complications and efficacy of spinal cord stimulation in patients with refractory angina. PACE, 17: 1751–1760.

DeJongste, M.J., Haaksma, J., Hautvast, R.W., Hillege, H.L., Meyler, P.W., Staal, M.J., Sanderson, J.E., and Lie, K.I. (1994b) Effects of spinal cord stimulation on myocardial ischaemia during daily life in patients with severe coronary artery disease. A prospective ambulatory electrocardiographic study. Br. Heart J., 71: 413–418.

DeJongste, M.J., Hautvast, R.W., Hillege, H.L., and Lie, K.I. (1994c) Efficacy of spinal cord stimulation as adjuvant therapy for intractable angina pectoris: a prospective, randomized clinical study. Working Group on Neurocardiology. J. Am. Coll. Cardiol., 23: 1592–1597.

DeJongste, M.J., Hautvast, R.V., and TerHorst, G.J. (1998) Spinal cord stimulation and the induction of c-fos and heat shock protein in the central nervous system of rats. Neuromodulation, 2: 27–32.

De Landsheere, C., Mannheimer, C., Habets, A., Guillaume, M., Bourgeois, I., Augustinsson, L.E., Eliasson, T., Lamotte, D., Kulbertus, H., Rigo, P. (1992) Effect of spinal cord stimulation on regional myocardial perfusion assessed by positron emission tomography. Am. J. Cardiol., 69: 1143–1149.

Di Pede, F., Zuin, G., Giada, F., Pinato, G., Turiano, G., Bevilacqua, M., Cazzine, R., and Raviele, A. (2001) Long term effects of spinal cord stimulation on myocardial ischemia and heart rate variability: results of a 48-hour ambulatory electrocardiographic monitoring. Ital. Heart J., 2(9): 690–695.

Egginton, S. and Hudlicka, O. (2000) Selective long-term electrical stimulation of fast glycolytic fibres increases capillary supply but not oxidative enzyme activity in rat skeletal muscles. Exp. Physiol., 85: 567–573.

Ekre, O., Eliasson, T., Norrsell, H., Wahrborg, P., and Mannheimer, C. (2002) Long-term effects of spinal cord stimulation and coronary artery bypass grafting on quality of life and survival in the ESBY study. Eur. Heart J., 23: 1938–1945.

Eliasson, T. (1994) Gothenburg, Thesis.

Eliasson, T. (2000) Spinal cord stimulation in angina pectoris and ischemic heart disease – a topical overview. Acta Chirurgica, Australia, 32: 61–65.

Eliasson, T., Albertsson, P., Hardhammar, P., Emanuelsson, H., Augustinsson, L.E., and Mannheimer, C. (1993a) Spinal cord stimulation in angina pectoris with normal coronary arteriograms. Coron. Artery Dis., 4: 819–827.

Eliasson, T., Albertsson, P., Hårdhammar, P., Emanuelsson, H., Augustinsson, L.-E., and Mannheimer, C. (1993b) Spinal cord stimulation in angina pectoris with normal coronary arteriograms. Coron. Artery Dis., 4: 819–827.

Eliasson, T., Augustinsson, L.E., and Mannheimer, C. (1996) Spinal cord stimulation in severe angina pectoris – presentation of current studies, indications and clinical experience. Pain, 65: 169–179.

Eliasson, T., Jern, S., Augustinsson, L.E., and Mannheimer, C. (1994) Safety aspects of spinal cord stimulation in severe angina pectoris. Coron. Artery Dis., 5: 845–850.

Eliasson, T., Mannheimer, C., Waagstein, F., Andersson, B., Bergh, C.H., Augustinsson, L.E., Hedner, T., and Larson, G. (1998) Myocardial turnover of endogenous opioids and calcitonin-gene-related peptide in the human heart and the effects of spinal cord stimulation on pacing-induced angina pectoris. Cardiology, 89: 170–177.

Emanuelsson, H., Mannheimer, C., Waagstein, F., and Wilhelmsson, C. (1987) Catecholamine metabolism during pacing-induced angina pectoris and the effect of transcutaneous electrical nerve stimulation. Am. Heart J., 114: 1360–1366.

Fallen, E.L. (1999) Commentary on spinal cord stimulation was effective in the treatment of chronic intractable angina pectoris. Evidence-based Cardiovascular Med., 3: 20.

Foreman, R.D. (1999) Mechanisms of cardiac pain. Annu. Rev. Physiol., 61: 143–167.

Foreman, R.D., Blair, R.W., Holmes, H.R., and Armour, J.A. (1999) Correlation of ventricular mechanosensory neurite activity with myocardial sensory field deformation. Am. J. Physiol., 276: 979–989.

Foreman, R.D., Linderoth, B., Ardell, J.L., Barron, K.W., Chandler, M.J., Hull, S.S., Jr., Terhorst, G.J., DeJongste, M.J., and Armour, J.A. (2000) Modulation of intrinsic cardiac neurons by spinal cord stimulation: implications for its therapeutic use in angina pectoris. Cardiovasc. Res., 47: 367–375.

Freedman, S.B. and Isner, J.M. (2001) Therapeutic angiogenesis for ischemic cardiovascular disease. J. Mol. Cell. Cardiol., 33: 379–393.

Gibbons, R.J., Chatterjee, K., Daley, J., Douglas, J.S., Fihn, S.D., Gardin, J.M., Grunwald, M.A., Levy, D., Lytle, B.W., O'Rourke, R.A., Schafer, W.P., Williams, S.V. (1999) ACC/AHA/ACP-ASIM guidelines for the management of patients with chronic stable angina: executive summary and recommendations. A Report of the American College of Cardiology/American Heart Association Task Force on Practice Guidelines (Committee on Management of Patients with Chronic Stable Angina). Circulation, 99: 2829–2848.

Gonzalez-Darder, J.M., Gonzalez-Martinez, V., and Canela-Moya, P. (1998) Cervical spinal cord stimulation in the treatment of severe angina pectoris. Neurosurg. Quarterly, 8: 16–23.

Greco, S., Auriti, A., Fiume, D., Gazzeri, G., Gentilucci, G., Antonini, L., and Santini, M. (1999) Spinal cord stimulation for the treatment of refractory angina pectoris: a two year follow-up. PACE, 22: 26–32.

Hautvast, R.W., Szabo, B.M., DeJongste, M.J.L., Hooijschuur, C.A.M., Lie, K.I., Staal, M.J., Meyler, W.J., Küther, R.F. and Zijlstra, G.J. (1993) Influence of spinal cord stimulation on left ventricular function in patients with refractory angina pectoris. 2nd International Symposium on Heart Failure – mechanisms and management.

Hautvast, R.W., Blanksma, P.K., DeJongste, M.J., Pruim, J., Van der Wall, E.E., Vaalburg, W., and Lie, K.I. (1996) Effect of spinal cord stimulation on myocardial blood flow assessed by positron emission tomography in patients with refractory angina pectoris. Am. J. Cardiol., 77: 462–467.

Hautvast, R.W., Ter Horst, G.J., DeJong, B.M., DeJongste, M.J., Blanksma, P.K., Paans, A.M., and Korf, J. (1997) Relative changes in regional cerebral blood flow during spinal cord stimulation in patients with refractory angina pectoris. Eur. J. Neurosci., 9: 1178–1183.

Hautvast, R., Brouwer, J., DeJongste, M., and Lie, K. (1998a) Effect of spinal cord stimulation on heart rate variability and myocardial ischemia in patients with chronic intractable angina pectoris – a prospective ambulatory electrocardiographic study. Clin. Cardiol., 21: 33–38.

Hautvast, R.W.M., DeJongste, M.J.L., Staal, M.J., Van Gilst, W.H., and Lie, K. (1998b) Spinal cord stimulation in chronic intractable angina pectoris: a randomized, controlled efficacy study. Am. Heart J., 136: 1114–1120.

Heberden, W. (1772) Some account of a disorder of the breast. Med. Trans., 2: 59–67.

Jessurun, G.A., DeJongste, M.J., and Blanksma, P.K. (1996) Current views on neurostimulation in the treatment of cardiac ischemic syndromes. Pain, 66: 109–116.

Jessurun, G., Meeder, J., and DeJongste, M. (1997a) Defining the problem of intractable angina. Pain Rev., 4: 89–99.

Jessurun, G., Ten Vaarwerk, I., DeJongste, M., Tio, R.A., and Staal, M.J. (1997b) Sequalae of spinal cord stimulation for refractory angina pectoris. Reliability and safety profile of long-term clinical application, Coron. Artery Dis., 8: 33–37.

Jessurun, G.A., Tio, R.A., De Jongste, M.J., Hautvast, R.W., Den Heijer, P., and Crijns, H.J. (1998) Coronary blood flow dynamics during transcutaneous electrical nerve stimulation for stable angina pectoris associated with severe narrowing of one major coronary artery. Am. J. Cardiol., 82: 921–926.

Jessurun, G.A., DeJongste, M.J., Hautvast, R.W., Tio, R.A., Brouwer, J., Van Lelieveld, S., and Crijns, H.J. (1999) Clinical follow-up after cessation of chronic electrical neuromodulation in patients with severe coronary artery disease: a prospective randomized controlled study on putative involvement of sympathetic activity. Pacing Clin. Electrophysiol., 22: 1432–1439.

Keefer, C.S. and Resnik, W.H. (1928) Angina pectoris: a syndrome caused by anoxemia of the myocardium. Arch. Int. Med., 41: 769.

Khogali, S.S., Miller, M., Rajesh, P.B., Murray, R.G., and Beattie, J.M. (1999) Video-assisted thoracoscopic sympathectomy for severe intractable angina. Eur. J. Cardiothorac. Surg., 16(Suppl 1): S95–S98.

Kidd, P.M. (1998) Integrative cardiac revitalization: bypass surgery, angioplasty and chelation. Benefits, risks and limitations. Altern. Med. Rev., 3: 4–17 Review.

Kim, C.K., Bartholomew, B.A., Mastin, S.T., Taasan, V.C., Carson, K.M., and Sheps, D.S. (2003) Detection and reproducibility of mental stress-induced myocardial ischemia with Tc-99m sestamibi SPECT in normal and coronary artery diseased populations. J. Nucl. Cardiol., 10: 56–62.

Kingma, J.G., Jr., Linderoth, B., Ardell, J.L., Armour, J.A., DeJongste, M.J., and Foreman, R.D. (2001) Neuromodulation therapy does not influence blood flow distribution or left-ventricular dynamics during acute myocardial ischemia. Auton. Neurosci., 91: 47–54.

Kraatz, E.G., Misfeld, M., Jungbluth, B., and Sievers, H.H. (2001) Survival after transmyocardial laser revascularization in relation to nonlasered perfused myocardial zones. Ann. Thorac. Surg., 71: 532–536.

Kujacic, V., Eliasson, T., Mannheimer, C., Jablonskiene, D., Augustinsson, L.-E., and Emanuelsson, H. (1993) Assessment of the influence of spinal cord stimulation (SCS) on left ventricular function in patients with severe angina pectoris: an echocardiographic study. Eur. Heart J., 14: 1238–1244.

Linderoth, B. and Foreman, R.D. (1999) Physiology of spinal cord stimulation: review and update. Neuromodulation, 2: 150.

Mannheimer, C. (1984) Gothenburg, Thesis.

Mannheimer, C. and Eliasson, T. (1995) *Spinal Cord Stimulation*. IIDietrich Steinkopff Verlag, Darmstadt.

Mannheimer, C., Carlsson, C.-A., Ericsson, K., Vedin, A., and Wilhelmsson, C. (1982) Transcutaneous electrical nerve stimulation in severe angina pectoris. Eur. Heart J., 3: 297–302.

Mannheimer, C., Carlsson, C.-A., Emanuelsson, H., Vedin, A., Waagstein, F., and Wilhelmsson, C. (1985) The effects of transcutaneous electrical nerve stimulation in patients with severe angina pectoris. Circulation, 71: 308–316.

Mannheimer, C., Carlsson, C.-A., Vedin, A., and Wilhelmsson, C. (1986) Transcutaneous electrical nerve stimulation (TENS) in angina pectoris. Pain, 26: 291–300.

Mannheimer, C., Augustinsson, L.-E., Carlsson, C.-A., Manhem, K., and Wilhelmsson, C. (1988) Epidural spinal electrical stimulation in severe angina pectoris. Br. Heart J., 59: 56–61.

Mannheimer, C., Emanuelsson, H., Waagstein, F., and Wilhelmsson, C. (1989) Influence of naloxone on the effects of high frequency transcutaneous electrical nerve stimulation in angina pectoris induced by atrial pacing. Br. Heart J., 62: 36–42.

Mannheimer, C., Emanuelsson, H., Larsson, G., Waagstein, F., Augustinsson, L.-E., Eliasson, T., and Nilsson, A. (1991) Myocardial release of endogenous opioids in the human heart and the effects of epidural spinal electrical stimulation in pacing-induced angina pectoris. J. Am. Coll. Cardiol., 17: 107.

Mannheimer, C., Eliasson, T., Andersson, B., Berg, H., Augustinsson, L.-E., Emanuelsson, H., and Waagstein, F. (1993a) Effects of spinal cord stimulation in angina pectoris induced by pacing and possible mechanisms of action. Br. Med. J., 307: 477–480.

Mannheimer, C., Eliasson, T., Andersson, B., Berg, H., Augustinsson, L.-E., Emanuelsson, H., and Waagstein, F. (1993b) Spinal cord stimulation (SCS) in pacing-induced angina pectoris. J. Am. Coll. Cardiol., 21: 324A.

Mannheimer, C., Eliasson, T., Augustinsson, L.-E., Blomstrand, C., Emanuelsson, H., Larsson, S., Norrsell, H., and Hjalmarsson, Å. (1998) Electrical stimulation versus coronary artery bypass grafting in severe angina pectoris. Circulation, 97: 1157–1163.

Mannheimer, C., Camici, P., Chester, M.R., Collins, A., DeJongste, M., Eliasson, T., Follath, F., Hellemans, I., Herlitz, J., Luscher, T., Pasic, M., Thelle, D. (2002) The problem of chronic refractory angina; report from the ESC Joint Study Group on the Treatment of Refractory Angina. Eur. Heart J., 23: 355–370.

Marber, M., Walker, D., and Yellon, D. (1993) Spinal cord stimulation or ischaemic preconditioning?. Br. Med. J., 307: 737.

Maseri, A. (1995) Chapter 4: the coronary circulation. In: A. Maseri (Ed.), *Ischemic Heart Disease* (pp. 71). Churchill Livingston, New York.

Melzack, R. and Wall, P.D. (1965) Pain mechanisms: a new theory. Science, 150: 971–979.

Meyler, W., De Jongste, M., and Rolf, C. (1994) Clinical evaluation of pain treatment with TENS in patients with different pain syndromes. Pain, 10: 22–27.

Mobilia, G., Zuin, G., Zanco, P., Di Pede, F., Pinato, G., Neri, G., Cargnel, S., Raviele, A., Ferlin, G., Buchberger, R. (1998) Effects of spinal cord stimulation on regional myocardial blood flow in patients with refractory angina. A positron emission tomography study. G. Ital. Cardiol., 28(10): 1113–1119.

Mouallem, M., Schwartz, E., and Farfel, Z. (2000) Prolonged oral morphine therapy for severe angina pectoris. J. Pain Symtom. Manage., 19: 393–397.

Mukherjee, D., Bhatt, D., and Roe, M.T. (1999) Direct myocardial revascularization and angiogenesis: how many patients might be eligible?. Am. J. Cardiol., 84: 598–600.

Mulcahy, D., Knight, C., Stables, R., and Fox, K. (1994) Lasers, burns, cuts, tingles and pumps: a consideration of alternative treatments for intractable angina. Br. Heart J., 71: 406–407.

Murphy, D. and Giles, K. (1987) Dorsal column stimulation for pain relief from intractable angina pectoris. Pain, 28: 365–368.

Murray, S., Carson, K., Ewings, P., Collins, P., and James, M. (1999) Spinal cord stimulation significantly decreases the need for acute hospital admission for chest pain in patients with refractory angina pectoris. Heart, 82: 89–92.

Norrsell, H., Eliasson, T., Mannheimer, C., Augustinsson, L.E., Bergh, C.H., Andersson, B., Waagstein, F., and Friberg, P. (1997) Effects of pacing-induced myocardial stress and spinal cord stimulation on whole body and cardiac norepinephrine spillover. Eur. Heart. J., 18: 1890–1896.

Norrsell, H., Eliasson, T., Albertsson, P., Augustinsson, L.E., Emanuelsson, H., Eriksson, P., and Mannheimer, C. (1998) Effects of spinal cord stimulation on coronary blood flow velocity. Coron. Artery Dis., 9: 273–278.

Norrsell, H., Pilhall, M., Eliasson, T., and Mannheimer, C. (2000) Effects of spinal cord stimulation and coronary artery bypass grafting on myocardial ischemia and heart rate variability: further results from the ESBY study. Cardiology, 94(1): 12–18.

Olausson, K., Magnusdottir, H., Lurje, L., Wennerblom, B., Emanuelsson, H., and Ricksten, S.E. (1997) Anti-ischemic and anti-anginal effects of thoracic epidural anesthesia versus those of conventional medical therapy in the treatment of severe refractory unstable angina pectoris. Circulation, 96: 2178–2182.

Palumbo, L.T. and Lulu, D.J. (1966) Anterior transtheoracic upper dorsal sympathectomy; current results. Arch. Surg., 92: 247–257.

Panza, J.A. (2002) Myocardial ischemia and the pains of the heart (Editorial). N. Engl. J. Med., 346: 1934–1935.

Parmley, W.W. (1997) Optimal treatment of stable angina, Cardiology, 88 Suppl 3, 27–31 Review.

Reynolds, J.L. (1974) A practical approach to the management of angina. Drugs, 8: 208–216.

Rosen, S., Paulesu, E., Frith, C., Frackowiak, S., Davies, G., Jones, T., and Camici, P. (1994) Central nervous pathways mediating angina pectoris. Lancet, 344: 147–150.

Ross, R. and Glomset, J.A. (1976) The pathogenesis of atherosclerosis (first of two parts). N. Engl. J. Med., 295: 369–377.

Sanderson, J.E., Brooksby, P., Waterhouse, D., Palmer, R.B.G., and Neubauer, K. (1992) Epidural spinal electrical stimulation for severe angina: a study of its effects on symptoms, exercise tolerance and degree of ischaemia. Eur. Heart J., 13: 628–633.

Sanderson, J., Ibrahim, B., Waterhouse, D., and Palmer, R. (1994) Spinal electrical stimulation for intractable angina – long-term clinical outcome and safety. Eur. Heart J., 15: 810–814.

Sanderson, J., Woo, K., Chung, H., Chan, W., Tse, L., and White, H. (1996) The effect of transcutaneous electrical nerve stimulation on coronary and systemic haemodynamics in syndrome X. Coron. Artery Dis., 7: 547–552.

Schoebel, F.C., Frazier, O.H., Jessurun, G.A., De Jongste, M.J., Kadipasaoglu, K.A., Jax, T.W., Heintzen, M.P., Cooley, D.A., Strauer, B.E., Leschke, M. (1997) Refractory angina pectoris in end-stage coronary artery disease: evolving therapeutic concepts. Am. Heart J., 134: 587–602.

Singh, B.N. (1983) Amiodarone: Historical development and pharmacologic profile, Am. Heart J., 106: 788–797 Review.

Strobos, M.A., Coenraads, P.J., De Jongste, M.J., and Ubels, F.L. (2001) Dermatitis caused by radio-frequency electromagnetic radiation. Contact Dermatitis, 44: 309.

Tanaka, S., Barron, K.W., Chandler, M.J., Linderoth, B., and Foreman, R.D. (2003) Role of primary afferents in spinal cord stimulation-induced vasodilation: characterization of fiber types. Brain Res., 959: 191–198.

TenVaarwerk, I., Jessurun, G., DeJongste, M., Andersen, C., Mannheimer, C., Eliasson, T., Tadema, W., and Staal, M. (1999) Clinical outcome of patients treated with spinal cord stimulation for therapeutically refractory angina pectoris. Heart, 82: 82–88.

Urano, H., Ikeda, H., Ueno, T., Matsumoto, T., Murohara, T., and Imaizumi, T. (2001) Enhanced external counterpulsation improves exercise tolerance, reduces exercise-induced myocardial ischemia and improves left ventricular diastolic filling in patients with coronary artery disease. J. Am. Coll. Cardiol., 37: 93–99.

Wannamethee, S.G., Shaper, A.G., and Walker, M. (2000) Physical activity and mortality in older men with diagnosed coronary heart disease. Circulation, 102: 1358–1363.

Wettervik, C., Claes, G., Drott, C., Emanuelsson, H., Lomsky, M., Radberg, G., and Tygesen, H. (1995) Endoscopic transthoracic sympathicotomy for severe angina. Lancet, 345: 97–98.

Wiener, L. and Cox, J.W. (1966) Influence of stellate ganglion block on angina pectoris and the post-exercise electrocardiogram. Am. J. Med. Sci., 252: 289–295.

Zamotrinsky, A., Afanasiev, S., Karpov, R.S., and Cherniavsky, A. (1997) Effects of electrostimulation of the vagus afferent endings in patients with coronary artery disease. Coron. Artery Dis., 8: 551–557.

Zamvar, V., Williams, D., Hall, J., Payne, N., Cann, C., Young, K., Karthikeyan, S., and Dunne, J. (2002) Assessment of neurocognitive impairment after off-pump and on-pump techniques for coronary artery bypass graft surgery: prospective randomised controlled trial. Br. Med. J., 30(325): 1268.

Zanger, D.R., Solomon, A.J., and Gersh, B.J. (2000) Contemporary management of angina: part II. Medical management of chronic stable angina. Am. Fam. Physician, 61: 129–138.

Electrical Stimulation and the Relief of Pain
Pain Research and Clinical Management, Vol. 15
Edited by Brian A. Simpson

CHAPTER 11

Spinal cord stimulation: mechanisms of action in neuropathic and ischaemic pain

Björn A. Meyerson* and Bengt Linderoth

Department of Clinical Neuroscience, Section of Neurosurgery, Karolinska Institute/Karolinska Hospital, S-171 76 Stockholm, Sweden

Abstract

In spite of having been extensively utilized for more than three decades in the management of various forms of chronic pain, spinal cord stimulation (SCS) is still poorly understood – more specifically, very little is known about why and how it acts. Originally, SCS was a spin-off from the gate-control theory which however does not suffice to explain its clinical effects. In the 1970s and 1980s many experimental studies were performed on intact, anaesthetized animals subjected to peripheral noxious (mechanical, thermal, electrical) stimuli. SCS was generally applied during short periods of time and with high intensity, and it was demonstrated that the nociceptive responses could be attenuated. However, considering that clinical SCS appears not to be efficacious for nociceptive pain, experiments on animal models of mononeuropathy appear more appropriate. SCS applied in such animals (rats) may suppress mechanical hypersensitivity (allodynia) and neuronal hyperexcitability in the spinal dorsal horn. These effects are associated with increased spinal release of gamma aminobutyric acid (GABA) and decreased release of excitatory amino acids. The anti-allodynic effect of SCS may be enhanced by intrathecal (i.t.) administration of $GABA_B$ agonists, adenosine, gabapentin, pregabalin and clonidine. This has led to clinical trials with the combination of SCS and i.t. baclofen. Evidence has been recently presented in favour of the involvement of a supraspinal mechanism in the SCS mode of action whereas data from other studies suggest that instead the role of segmental spinal mechanisms is pivotal. There are also somewhat conflicting experimental data on the possible effect of SCS on C fibre-mediated nociception. The mechanisms involved in the effect of SCS on pain due to peripheral tissue ischaemia have been subjected to only a few experimental studies in patients and in animals. Such pain is predominantly nociceptive and there is much evidence that its alleviation is secondary to a stimulation-induced reduction of the ischaemia resulting from a vasodilatory effect. A peripheral vasodilatation could be produced by either an antidromic activation of primary afferents or a sympathetically mediated vasodilatation. Animal data indicate that both mechanisms may be responsible and that the former presumably acts via a peripheral release of calcitonin gene related peptide (CGRP), and the latter may operate more or less depending upon the activity level of the sympathetic efferent control. It is concluded that a better understanding of the mode of action of SCS when applied either for neuropathic or ischaemic pain is a prerequisite for the further advancement of the method as well as for the development of stringent patient selection criteria.

Keywords: Spinal cord stimulation; Neuropathic pain; Ischaemic pain; GABA; Adenosine; Microdialysis; Mechanisms

*Correspondence to: Dr. B.A. Meyerson. Phone: + 46 8 5177 4749; Fax: + 46 8 307091; E-mail: bjorn.meyerson@ks.se

1. Background

In the most cited paper in modern pain literature, that on the gate-control theory, the authors suggested that the therapeutic implication of their model would be to selectively activate large fibres for the control of pain (Melzack and Wall, 1965). Actually, Wall and Sweet (see White and Sweet, 1969) had already in October 1965 treated a patient suffering from pain due to median nerve injury with stimulation of the nerve via an implanted electrode. We are also told that Wall and Sweet tested the theory by sticking needle electrodes into their own infraorbital nerves and observed that low-intensity stimulation produced analgesia to pin prick in the territory of the nerve. It should be noted, however, that the idea that pain may occur as a result of imbalance between large and fine fibre systems had also been much discussed by several previous researchers. Thus, Head and Thompson (1906) argued that discriminative sensations, such as touch, normally exert an inhibitory influence on the impulses subserving pain. Head further postulated that facilitation or inhibition of sensory impulses occurs in the posterior horn before they are relayed to secondary neurons. The notion that epicritic sensibility exerts an inhibitory influence over protopathic sensibility was the basis for trials with sensory thalamic stimulation already performed in 1962 in Paris by Mazars and colleagues (1973, 1975b). There is reason in this context also to refer to Noordenbos (1959) who described the inhibitory influence of fast on slow fibres as 'fast blocks slow'. Another example of an early account of interaction between coarse and thin fibres is a publication by Zotterman (1939) who postulated that hyperalgesia may be due to absence of impulses rapidly conducted to the brain.

Although one may argue that the basics of the gate-control theory were not that novel, it was based on experiments using modern electrophysiological techniques and these findings were well synthesized and presented in a form representing a new conceptualisation of pain. The theory was subsequently much criticized but its simplicity has

made it useful as a framework for understanding the dynamics of pain generation and pain control. Moreover, its clinical implications have been of tremendous importance since it triggered the development of various forms of electric stimulation as a new treatment modality. In modern pain research, interest is focussed on the pivotal role of the profound plasticity of the nervous system in the generation and maintenance as well as for the modulation of pain. In retrospect, the gate concept for pain control therefore appears to provide a relatively static and mechanistic model that does not account for the dynamics of the pathophysiology of chronic pain.

The first trials with spinal cord stimulation (SCS) were reported by Shealy and colleagues (1967). Experiments in cats had shown that in the awake state stimulation of the dorsal aspect of the spinal cord could block reactions to peripheral painful stimuli. In a sense, the relevance of the gate-control theory for its clinical application in the form of SCS is paradoxical since it was based on animal experiments in which peripheral noxious stimuli were employed similar to the case with Shealy's cats. One would thus expect that SCS could be useful also for nociceptive, acute and chronic pain, while clinical experience has taught us that it is effective only for some neuropathic forms of pain. Transcutaneous nerve stimulation (TENS) was introduced shortly after SCS but was at that time merely utilized for screening patients for SCS. In a sense, TENS may be seen as a more direct application of the gate concept since it is also effective for nociceptive forms of pain, particularly when applied with low-frequency, high-intensity stimuli.

Today it is also known that SCS may effectively relieve ischaemic pain of peripheral origin and angina pectoris. This seems paradoxical since such pains are principally of a nociceptive character. However, the effect in these conditions is conceivably secondary to a decrease of the tissue ischaemia produced by the stimulation and subserved by mechanisms different from those involved in relief of neuropathic pain. It was first reported by Cook and colleagues in 1976 that SCS may effectively relieve pain associated with disturbed peripheral circulation due to arterio-sclerosis or to diabetic vasculopathy (for review see, e.g. Augustinsson et al., 1997). In particular the ischaemic pain that is present in conditions with peripheral vasospasm (Raynaud's phenom-enon, Buerger's disease, scleroderma) may respond positively to SCS (for reviews, see e.g. Herreros et al., 1994; Horsch and Claeys, 1995). It should be pointed out that besides the relief of ischaemic pain SCS has also been demonstrated to exert beneficial effects on the ischaemic condition *per se* (for reviews, see e.g. Augustinsson et al., 1995; Linderoth et al., 1995).

Despite the extensive practice of SCS for more than three decades and the growing interest in its application for new indications, our knowledge and understanding of the physiological and biochemical mechanisms involved are still frag-mentary, and this has probably hampered the further development and dissemination of the method. Not until recent years have some novel experimental data accumulated which have shed some light on the possible mode of action of SCS both in neuropathic pain and in angina pectoris (for reviews, see Roberts and Rees, 1994; Linderoth and Foreman, 1999; Linderoth and Meyerson, 2000; Meyerson and Linderoth, 2000).

There is evidence indicating that the mechan-isms involved, when SCS is applied for pain in ischaemic tissue and for neuropathic pain, are fundamentally different (e.g. Linderoth and Meyerson, 1995) and therefore they will be discussed separately.

2. Mode of action in neuropathic pain

2.1. Observations and experimental findings in man

Anecdotal observations reported even in the first clinical studies of SCS indicated that the treatment was inefficacious for chronic and acute, as well as experimentally induced, nociceptive pain. Thus, in a patient who is effectively treated for chronic sciatic pain a new pain resulting from a fracture of the same leg was not alleviated by the stimulation (Nashold et al., 1972). It is also known that SCS does not influence the pain from ischaemic ulcers although the resting, deep pain may be effectively relieved as a result of peripheral vasodilatation. However, in clinical practice the question of whether SCS may, at least to some extent, alleviate nociceptive pain still appears to be a controversial issue. In many published series of patients subjected to SCS, 'low back pain' is a common indication although its responsiveness is yet to be fully established (e.g. Barolat, 1999). Most authors contend that SCS predominantly influences the 'radiating pain component' or 'pain in the leg' which represents lumbosacral rhizopathy (North et al., 1993) but there are also those who claim that the pain component confined to the axial, lumbar portion of the back may be alleviated (Barolat et al., 2001; Ohnmeiss and Rashbaum, 2001; for discussion, see North and Guarino, 1999). It is most probable that this latter pain is essentially nociceptive but relevant studies fail to supply detailed mappings of the stimulation-induced paraesthesiae to confirm that it is possible with this form of stimulation to provoke paraesthesiae in midline structures. Moreover, in these studies it is difficult to identify precisely the patient selection criteria since the relative severity and extension of pain in the lower back and pain associated with rhizopathy, respectively, are poorly described. Hardly any attempts have been made to identify and analyze the low back pain components as being nociceptive or neurogenic.

A few studies have been performed on patients addressing the issue of the modulatory effect of SCS on somatosensory functions, in particular acute nociception. In the first clinical reports on the applications of SCS, it was stated that the threshold of cutaneous-induced pain may be ele-vated (Shealy et al., 1967) but this finding could not be reproduced by others (Nashold et al., 1972). In 1975, Lindblom and Meyerson studied the perception of cutaneous mechanical pain induced by the use of a calibrated flat forceps in patients undergoing SCS treatment. The stimulus was applied in regions both inside and outside the field of SCS-produced paraesthesiae. The thresholds were significantly increased only in sites displaying hyperalgesia and allodynia. In normal skin, there was no effect on the thresholds, though the painful stimulus was applied in an area covered by the paraesthesiae. Doerr et al. (1978) studied the effect of SCS on perception and pain thresholds using electrical stimulation of the skin. They found that only after long-term SCS was there a significant increase of both thresholds, but this effect did not relate to the relief of the spontaneous pain treated by the SCS.

A possible effect on heat pain thresholds has been studied employing the quantitative sensory testing (QST) technique (Lindblom and Meyerson, 1976a). In that study, there was no alteration of thresholds in normal skin but, when tested in areas of thermal hyperalgesia, the abnormally low thresholds were elevated towards normal levels and the warmth–cold difference limen (range of perceived sensation) was normalized. The findings of Lindblom and Meyerson have been challenged by Marchand and co-workers (1991, 1993) who reported that SCS could alter the ratings of cutaneous heat pain induced by a contact thermode. There was an elevation of the heat pain threshold from 48.5° before to 49.4°C after SCS. The testing was performed in normal skin and it is unlikely that the minute threshold increase of heat threshold of approximately 1°C reflects an anti-nociceptive effect corresponding to that on severe clinical pain.

It is reasonable to assume that the SCS-induced paraesthesiae can interfere with the perception of tactile vibratory stimuli applied also to normal skin. In fact, it has been shown that SCS causes an increase of these thresholds as well as of the perception of supra-threshold tactile stimuli (Lindblom and Meyerson, 1976b). This is presumably the reason why some patients may experience a slight disturbance of gait when the SCS-produced paraesthesiae are felt in the legs.

The experimentally demonstrated time-course of the changes of both threshold and supra-threshold sensations evoked by tactile and vibratory stimuli during SCS, and the fact that these changes may be present also outside the area of paraesthesiae, indicate that SCS influences mechanoreceptive functions by producing a central inhibitory state.

Although it is universally accepted that the presence of paraesthesiae, indicating the activation of the dorsal columns (DCs), is a prerequisite for pain relief, it has also been argued that the tingling and vibratory sensations are merely epiphenomena and that the therapeutic effects could instead be exerted via the activation of pathways other than the DC. One possible stimulation target could be the dorsolateral funiculus (DLF), which is known to contain descending pain controlling pathways. However, most of the fibres in the DLF are relatively thin and therefore have a high threshold. In a recent morphometric study (Feirabend et al., 2002) it was concluded that it is unlikely that even the largest DLF fibres are recruited by SCS. An alternative would be a conduction block of the spinothalamic fibres partly as a result of 'collision' between impulses mediating pain and the activation produced by the SCS (Larson et al., 1974; Campbell, 1981; Campbell et al., 1990). However, this explanation seems less likely in view of the fact that therapeutic SCS is never perceived as painful, which would be expected with activation of spinothalamic pathways, and also the majority of these fibres are thin and have a high activation threshold. Moreover, nociceptive transmission in the spinal cord is not blocked or substantially attenuated by SCS since the perception of acute or experimentally induced nociceptive pain is spared (Lindblom and Meyerson, 1975, 1976a; see also Price, 1991). A strong support for the crucial role of the DC in SCS is the fact that the treatment generally fails in patients suffering from pain associated with extensive deafferentation due to degeneration after an extensive peripheral nerve lesion or direct injury of the DC fibres. Furthermore, it is well known that SCS should always be applied ipsilaterally to the pain.

The possibility that SCS may inhibit also nociceptive input at a segmental spinal level is substantiated by the finding in patients that the stimulation may depress a nociceptive flexor reflex (Garcia-Larrea et al., 1989). Electrical stimuli applied to the sural nerve territory induce a contraction of the biceps femoris when the intensity of the stimulation is perceived as a 'pricking' pain sensation. This flexor response, generally referred to as RIII (Willer, 1977), appears with a latency of about 80 ms and conceivably represents the activation of Aδ afferent fibres. It has been demonstrated that this reflex may be attenuated by SCS and that the effect is correlated with the clinical pain relieving effect. However, the observed RIII suppression was short-lasting and in only a few of the patients tested did it persist for more than 10 min after cessation of the SCS. These findings appear to be clinically useful as an objective correlate to the pain relieving effect of SCS but are difficult to explain in view of the fact that SCS is otherwise mostly effective for neurogenic forms of pain and furthermore does not influence either novel acute pain or evoked, experimental pain resulting from Aδ-fibre activation. It should also be emphasized that the inhibited RIII reflex does not represent C fibre activation. Moreover, it should be noted that the reflex attenuation during SCS might be due to an effect on motor neuron excitability, since it has been shown that SCS when applied for spasticity may also influence the so-called H-reflex (Feeney and Gold, 1980).

2.2. Neurophysiological mechanisms studied in normal animals

Following the initial animal experiments by Shealy numerous studies were performed in the subsequent decade aiming at the elucidation of the mechanisms involved in the SCS pain relieving effect. A typical, early study was that of Handwerker and colleagues (1975) published in the second issue of the first volume of Pain in 1975. In the rat they demonstrated complete suppression of dorsal horn

(DH) neuronal activity evoked by heating the hindpaw during acute stimulation of the DCs (Fig. 1). With the use of graded noxious electrical peripheral stimulation activating polymodal DH neurons (Feldman, 1975), it could be shown that SCS had a selective presynaptic inhibitory effect on Aδ and C fibre activity. It was also demonstrated that inhibition could be induced by activation of low-threshold fibres originating from the fringe of the nociceptor receptive field, and these fibres conceivably project to the DCs (Hillman and Wall, 1969). In a study by Dubuisson (1989), it was shown that SCS in cats induced activation of DH cells in lamina 1 through 3 consistent with direct excitatory synaptic input from DC collaterals. The deeper cells, conceivably of a wide-dynamic-range (WDR) type, in lamina 4–5 responding to noxious peripheral input were also inhibited. This effect was assumed to involve a network of interneurons, in or near the substantia gelatinosa.

It has generally been assumed that stimulation of the DC gives rise to antidromic activation involving collaterals which, in the DH, indirectly via interneurons or directly via pre- or post-synaptic activation, may inhibit second-order nociceptive neurons. As discussed by Foreman and co-workers (1976) and by Willis (1985), antidromic activation of DC pathways originating from DH cells in lamina 3–4 and terminating in the DC nuclei may be of importance.

More recently, Chandler et al. (1993) and Foreman (1995) have conducted studies on the SCS effects on cardiac pain but applicable to somatic nociceptive pain. Spinothalamic tract cells were peripherally activated by bradykinin or pinch and found to be inhibited by SCS. Further analysis revealed that SCS preferentially suppressed high-threshold, nociceptive-specific cells rather than WDR cells.

In addition to the notion of a specific inhibitory effect of SCS on nociceptive DH neurons, a more direct block of transmission of pain signals in the spinothalamic tract has been proposed. In a study by Larson and colleagues (1974), it was reported that in some patients with intense

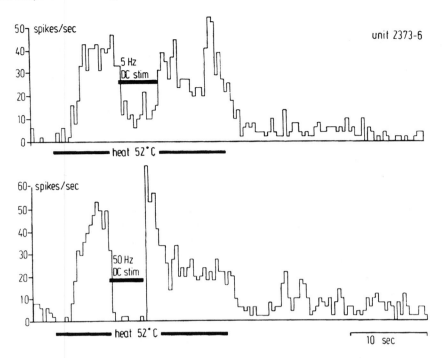

Fig. 1. Recordings from DH class 2 neurons (WDR) in cat. Discharge in response to radiant heat stimulation of the skin. Electrical stimulation of high intensity was applied to the DC at the L2 level. The suppressive effect was segmental since the spinal cord rostral to the stimulation was blocked. Apart from the original work of Shealy in 1967, this is the first experimental study in animals aiming at elucidating the mechanisms of pain relief with SCS. It is also a typical example of the type of experimental design that was employed in the field during the 1970s and 1980s. (From Handwerker, Iggo and Zimmermann, 1975, with permission.)

pain very high-intensity stimulation was required and in experiments on monkeys SCS was found to abolish evoked potentials. On the basis of these observations it was concluded that SCS produces local changes in the spinal cord resulting in a block of neuronal transmission. It was also proposed that pain relief was the result of 'collision' between impulses mediating pain and those induced by SCS (Campbell, 1981). This idea led to trials in which the stimulating electrode was applied on the ventral aspect of the cord that, however, never proved to be successful.

It should be noted that, at variance with the time course of the clinical application of SCS, the stimulation in virtually all animal experiments until the early 1990s was applied for short periods of time (milliseconds or seconds) and with single, conditional (e.g. Emmers and Ruderman, 1974) or short trains of pulses, often with high intensity.

Moreover, the observed inhibitory effects were present only concomitantly with the SCS while clinical pain relief typically outlasts therapeutic stimulation. Only a few animal studies have recorded longer periods (up to 30 min) of post-SCS inhibition of DH nociceptive discharge (Lindblom et al., 1977; Rees and Roberts, 1989). In a study on cats by Pearl and Anderson (1977) it was found that low-intensity SCS, applied for up to 10 min, did not influence responses in the nucleus reticularis gigantocellularis evoked by peripheral C fibre electrical activation.

In a few studies on intact animals the effect of SCS on the flexor reflex has been examined and these results have been contradictory. Thus, it was reported to be partially but consistently attenuated by Saadé et al. (1985; see also below), whereas McMillan and co-workers (1986) found it instead to be moderately facilitated.

Recently, the effect of SCS on long-term-potentiation (LTP) has been investigated (Wallin et al., 2003). It was found that the duration of the LTP response to C fibre activation was significantly decreased, from about 6 h to about 30 min. It should be noted that only the sensitized C fibre response was influenced while neither the normal C- nor Aβ-functions were affected.

To the best of our knowledge there are only two studies involving acute, nociceptive pain in which SCS has been applied in intact, awake animals. Actually, Shealy and colleagues in 1967 reported that SCS applied in cats produced a profound generalized analgesia to intense noxious stimuli. In a recent study, we have applied SCS, via a permanently implanted electrode, in rats pre-treated by carrageenan (CAR) injected in a hind-paw (Cui et al., 1999). This manoeuvre produces oedema and local tenderness resulting in a decreased withdrawal and/or localizing threshold to mechanical stimuli indicative of hyperalgesia/allodynia. Behavioural changes and local signs of inflammation and inflammatory pain may last for about 7 days and therefore the noxious nature of CAR may represent subacute rather than acute pain. There is evidence that at least the initial phase of the hyperalgesia following CAR-induced hind paw inflammation is related to sensitization of nociceptors as well as to activation of previously unresponsive afferents (Kocher et al., 1987). It was found that in the acute phase, 3 h after the injection, SCS *enhanced* the CAR-induced hyperalgesia and oedema. In contrast, in the subacute phase at 3–5 days after the injection, SCS instead *suppressed* the hyperalgesia although the oedema was still increased. It should be noted, however, that this suppressive effect on the hyperalgesia was very short-lasting and did not exhibit the protracted post-stimulatory SCS effect that we have previously demonstrated on tactile allodynia as a result of peripheral nerve injury (see below). Circumstantial evidence suggests that the oedema augmentation by SCS in the acute phase may be the result of enhanced vasodilatation with fluid extravasation. The attenuation of hyperalgesia in the subacute phase may be due to an inhibitory effect of SCS on A fibre-mediated WDR neuronal hyperactivity but a direct effect on sensitized nociceptive-specific second-order neurons cannot be excluded. It may be questioned whether CAR-induced effects are indeed relevant for the chronic, nociceptive forms of pain commonly encountered in clinical practice and sometimes considered for SCS treatment (e.g. axial pain confined to the lumbar region). It should be emphasized that this study cannot be considered as a final proof that SCS may also influence chronic, C fibre-mediated nociceptive pain and further experimental studies performed on more appropriate pain models are needed.

2.3. Neurophysiological mechanisms studied in animal models of neuropathic pain

It is evident today that most of the experimental SCS studies performed during the 1970s and 1980s are of limited relevance: they were performed on anaesthetized but otherwise intact animals; purely noxious and phasic peripheral stimuli were used; the SCS parameters were set as generally used in electrophysiological experiments; SCS was often applied for short periods of time. Thus, it appears that the experiments were not designed to mimic the clinical features of SCS, for example: the preferential effect on neuropathic versus nociceptive chronic pain; low-intensity stimulation just above the threshold for inducing paraesthesiae; application of SCS during relatively long periods of time (10–30 min). Nevertheless these earlier studies provided valuable data on the 'normal' physiology related to SCS, and they further constitute a basis for designing experiments with the use of more adequate animal models.

A major problem is the choice of animal models of pain relevant for experimental SCS studies. Although a number of different models claiming to represent neuropathic pain has been introduced in recent years, and although these animals all exhibit behavioural signs that may be interpreted as *evoked* pain there is no evidence suggesting that they suffer on-going, *spontaneous* pain. Clinical observations suggest that there is no clear correlation between spontaneous pain and any kind of abnormal evoked pain or sensory abnormality. Thus, it has been reported that the thresholds in cold, tactile and pinch allodynia responded differently to various forms of treatment in spite of good relief of the spontaneous pain (Lindblom, 1985).

Until very recently, models of mononeuropathy produced according to Bennett and Xie (1988) and Seltzer and colleagues (1990) were the most commonly used in research on neuropathic pain. A common feature of these models is that following the partial nerve lesion the animals develop hypersensitivity to both tactile and thermal innocuous stimuli applied to the nerve-injured hind-paw. In the last decade, in a series of studies, we have employed these models as well as another more recently developed one (Gazelius et al., 1996). In rats with mononeuropathy, we have implanted a miniature spinal cord electrode permitting stimulation in the freely moving animal with parameters similar to those utilized clinically. We have focussed on the SCS effect on tactile allodynia using von Frey filaments. After 10–20 min of SCS a substantial portion of the animals exhibit a marked tendency towards normalization of the abnormally low tactile thresholds in the nerve-lesioned hind-paw (Meyerson et al., 1995; Fig. 2). The threshold elevation persists for up to 40 min after cessation of the SCS. This effect on tactile allodynia is in fact very similar to what is seen in the clinic and systematically assessed in the study by Lindblom and Meyerson (1975) referred to above.

There is a good deal of evidence that the phenomenon of tactile allodynia is mediated mainly via low-threshold $A\beta$ fibres (Campbell et al., 1988; Woolf and Doubell, 1994) and that it represents a central state of hyperexcitability (e.g. Bennett, 1993). The plasticity changes in the spinal cord following peripheral nerve injury are manifested by persistently augmented responsiveness and a high degree of spontaneous discharge of DH

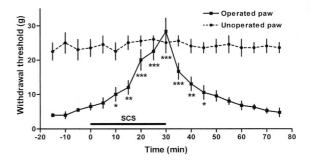

Fig. 2. Experiments performed in rats with partial injury of the left sciatic nerve and exhibiting increased sensitivity to innocuous tactile stimuli (von Frey filaments) applied to the nerve-injured paw ('allodynia'). SCS was applied for 10 min with an intensity 2/3 of that evoking a motor response in the awake, freely moving animal. The marked anti-allodynic effect is represented by the increase in paw withdrawal thresholds. Note that the SCS effect significantly outlasted the stimulation session. (From Meyerson et al., 1995, unpublished.)

neurons. It appears that these changes of excitability affect WDR more than nociceptive-specific neurons (Sotgiu et al., 1995). It has been demonstrated that SCS may induce a significant and long-lasting suppression of both the exaggerated principal response as well as the after-discharges recorded from DH lamina 3–5 neurons in nerve-lesioned rats (Yakhnitsa et al., 1999; Fig. 3). In the clinical setting, this suppression of WDR cell activity could correspond to the beneficial effect of SCS not only on the allodynia but also on the spontaneous neuropathic pain.

The classical flexor reflex has been a commonly studied marker of a nociceptor event predominantly representing C fibre activation though it comprises also an early response component, which in the rat appears with a latency of about 12 ms. Conceivably, this initial response is mediated via $A\beta$ fibres. After partial sciatic nerve injury the threshold for eliciting this reflex in lightly anaesthetized animals was significantly decreased and SCS produced an increase of the threshold of the early component, but not of the late one, corresponding to the activation of $A\beta$ and C fibres, respectively. Conversely, SCS had no effect on the reflex recorded in the non-nerve

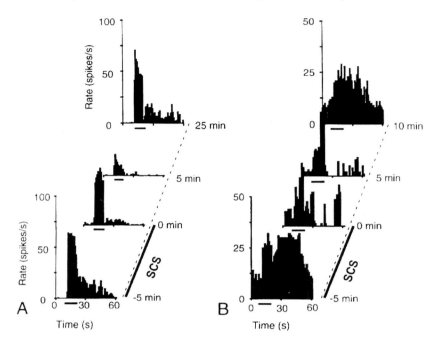

Fig. 3. Peristimulus time histograms of press-evoked responses recorded from two WDR DH neurons in a nerve-injured rat with tactile allodynia. SCS was applied with 'clinical' parameters for 5 min. Responses before SCS are depicted in the bottom graphs and time after cessation of SCS is shown to the right. Bars under each histogram represents duration of applied paw pressure. Note that the pressure was gentle and innocuous. (From Yakhnitsa et al., 1999, with permission.)

injured leg (Meyerson et al., 1995; Ren et al., 1996).

The behavioural phenomenon of autotomy (scratching, licking and biting the affected limb), following sciatic nerve or spinal root section, has been considered as another model of neuropathic (deafferentation) pain, though its clinical relevance has been challenged (Gybels and Kupers, 1991). Rats subjected to sciatic nerve axotomy have been subjected to daily 30-min sessions of SCS applied for 10 days and it was demonstrated that there was a long-lasting (70 days) reduction of both the occurrence and severity of autotomy. This effect was particularly more prominent if the SCS treatment period was started a few days before the nerve section (Gao et al., 1996). That latter finding suggests that pre-emptive SCS may have a priming effect on spinal cord excitability similar to the effects of pre-emptive modulation of the GABAergic system on the incidence of signs of mononeuropathy (Cui et al., 1997c).

2.4. Spinal and/or supraspinal site of action?

In the early experimental studies in the 1970s and early 1980s on the mode of action of SCS interest was already focussed on the issue of segmental versus supraspinal mechanisms. It is well known that the presence of paraesthesiae in the painful area, indicating the activation of the DCs, is a prerequisite for pain relief. For obvious reasons supraspinal centres are involved as the orthodromic activation of the DCs is relayed via the DC nuclei and projected onto nuclei in the brain stem, to the sensory thalamus and to the cortex. However, it cannot be excluded that the tingling and vibratory sensations evoked by SCS are merely epiphenomena, and that the therapeutic effects are instead exerted via the activation of other pathways than the DCs. As will be further discussed below it should be noted that peripheral vasodilatation may be produced by SCS applied with an intensity subthreshold for evoking paraesthesiae (Linderoth, 1995).

In some studies the site of nociceptive control has been allocated to high CNS centres. Larson and colleagues (1974) concluded from studies on both monkeys and patients that, although SCS seemed to block neuronal transmission also on the spinal level, prolonged alteration of the cortical-evoked potentials following SCS pointed to a supraspinal mechanism behind the pain relief. Nyquist and Greenhoof (1973) demonstrated depressed activity in the centro-median nucleus in response to SCS in cats and drew the conclusions that pain inhibition may take place also at the thalamic level. Bantli and colleagues (1975) observed attenuation of evoked potentials following SCS in the postero-lateral and the medial thalamus, and in the primary sensory area of the macaque monkey. Support for the involvement of supraspinal gating mechanisms has also been provided by Roberts and Rees (1994) who reported that SCS in the rat excites cells in the anterior pretectal nucleus from where a profound and long-lasting inhibition of nociceptive DH-neurons may be produced. This effect was shown to be mediated via the DLF. Contrary to these findings is the observation by Dubuisson (1989) that the inhibitory effect of SCS on nociceptive-specific DH neurons was abolished by a section of the DC caudally to the stimulation site.

In a series of publications Saadé and co-workers (Saadé et al., 1985, 1986, 1999) have reported on experiments in decerebrated and in intact animals (cat, rat) in which it was demonstrated that the flexor reflex as well as nociceptive evoked neuronal evoked activity could be effectively inhibited by SCS also after DC lesions. Therefore, they concluded that the pain relieving effect of SCS is principally mediated via a DC-brain stem-spinal loop. Their findings are at variance with our observations, referred to above, that the C-fibre component of the flexor reflex is not influenced by SCS (see also Wallin et al., 2003). Moreover, the normalization of the threshold of the early $A\beta$-fibre response in nerve-injured rats following SCS was found to be retained after spinal cord section rostral to the site of stimulation (Ren et al., 1996).

In a recent study, *chronic* and selective DC lesions were performed in two different models of neuropathy and it was demonstrated that SCS applied at the level of the DC nuclei, i.e. above the lesions, still suppressed behavioural signs of neuropathy (tactile allodynia and thermal hyperalgesia) (El-Khoury et al., 2002). These results were interpreted as giving further support to the authors' notion that SCS is predominantly dependent on the activation of supraspinal mechanisms. One may argue that perhaps the application of SCS to the second-order lemniscal neuronal pathway is not a true model of the clinical application of stimulation of the DCs but for obvious reasons that would not have been possible in a model with chronic DC section. In an ongoing study, performed on a lightly anaesthetized rat model of mononeuropathy, *acute*, selective DC lesions were produced between the site of SCS and that of the neuronal recordings. It was found that under these conditions the inhibiting effect on evoked responses to innocuous peripheral stimuli was almost totally abolished (Yakhnitsa et al., 1998, 1999, 2003, in preparation).

It is obvious that there are somewhat conflicting data as to the possible effect of SCS on C fibre-mediated pain and the relative importance of spinal segmental versus supraspinal mechanisms. The situation is further complicated by the fact that, in both men and experimental models of neuropathy, there are apparently two forms of tactile allodynia, dynamic and static, which are mediated by $A\beta$ and C fibres, respectively (Ochoa and Yarnitsky, 1993; Field et al., 1999) and that there may be a presynaptic interaction between these two systems. It has also been demonstrated that tactile allodynia, without specification, is principally mediated via the DCs and dependent also on supraspinal processing while thermal hyperalgesia seems to be related to the C-fibre system and involving both spinal and supraspinal circuits (Bian et al., 1998; Ossopov et al., 1999; Sun et al., 2001; for discussion, see Saadé et al., 2002).

A problem with assigning the mode of action exclusively to segmental, spinal mechanisms activated by antidromic activity in the DC acting directly, or rather indirectly, on WDR neurons is that one would expect enhancement rather than suppression of peripheral hypersensitivity (tactile-thermal allodynia, hyperalgesia). A possible alternative would be that the SCS effect is more dependent on the activation of post-synaptic DC fibres enabling the involvement of interposed inhibitory interneurons

2.5. Transmitters and receptor-related mechanisms

Data from humans on biochemical correlates to SCS are sparse and contradictory (for review, see Linderoth et al., 1993). These studies have been performed with analyses of lumbar cerebrospinal fluid (CSF) collected from patients during stimulation. However, this approach is problematic in that transient changes of relevant substances may be missed when collected via a single lumbar puncture, local release may not be reflected in changes in the CSF, changes in concentration of substances may be distorted by their rapid turnover, etc.

There is no convincing evidence for the involvement of opioid mechanisms in the effects of SCS. As early as 1977 it was reported that in patients endorphins were not influenced by SCS and the pain relieving effect could not be reversed by the opiate antagonist naloxone (Meyerson et al., 1977). It is worth mentioning also that in 1980 Sinclair and co-workers documented that in cats SCS-induced inhibition of WDR neuronal responses to noxious stimuli was not altered by naloxone (Sinclair et al., 1980). There is merely a single study on patient CSF where weak support for a role of opioids in the SCS effect was obtained (Tonelli et al., 1988).

It is surprising that the possible relationship between SCS and the release of monoamines has attracted relatively little interest considering the demonstrated existence of monaminergic pain-controlling pathways in the DLF. Data derived from studies in humans are sparse, and partly contradictory, and the same applies to a few studies performed on intact animals. Therefore, no conclusion can be presently drawn about the role of monoamines in therapeutic SCS.

The role of the neuropeptide substance P (SP) as a primary neuromodulator released from the nociceptive afferent terminals is well established. However, SP is present also in some descending pathways which exert a modulatory influence on pain transmission at the spinal level and it is well known that SP administered in certain loci in the CNS has antinociceptive properties. In fact, the SP content in human CSF appears to increase as a result of therapeutic SCS (Meyerson et al., 1985). There is also some evidence that SCS may augment the spinal release of SP as assessed by microdialysis in DH of cats (Linderoth et al., 1992). It was concluded that this release is controlled by descending pathways rather than by primary afferent activity.

In recent years some studies performed on animal models of mononeuropathy have shed some light on the possible involvement of several transmitter/modulator systems. It should be appreciated that nerve injury induces very complex changes in the spinal transmitter/modulator systems and therefore acute experiments performed on intact animals may not be appropriate for the study of neurochemical correlates of SCS.

Much interest has focussed on the gamma aminobutyric acid (GABA) system and in recent years robust data have accumulated on its pivotal role in the mode of action of SCS. Thus, it was demonstrated that in intact cats, SCS-induced inhibition of spinothalamic tract neurons could be counteracted by the $GABA_A$ antagonist bicuculline (Duggan and Foong, 1985). We have further explored the possible role of GABA in SCS. Using microdialysis in the DH of rats it was first shown that SCS induced GABA release (Linderoth et al., 1994a). Subsequently it was demonstrated in rat models of mononeuropathy that the extracellular release of GABA was significantly lower in those displaying tactile allodynia following sciatic nerve injury than in intact animals, indicating a dysfunction of the spinal GABA system caused by the nerve injury (Stiller et al., 1996). Moreover, SCS resulted in an increase of GABA release in animals which in preceding behavioural experiments had responded to SCS by a normalization of the withdrawal thresholds. It was also demonstrated that the increased release of GABA induced by SCS attenuated the release of the excitatory amino acids glutamate and aspartate (Cui et al., 1997a). It should also be noted that one laboratory (Simpson et al., 1993) has reported the release of the inhibitory amino acid glycine in the spinal cord of *intact* rabbits after a 90-min period of experimental SCS. The development of allodynia after peripheral nerve injury seems to be related to dysfunction of the spinal GABA systems, and SCS may act by restoring normal GABA levels in the DH. In behavioural studies it was demonstrated that the allodynia-suppressive effect of SCS could be counteracted by intrathecal injection of a $GABA_B$ antagonist whereas the $GABA_A$ antagonist bicuculline was less effective. Conversely, intrathecal administration of GABA or a $GABA_B$ agonist, baclofen, markedly enhanced the effect of SCS (Cui et al., 1996). This combined effect of the drug and SCS could be counteracted by a $GABA_B$ receptor antagonist.

Recent animal and human studies indicate also that the central neuromodulator adenosine could be involved in the SCS effect (Cui et al., 1997b). It seems actually to exert a synergistic effect with SCS on experimental allodynia, mediated by $GABA_B$ receptor activation and simultaneous activation of the adenosine A-1 receptor. Furthermore, both an adenosine A-1 agonist and the $GABA_B$ agonist baclofen can be used in 'subclinical' doses to potentiate the effect on SCS in previously unresponsive rats, thereby transforming them into responders (Cui et al., 1998). A recently completed clinical study has confirmed that in some patients intrathecal baclofen, administered in low doses via an implanted pump, may significantly enhance the analgesic effect of SCS (Meyerson et al., 1997; Lind et al., 2003, submitted).

It has also been shown that, similar to the effect of baclofen and adenosine, i.t. gabapentin, pregabapentin and clonidine, in doses that alone have no effect, can transform non-SCS responding rats with mononeuropathy into responders (Wallin et al., 2002; Schechtmann et al., 2003, submitted). The mechanisms of action of gabapentin are poorly understood but it is likely that it influences the Ca^{2+} channels thereby attenuating the glutaminergic transmission (Shimoyama et al., 2000). Further, it cannot be excluded that it also interacts with the GABA system (Taylor et al., 1998). The mode of action of clonidine is complex but it may nevertheless perhaps tell us something about the mechanisms involved in SCS. It has since long been assumed that the analgesic effect of clonidine is attributed to its anti-sympathetic effect. However, the group of Eisenach has shown that the analgesic, and anti-allodynic, effect is associated with increased spinal release of acetylcholine and mediated by muscarinic, and to some extent nicotinic, receptors (Eisenach et al., 1996; Pan et al., 1999). These findings call for a study of a possible role of the cholinergic spinal system in the effects of SCS.

A synthesis of the possible mode of action of SCS in neuropathic pain is shown schematically in Fig. 4.

3. Mode of action in pain caused by peripheral tissue ischaemia

A reduction of the nociceptive pain in peripheral ischaemia could in principle be accomplished in two different ways. The first alternative is that the stimulation produces an inhibition of the nociceptive influx; a second possible mode of action is that pain relief is secondary to a stimulation-induced reduction of the tissue ischaemia.

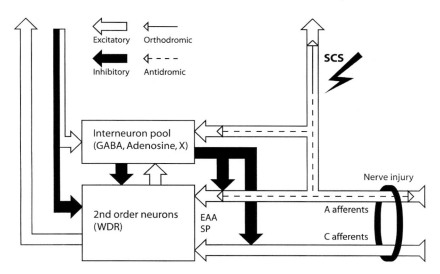

Fig. 4. Schematic representation of the possible mode of action of SCS in neuropathic pain based on present knowledge derived predominantly from experiments performed on animal (rat) models of mononeuropathy. Both segmental and supraspinal mechanisms are represented. Possible supraspinal relays are not included because of insufficient knowledge about the organisation of a proposed supraspinal loop. Broken arrow lines represent antidromic, and full line arrows orthodromic activation in the DCs, their collaterals and in primary A-afferents. The diagram does not depict the possible SCS activation of the dorsolateral columns. It is conceivable that numerous transmitters and modulators are involved in the modulation exerted by interneurons (represented by 'X'). Descending control of second order neurons is here represented as inhibitory only, although there is evidence suggesting also a facilitatory supraspinal input. (SP – substance P; EAA – excitatory amino acids: glutamate, aspartate.)

3.1. SCS blocks ischaemic pain?

That the alleviation of ischaemic pain is the result of a block of transmission of noxious impulses transmitted via the DH to the brain via the spinothalamic tracts, has been advocated by the group at Oklahoma University (for review see, e.g. Foreman, 1995). Ischaemic deep aching pain is mainly nociceptive (Bonica, 1990; Seijo, 1994). Superficial pain components, e.g. pain from ischaemic ulcers and from the borders of gangrenous areas, and transient pain during changing of bandages are largely unaffected by stimulation. This indicates that blocking of the pain signal cannot be the exclusive mechanism. Neuropathic pain may respond within 10 min of stimulation while it often takes several days of protracted SCS therapy before ischaemic pain in arterial occlusive disease is significantly affected. This suggests that a period of time is required to reverse the pain-producing local processes (e.g. normalize tissue pH). This process is more rapid in pure vasospastic conditions with no occlusive vessel wall pathology and here the effect is possibly achieved by diminishing vasoconstrictor tone. In angina pectoris (see Chapter 10) the pain alleviation is also rapid (minutes). Although the coverage with paraesthesiae is important also in ischaemic pain, it seems to be more critical for the effect in neuropathic conditions. In ischaemia, extra-segmental effects are more common, and furthermore even subliminal SCS can induce peripheral vasodilatation (Linderoth, 1995; Linderoth and Meyerson, 1995).

3.2. SCS primarily affects peripheral ischaemia?

In both experimental and clinical studies it has been demonstrated that SCS induces an increase in peripheral blood flow predominantly in the smaller arterioles and capillaries, both in the thermoregulatory and in the nutritive systems

(Broseta et al., 1986; Jacobs et al., 1988; Jacobs et al., 1990; Galley et al., 1992; for reviews see, e.g. Groth, 1985; Herreros et al., 1994; Horsch and Claeys, 1995; Linderoth, 1995). Also the larger vessels may be affected. In principle, this could represent an epiphenomenon – like the paraesthesiae discussed above – but available clinical observations strongly favour the notion that the reversal of the ischaemia is a critical factor for the alleviation of ischaemic pain.

The mechanisms whereby SCS may reduce ischaemia have been much discussed. There are two principally different modes of action: (1) SCS increases or redistributes blood flow locally; and/or (2) SCS alters cell metabolism in such a way that oxygen demand is decreased. The first alternative is compatible with a peripheral vasodilatation as referred to above; the second is supported by experimental findings of a cell protective effect of SCS when local blood flow is totally shut-off in a skin flap (e.g. Gherardini et al., 1999) and when cardiac ischaemia is diminished without an increase in flow or a redistribution in the coronary circulation (for review see, e.g. Eliasson et al., 1996). This issue however is controversial (for further discussion see Chapter 10).

In order to induce a peripheral flow increase, SCS has been proposed to either: (1) activate the afferent system antidromically with a possible release of vasoactive compounds affecting the peripheral vessels; or (2) depress sympathetically mediated vasoconstriction.

3.2.1. The antidromic hypothesis

This idea postulates that the vasodilatation produced by SCS would depend on the same mechanisms that account for the marked vascular response evoked by antidromic activity recruiting also small diameter fibres systems by high-intensity stimulation of dorsal roots or peripheral nerves. This concept is actually based on old observations made by Bayliss (1901) and subsequently confirmed by others (e.g, Hinsley and Gasser, 1930). Hilton and Marshall (1980) proposed that the

effect was mainly due to a release of prostacyclin from thin nerve fibres but others have suggested other substances like SP and calcitonin gene related peptide (CGRP) (for review see Linderoth et al., 1992). One problem with this hypothesis is that the high amplitude of stimulation needed to recruit Aδ and C fibres involved in antidromic vasodilatation would be too painful to be clinically useful.

The 'antidromic SCS hypothesis' has been subjected to study in a series of experiments (Linderoth, 1989; Linderoth et al., 1991a). Anaesthetized rats were submitted to SCS applied with parameters similar to those used in the clinic (frequency 50 Hz; pulse width 0.2 ms; SCS intensity 66% of motor threshold (MT)). The peripheral microcirculation in the hind paws was investigated by laser Doppler technique. In the initial experiments various pathways suggested to mediate this peripheral vasodilatation were eliminated surgically. These studies indicated that neither antidromic activation of primary afferents nor recruitment of small diameter fibres was mandatory for the SCS-induced vasodilatation with low-amplitude SCS.

Contradictory results have been reported by the group at Oklahoma University who tried to replicate the Karolinska findings using somewhat higher stimulation intensity (about 90% of MT) (Croom et al., 1996, 1997). The vasodilatation was abolished if the T12-L5 roots were transected. Furthermore, the flow response was attenuated if a CGRP receptor antagonist (CGRP-8-37) was given intravenously just before SCS. A similar suppressive effect could be induced by the nitric oxide (NO) synthase inhibitor L-NAME demonstrating that the effect involves nitric oxide. The authors concluded that SCS – just below discomfort level – may induce antidromic vasodilatation via the fast A-delta fibres releasing CGRP without actually causing a painful sensation (Croom et al., 1998). That some fibres from the A-delta group are transmitting also non-noxious information has been previously reported (e.g. Adriansen et al., 1983).

Complementary information was provided in a recent collaborative study between the two groups (Tanaka et al., 2003) where antidromic compound action potentials were recorded in the tibial nerve during experimental SCS applied with different amplitudes in the rat. Topical application of capsaicin on the nerve did not alter the vasodilatation observed with SCS at 30 and 60% of MT but considerably shortened the duration of the effect obtained at 90% of MT. From these observations it was concluded that the vasodilatation up to 60% of MT was subserved solely by large diameter myelinated fibres, but at and above the intensity 90% of MT also thin unmyelinated fibres participated.

There are several vasoactive substances which may be released by electrical afferent stimulation such as TENS and SCS. At present there is evidence only for CGRP release having a possible mediating role in the peripheral vasodilatation that occurs during SCS delivered with high- but subthreshold for pain-intensity. These observations are corroborated by findings in a recent study of survival of ischaemic neurovascular skin flaps in the rat where SCS at 60 or 90% of MT, given during 30 min prior to a 12 h total shut-off of flap circulation, significantly increased flap survival. Administration of a CGRP antagonist immediately prior to stimulation with 90% of MT decreased the flap survival rate significantly from 87 to 37% (Gherardini et al., 1999).

3.2.2. SCS alters autonomic activity

In view of the well-documented vasodilatory effect of SCS there is reason to assume that it may alter the functioning of the autonomic system, either the sympathetic or parasympathetic or both. In patients submitted to SCS, Meglio et al. (1986) monitored various autonomic reflexes and cardiac activity and recorded a decrease in heart rate although peripheral blood flow increased simultaneously. Another finding was that sympathetic reflexes tested during stimulation seemed to decrease in amplitude.

Augustinsson and colleagues (1982) reviewed various types of electrostimulation and the resulting autonomic effects. They confirmed the beneficial effect of SCS on detrusor dyssynergia in multiple sclerosis, an increase in peripheral circulation in vasculopathic cases and also observed changes in bowel activity with both cervical SCS and abdominal TENS. That TENS *per se* can exert beneficial effects on ischaemia and ulcer healing in peripheral arterial occlusive disease has been observed by Eriksson and Skoglund (1988). In general, the stimulation-induced changes in skin temperature and oxygen tension have been related to the paraesthesiae evoked by the SCS, being more pronounced in the parts of the body where the tingling is strongest (e.g. Sciacca et al., 1986). However, increases in skin temperature have also been observed in limbs where no paraesthesiae were experienced and with SCS applied with an intensity which was subthreshold for paraesthesiae (cf. Linderoth, 1995).

It is well known that sympathetic blocks and sympathectomy can be effective in ischaemic pain conditions, at least temporarily.

In a series of experiments we eliminated sympathetic outflow to the monitored vascular beds in the following ways: (1) sectioning of ventral roots supplying the examined area (Linderoth et al., 1991b); (2) Sectioning of the sciatic nerve (Linderoth, 1989); (3) Bilateral lumbar sympathectomy performed 1 week before SCS (Linderoth et al., 1991b). Each of these manoeuvres abolished the vasodilatory response otherwise induced by SCS and by themselves resulted in an increase in hind limb microcirculation. Furthermore, 'chemical sympathectomy', using the ganglion blocker hexamethonium or by pretreating the animals with guanethidine, totally abolished the vasodilatory effects of SCS (Linderoth et al., 1991a).

In separate experiments (Linderoth et al., 1994b) selective pharmacological blocking of autonomic transmission was utilized, both on the ganglionic and on the neuro-effector levels. From these experiments it was evident that inhibition of transmission via muscarinic receptors had little effect on the stimulation-induced vasodilatation, whereas administration of a nicotinic receptor antagonist could abolish the SCS response. Blocking alpha-adrenergic transmission decreased the effect in both vascular beds studied (hind-paw skin and hamstring muscle) and this seemed to be mainly a result of inhibition of alpha-1-adreno-receptor-mediated influence on the microcirculation. Thus, these studies favour the view that SCS induces peripheral vasodilatation by suppressing sympathetic vasoconstrictor activity mainly exerted via nicotinic receptors in the ganglia and alpha-1-adrenoreceptors at the neuro-effector junction.

The critical role of the sympathetic system in the effect of SCS on the peripheral circulation has been challenged by the Oklahoma group (Croom et al., 1998) using a slightly higher SCS amplitude than that of the Karolinska group. The interpretation of their experiments was that the peripheral vasodilatation demonstrable in animals during SCS can occur through mechanisms that are independent of the sympathetic outflow (see discussion above on antidromic mechanisms).

Thus, there appears to exist a controversy regarding the relative contributions of SCS-induced sympathetic inhibition and of antidromic activation of vasodilatory mechanisms. A recent collaborative study has specifically focussed on this problem. It was suspected that the activation level of the sympathetic system could have a decisive influence on whether its inhibition, or the antidromic components, would demonstrate themselves in the net effect. The temperatures of the preparations (and of the labs) in Stockholm and Oklahoma seemed to differ to some extent. The study was thus designed to explore whether sympathetic activation by cooling of the examined limb of the animal would change the participation of autonomic mechanisms and antidromic activation in the SCS-induced response (Tanaka et al., 2003). The experiments demonstrated that in these Oklahoma Sprague-Dawley rats antidromic

mechanisms dependent on CGRP release dominated when sympathetic activation was low, but with SCS at 90% of MT and with the hind limb cooled sympathetic inhibition played a crucial role, especially in the persistence of the vasodilatory response after the first peak. This outcome calls for further investigation of possible differences in genetically determined sympathetic activation levels between different strains of rats.

3.3. Conclusions on SCS effects on ischaemic pain

The mechanisms underlying the effects of SCS on pain due to ischaemia in the extremities, whether resulting from occlusive vascular disease or vasospasm, are different from those acting in neuropathic pain. A rebalancing of oxygen need and supply, i.e. the relief of the net ischaemia, seems to be the pivotal factor. An SCS-induced vasodilation in a situation with low sympathetic vasoconstrictor tone may occur as a result of antidromic activation, whereas with a high level of sympathetic activity, say in a cold milieu, a stimulation-induced sympathetic inhibition may contribute. This dual mechanism concept is consistent with theories about the causal mechanisms in a disease condition which often responds well to SCS: the Raynaud's syndrome. It has been proposed that in this condition there is an increased sensitivity or increased density of alpha-adrenergic receptors (Freedman et al., 1989), which may be combined with dysfunction in the CGRP-system (Bunker et al., 1990). Consequently, a stimulation-induced 'normalization' of the function in each system could constitute the background to the efficacy of SCS in this condition.

Possible mechanisms of action of SCS in peripheral ischaemia are shown schematically in Fig. 5.

4. SCS in pain conditions with dysautonomy

SCS therapy is often effective in complex regional pain syndromes (CRPS) (e.g. Barolat et al., 1989; Kumar et al., 1997; Kemler et al., 1999, 2000a).

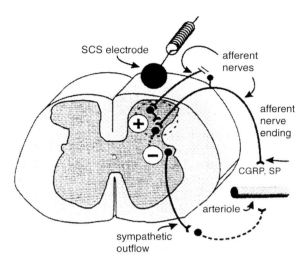

Fig. 5. Schematic representation of possible mechanisms involved in the SCS effect on peripheral tissue ischaemia. There is much evidence that the relief of pain due to ischaemia is secondary to the peripheral vasodilatation produced by SCS. In principle, the SCS effect can be exerted by two separate, or combined, mechanisms: (1) antidromic activation of primary A-afferents leading to peripheral release of vasodilatatory substances; (2) inhibition of sympathetic efferent activity resulting in decrease in nicotinic sympathetically maintained vasoconstrictor tone. (From Linderoth and Foreman, 1999, with permission.)

In principle, SCS could affect pain syndromes related to sympathetic hyperactivity in at least three ways. The first is by a direct action on the central hyperexcitability as discussed in a previous section of this chapter. Secondly, the direct-coupling hypothesis (Michaelis, 2000) implies that new, direct abnormal contacts develop between peripheral sympathetic and damaged somatosensory fibres. This would imply that central inhibition of sympathetic efferent activity, as indicated above, could exert a beneficial net effect on the pain condition. The same would be valid for abnormal couplings, 'sympathetic sprouting baskets', in the dorsal root ganglia (e.g. Jänig et al., 1996).

The third possibility involves the indirect-coupling concept, which means that the damaged sensory neurons would develop sensitivity to even mild degrees of hypoxia so that a moderate sympathetic hyperactivity with peripheral vasoconstriction could excite the neurons after lesions (Häbler et al., 2000; Michaelis, 2000). Both types of coupling seem plausible but the indirect-coupling hypothesis gets no support in a recent study by Kemler and colleagues (2000b) where SCS therapy in RSD cases did not result in peripheral vasodilatation. The non-autonomic, antidromic activation mechanisms discussed above could, however, contribute to the beneficial effects of SCS if the indirect coupling hypothesis is valid. Further research is demanded to elucidate the role of SCS in dysautonomic pain syndromes.

5. Conclusions

The research on mechanisms discussed in this chapter clearly indicates that the background to the beneficial effects of SCS in different pain syndromes is complex and varying between the conditions. At present only a small part of the action mechanisms of SCS has been unravelled. Increased knowledge about the underlying mechanisms will form the basis for further development and refinement of stimulation therapy; in fact it has done so already. SCS has the benefits of few side-effects in comparison with pharmacotherapy and may be looked upon as a technique to activate the endogenous biochemical delivery systems in the body by artificially activating neural circuits leading to effects both locally and in remote areas. It should be evident after reading this chapter that our knowledge at present is fragmentary and the key for the future is further research on pain mechanisms and how these may be modulated.

References

Adriansen, H., Gybels, J., Handwerker, H.O., and Van Hees, J. (1983) Response properties of thin myelinated (A-delta) fibers in human skin nerves. J. Neurophysiol., 49: 111–122.

Augustinsson, L.E., Carlsson, C.A., and Fall, M. (1982) Autonomic effects of electrostimulation. Appl. Neurophysiol., 45: 185–189.

Augustinsson, L.E., Linderoth, B., Mannheimer, C. and Eliasson, T. (1995) Spinal cord stimulation in cardiovascular disease. In: P. Gildenberg (Ed.), Neurosurgery Clinics of North America. pp. 157–166.

Augustinsson, L.E., Linderoth, B., Eliasson, T., and Mannheimer, C. (1997) Spinal cord stimulation in peripheral vascular disease and angina pectoris. In: P. Gildenberg, and R. Tasker (Eds.), Textbook of Stereotactic and Functional Neurosurgery (pp. 1973–1978). McGraw-Hill, New York.

Bantli, H., Bloedel, J.R., and Thienprasit, P. (1975) Supraspinal interactions resulting from experimental dorsal column stimulation. J. Neurosurg., 42: 296–300.

Barolat, G. (1999) A prospective multicenter study to assess the efficacy of spinal cord stimulation utilizing a multi-channel radio-frequency system for the treatment of intractable low back and lower extremity pain. Neuromodulation, 2: 179–183.

Barolat, G., Schwartzman, R., and Woo, R. (1989) Epidural spinal cord stimulation in the management of reflex sympathetic dystrophy. Stereotact. Funct. Neurosurg., 53: 29–39.

Barolat, G., Oakley, J.C., Law, J.D., North, R.B., Ketcik, R.N., and Sharan, A. (2001) Epidural spinal cord stimulation with a multiple electrode paddle lead is effective in treating intractable low back pain. Neuromodulation, 4: 59–66.

Bayliss, W.M. (1901) On the origin from the spinal cord of the vasodilator fibers of the hind-limb and on the nature of these fibers. J. Physiol., 26: 173–209.

Bennett, G. (1993) An animal model of neuropathic pain: a review. Muscle Nerve, 16: 1040–1048.

Bennett, G.J. and Xie, Y.K. (1988) A peripheral mononeuropathy in rat produces disorders of pain sensation like those seen in man. Pain, 33: 87–107.

Bian, D., Ossopov, H., Zhong, C.M., Malan, T.P., and Porreca, F. (1998) Tactile allodynia, but not thermal hyperalgesia, of hindlimbs is blocked by spinal transection in rats with nerve injury. Neurosci. Lett., 241: 79–82.

Bonica, J.J. (1990) Pain due to vascular disease. In: J.J. Bonica (Ed.), *The Management of Pain* (pp. 502–537). Lea & Febiger, Philadelphia.

Broseta, J., Barbera, J., De Vera, J.A., Barcia-Salorio, J.L., Garcia-March, G., Gonzalez-Darder, J., Rovaina, F., and Joanes, V. (1986) Spinal cord stimulation in peripheral arterial disease. J. Neurosurg., 64: 71–80.

Bunker, C.B., Terenghi, G., Springall, D.R., Polak, J.M., and Dowd, P.M. (1990) Deficiency of calcitonin gene-related peptide in Raynaud's phenomenon. Lancet, 336: 336.

Campbell, J.N. (1981) Examination of possible mechanisms by which stimulation of the spinal cord in man relieves pain. Appl. Neurophysiol., 44: 181–186.

Campbell, J., Raja, S., Meyer, R., and Mc Kinnon, S. (1988) Myelinated afferents signal the hyperalgesia associated with nerve injury. Pain, 32: 89–94.

Campbell, J.N., Davis, K.D., Meyer, R.A., and North, R.B. (1990) The mechanism by which dorsal column stimulation affects pain: evidence for a new hypothesis. Pain Suppl., 5: 228.

Chandler, M.J., Brennan, T.J., Garrison, D.W., Kim, K.S., Schwartz, P.J., and Foreman, R.D. (1993) A mechanism of cardiac pain suppression by spinal cord stimulation: implications for patients with angina pectoris. Eur. Heart J., 14: 96–105.

Cook, W.W., Oygar, A., Baggenstos, P., Pacheco, S., and Kleriga, E. (1976) Vascular disease of extremities: electrical stimulation of spinal cord and posterior roots. N.Y. State J. Med., 76: 366–368.

Croom, J.E., Barron, K.W., Chandler, M.J., and Foreman, R.D. (1996) Cutaneous blood flow increases in the rat hindpaw during dorsal column stimulation. Brain Res., 728: 281–286.

Croom, J.E., Foreman, R.D., Chandler, M.J., and Barron, K.W. (1997) Cutaneous vasodilatation during dorsal column stimulation is mediated by dorsal roots and CGRP. Am. J. Physiol., 272: H950–H957.

Croom, J.E., Foreman, R.D., Chandler, M.J., and Barron, K.W. (1998) Reevaluation of the role of the sympathetic nervous system in cutaneous vasodilatation during dorsal spinal cord stimualtion: are multiple mechanisms active?. Neuromodulation, 1: 91–101.

Cui, J.G., Linderoth, B., and Meyerson, B.A. (1996) Effects of spinal cord stimulation on touch-evoked allodynia involve GABAergic mechanisms. An experimental study in the mononeuropathic rat. Pain, 66: 287–295.

Cui, J.G., O'Connor, W.T., Ungerstedt, U., Linderoth, B., and Meyerson, B.A. (1997a) Spinal cord stimulation attenuates augmented dorsal horn release of excitatory amino acids in mononeuropathy via a GABAergic mechanism. Pain, 73: 87–95.

Cui, J.G., Sollevi, A., Linderoth, B., and Meyerson, B.A. (1997b) Andosine receptor activation suppresses tactile hypersensitivity and potentiates effect of spinal cord in mononeuropathic rats. Neurosci. Lett., 223: 173–176.

Cui, J.-G., Linderoth, B., and Meyerson, B.A. (1997c) Incidence of mononeuropathy in rats is influenced by pre-emptive alteration of spinal excitability. Eur. J. Pain, 1: 53–59.

Cui, J.G., Meyerson, B.A., Sollevi, A., and Linderoth, B. (1998) Effects of spinal cord stimulation on tactile hypersensitivity in mononeuropathic rats is potentiated by $GABA_B$ and adenosine receptor activation. Neurosci. Lett., 247: 183–186.

Cui, J.-G., Meyerson, B., and Linderoth, B. (1999) Opposite effects of spinal cord stimulation in different phases of carrageenan-induced hyperalgesia. Eur. J. Pain, 3: 365–374.

Doerr, M., Krainick, J., and Thoden, U. (1978) Pain perception in man after long term spinal stimulation. J. Neurol., 217: 261–270.

Dubuisson, D. (1989) Effect of dorsal-column stimulation on gelatinosa and marginal neurons of cat spinal cord. J. Neurosurg., 70: 257–265.

Duggan, A.W. and Foong, F.W. (1985) Bicuculline and spinal inhibition produced by dorsal column stimulation in the cat. Pain: 249–259.

Eisenach, J.C., De Kock, M., and Klimscha, W. (1996) Alpha(2)-adrenergic agonists for regional anesthesia. A clinical review of clonidine. Anesthesiology, 85: 655–674.

Eliasson, T., Augustinsson, L.E., and Mannheimer, C. (1996) Spinal cord stimulation in severe angina pectoris—presentation of current studies, indications and clinical experience. Pain, 65: 169–179.

El-Khoury, C., Hawwa, M., Baliki, S.F., Atweh, S.F., Jabbur, S.V., and Saadé, N.E. (2002) Attenuation of neuropathic pain by segmental and supraspinal activation of the dorsal column system in awake rats. Neuroscience, 112: 541–553.

Emmers, R. and Ruderman, M.J. (1974) Inhibition at the T-cells of the spinothalamic tract: a neurophysiological basis for electrically induced analgesia. Proc. Soc. Exp. Biol. Med., 145: 1310–1316.

Eriksson, A. and Skoglund, C.R. (1988) Effects of TNS on pain, skin circulation and wound healing in cases of peripheral vascular disease. Läkartidningen, 85: 1237–1241. Abstract in English.

Feeney, D.M. and Gold, G.N. (1980) Chronic dorsal column stimulation: effects on H-reflex and symtoms in a patient with multiple sclerosis. Neurosurgery, 6: 564–566.

Feirabend, H.K.P., Choufoer, S., Ploeger, S., Holsheimer, J., and Van Gool, J.D. (2002) Morphometry of human superficial dorsal and dorsolateral column fibres: significance to cord stimulation. Brain, 125: 1137–1149.

Feldman, R.A. (1975) Patterned response of lamina V cells: cutaneous and dorsal funicular stimulation. Physiol. Behav., 15: 79–84.

Field, M.J., Bramwell, S., Hughes, J., and Singh, L. (1999) Detection of static and dynamic components of allodynia in rat model of neuropathic pain: are they signalled by distinct primary neurons?. Pain, 83: 303–311.

Foreman, R.D. (1995) Neurophysiological mechanisms of pain relief by spinal cord stimulation in angina pectoris. In: S. Horsch, and I. Claeys (Eds.), *Spinal Cord Stimulation: An Innovative Method in the Treatment of PVD and Angina* (pp. 155–164). Steinkopff Verlag, Darmstadt.

Foreman, R.D., Beall, J.E., Applebaum, A.E., Coulter, J.D., and Willis, W.D. (1976) Effects of dorsal column stimulation on primate spinothalamic tract neurons. J. Neurophysiol., 39: 534–546.

Freedman, R.R., Sabharwal, S.C., Desai, N., Wenig, P., and Mayes, M. (1989) Increased alfa-adrenergic responsiveness in idiopathic Raynaud's disease. Arthrit. Rheum., 32: 61–65.

Galley, D., Rettori, R., Boccalon, H., Medvedowsky, A., Lefebvre, J.M., Sellier, F., Chauvreau, C., Serise, J.M., and Pieronne, A. (1992) Electrical stimulation of the spinal cord in arterial diseases of the legs. A multicenter study of 244 patients. J. Mal. Vasc., 17: 208–213.

Gao, X., Ren, B., Linderoth, B., and Meyerson, B. (1996) Daily spinal cord stimulation suppresses autotomy behaviour in rats following peripheral deafferentation, Neuroscience, 463–470.

Garcia-Larrea, L., Sindou, M., and Mauguière, F. (1989) Nociceptive flexion reflexes during analgesic neurostimulation in man. Pain, 39: 145–156.

Gazelius, B., Cui, J.-G., Svenssson, M., Meyerson, B., and Linderoth, B. (1996) Photochemically induced ischemic lesion of the rat sciatic nerve. A novel method providing high incidence of mononeuropathy. NeuroReport, 7: 2619–2623.

Gherardini, G., Lundeberg, T., Cui, J.-G., Eriksson, S.V., Trubek, S., and Linderoth, B. (1999) Spinal cord stimulation improves survival in ischemic skin flaps: an experimental study of the possible mediation via the calcitonin gene-related peptide. Plast. Reconstr. Surg., 103: 1221–1228.

Groth, K. (1985) Spinal cord stimulation for the treatment of peripheral vascular disease. In: H. Fields, R. Dubner, and F. Cervero (Eds.), *Advances in Pain Research and Therapy* (pp. 861–870). Raven Press, New York.

Gybels, J. and Kupers, R. (1991) Significance of autotomy scratching after peripheral nerve injury. In: J. Besson, and G. Guilbaud (Eds.), *Lesions of Primary Afferent Fibers as a Tool for the Study of Clinical Pain* (pp. 101–116). Elsevier, Amsterdam.

Häbler, H.-J., Eschenfelder, S., Brinker, H., Grunow, B., Liu, X., and Jänig, W. (2000) Neurogenic vasoconstriction in the dorsal root ganglion may play a crucial role in sympathetic-afferent coupling after spinal nerve injury. In: M. Devor, M.C. Rowbotham, and Z. Wiesemfeld-Hallin (Eds.), *Progress in Pain Research and Management* (pp. 661–667). IASP Press, Seattle.

Handwerker, H.O., Iggo, A., and Zimmermann, M. (1975) Segmental and supraspinal actions on dorsal horn neurons responding to noxious and non-noxious skin stimuli. Pain, 1: 147–165.

Head, H. and Thompson, T. (1906) The grouping of afferent impulses within the spinal cord. Brain, 29: 537–741.

Herreros, J., Lazorthes, Y., Boccalon, H., Galley, D., and Broggi, G. (1994) *Spinal Cord Stimulation for Peripheral Vascular Disease.* Editorial Libro del Ano, Madrid.

Hillman, P. and Wall, P.D. (1969) Inhibitory and excitatory factors influencing the receptive fields of Lamina V spinal cord cells. Exp. Brain Res., 9: 284–306.

Hilton, S.M. and Marshall, J.M. (1980) Dorsal root vasodilatation in cat skeletal muscle. J. Physiol., 299: 277–288.

Hinsley, J.H. and Gasser, H.S. (1930) The component of the dorsal root mediating vasodilatation and the Sherrington contracture. Am. J. Physiol., 679–689.

Horsch, S. and Claeys, I. (1995) *Spinal Cord Stimulation: An Innovative Method in the Treatment of PVD and Angina.* Steinkopff-Verlag, Darmstadt.

Jacobs, M.J., Jörning, P.J.G., Joshi, S.R., Kitslaar, P.J.E.H.M., Slaaf, D.W., and Reneman, R.S. (1988) Epidural spinal cord electrical stimulation improves microvascular blood flow in severe limb ischemia. Ann. Surg., 207: 179–183.

Jacobs, M.J., Jörning, P.J., Beckers, R.C., Ubbink, D.T., van Kleef, M., Slaaf, D.W., and Reneman, R.S. (1990) Foot salvage and improvement of microvascular blood flow as a result of epidural spinal cord electrical stimulation. J. Vasc. Surg., 12: 354–360.

Jänig, W., Levine, J.D., and Michaelis, M. (1996) Interactions of sympathetic and afferent neurons following nerve injury and tissue trauma. Prog. Brain Res., 113: 161–184.

Kemler, M.A., Barendse, G.A.M., Van Kleff, M., Van Den Wildenberg, F.A.J.M., and Weber, W.E.J. (1999) Electric spinal cord stimulation in reflex sympathetic dystrophy: retrospective analysis of 23 patients. Neurosurgery, 90(Suppl.): 79–83.

Kemler, M.A., Barendse, G.A.M., Van Kleff, M., De Vet, H.C.W., Rijks, C.P.M., Furneé, C.A., and Van Den Wildenberg, F.A.J.M. (2000a) Spinal cord stimulation in patients with reflex sympathetic dystrophy. N. Eng. J. Med., 343: 618–624.

Kemler, M.A., Barendse, G.A.M., Van Kleff, M., and oude Egbrink, M.G.A. (2000b) Pain relief in complex regional pain syndrome due to spinal cord stimulation does not depend on vasodilatation. Anesthesiology, 92: 1653–1660.

Kocher, L., Anton, F., Reeh, P.W., and Handwerker, H.O. (1987) The effect of carrageenan-induced inflammation on the sensitivity of unmyelinated skin receptors in the rat. Pain, 29: 363–373.

Kumar, K., Nath, R.K., and Toth, C. (1997) Spinal cord stimulation is effective in the management of reflex sympathetic dystrophy. Neurosurgery, 40: 503–508.

Larson, S.J., Sances, A., Riegel, D.H., Meyer, G.A., Dallmann, D.E., and Swiontek, T. (1974) Neurophysiological effects of dorsal column stimulation in man and monkey. J. Neurosurg., 41, 217–223.

Lind, G., Meyerson, B.A., and Linderoth, B. (2003) Intrathecal baclofen enhances benefit from spinal cord stimulation. (Submitted).

Lindblom, U. (1985) Assessment of abnormal evoked pain in neurological pain patients and its relation to spontaneous pain: a descriptive and conceptual with some analytical results. In: H.L. Fields, and F. Cervero (Eds.), Advances in Pain Research and Therapy (pp. 409–423). Raven Press, New York.

Lindblom, U. and Meyerson, B.A. (1975) Influence on touch, vibration and cutaneous pain of dorsal column stimulation in man. Pain, 1: 257–270.

Lindblom, U. and Meyerson, B.A. (1976a) Mechanoreceptive and nociceptive thresholds during dorsal column stimulation in man. In: J. Bonica, and D. Albe-Fessard (Eds.), Advances in Pain Research and Therapy (pp. 469–474). Raven Press, New York.

Lindblom, U. and Meyerson, B. (1976b) On the effect of electrical stimulation of the dorsal column system on secondary thresholds in patients with chronic pain. In:

A. Iggo, and O. Illyinsky (Eds.), Somatosensory and Visceral Receptor Mechanisms (pp. 237–241). Elsevier, Amsterdam.

Lindblom, U., Tapper, D.N., and Wiesenfeldt, Z. (1977) The effect of dorsal column stimulation on the nociceptive response of dorsal horn cells and its relevance for pain suppression. Pain, 4: 133–144.

Linderoth, B. (1989) Is vasodilatation following dorsal column stimulation mediated by antidromic activation of small diameter afferents?. Acta Neurochir., Suppl. (Wien): 46.

Linderoth, B. (1995) Spinal cord stimulation in ischemia and ischemic pain: possible mechanisms of action. In: S. Horsch, and L. Claeys (Eds.), Spinal Cord Stimulation. An Innovative Method in the Treatment of PVD and Angina (pp. 19–35). Steinkopff Verlag, Darmstadt.

Linderoth, B. and Foreman, R.D. (1999) Physiology of spinal cord stimulation: review and update. Neuromodulation, 2: 150–164.

Linderoth, B. and Meyerson, B.A. (1995) Dorsal column stimulation: modulation of somatosensory and autonomic function. Seminars in The Neurosciences, 7: 263–277.

Linderoth, B. and Meyerson, B. (2000) Spinal cord stimulation. Mechanisms of action. In: K. Burchiel (Ed.), Pain Surgery (pp. 505–526). Thieme, New York.

Linderoth, B., Fedorcsak, I., and Meyerson, B.A. (1991a) Peripheral vasodilatation after spinal cord stimulation: animal studies of putative effector mechanisms. Neurosurgery, 28: 187–195.

Linderoth, B., Gunasekera, L., and Meyerson, B.A. (1991b) Effects of sympathectomy on skin and muscle microcirculation during dorsal column stimulation: animal studies. Neurosurgery, 29: 874–879.

Linderoth, B., Gazelius, B., Franck, J., and Brodin, E. (1992) Dorsal column stimulation induces release of serotonin and substance P in the cat dorsal horn. Neurosurgery, 31: 289–297.

Linderoth, B., Stiller, C.O., Gunasekera, L., O'Connor, W.T., Franck, J., Gazelius, B., and Brodin, E. (1993) Release of neurotransmitters in the CNS by spinal cord stimulation: survey of present state of knowledge and recent experimental studies. Stereotact. Funct. Neurosurg., 61: 157–170.

Linderoth, B., Stiller, C.O., Gunasekera, L., O'Connor, W.T., Ungestedt, U., and Brodin, E. (1994a) Gamma-aminobutyric acid is released in the dorsal horn by electrical spinal cord stimulation: an in vivo microdialysis study in the rat. Neurosurgery, 34: 484–489.

Linderoth, B., Herregodts, P., and Meyerson, B. (1994b) Sympathetic mediation of peripheral vasodilatation induced by spinal cord stimulation: animal studies of the role of cholinergic and adrenergic receptor subtypes. Neurosurgery, 35: 711–719.

Linderoth, B., Gheradini, G., Ren, B., and Lundeberg, T. (1995) Pre-emptive spinal cord stimulation reduces ischemia in an animal model of vasospasm. Neurosurgery, 37: 266–272.

Marchand, S. (1993) Nervous system stimulation for pain relief (Commentary). APS J., 2: 103–106.

Marchand, S., Bushnell, M., Molina-Negro, P., Martinez, S., and Duncan, G. (1991) The effects of dorsal column stimulation on measures of clinical and experimental pain in man. Pain, 45: 249–257.

Mazars, G.J. (1975) Intermittent stimulation of nucleus ventralis posterolateralis for intractable pain. Surg. Neurol., 4: 93–95.

Mazars, G., Merienne, S., and Cioloca, C. (1973) Stimulations thalamiques intermittentes antalgiques. Rev. Neurol. (Paris), 128: 273–279.

McMillan, J.A., Moudy, A.M., and Griffith, H.S. (1986) Dorsal column stimulation does not inhibit segmental nociceptive reflexes of hind limbs. Exp. Neurol., 93: 522–530.

Meglio, M., Cioni, B., Rossi, G.F., Sandric, S., and Santarelli, P. (1986) Spinal cord stimulation affects the central mechanisms of regulation of the heart rate. Appl. Neurophysiol., 49: 139–146.

Melzack, R. and Wall, P.D. (1965) Pain mechanisms: a new theory. Science, 150: 971–979.

Meyerson, B.A., Boethius, J., Terenius, L., Wahlström, A. 1977. 'Endorphine mechanisms in pain relief with intracerebral and dorsal column stimulation.' In 3rd Meeting of the European Society for Stereotactic and Functional Neurosurgery, Freiburg.

Meyerson, B.A., Brodin, E., and Linderoth, B. (1985) Possible neurohumoral mechanisms in CNS stimulation for pain suppression. Appl. Neurophysiol., 48: 175–180.

Meyerson, B.A., Cui, J.-G., Yakhnitsa, V., Solveli, A., Segerdahl, M., Stiller, C.-O., O'Connor, W.T., and Linderoth, B. (1997) Modulation of spinal pain mechanisms by spinal cord stimulation and the potential role of adjuvant pharmacotherapy. Stereotact. Funct. Neurosurg., 68: 129–140.

Meyerson, B.A. and Linderoth, B. (2000) Mechanisms of spinal cord stimulation in neuropathic pain. Neurol. Res., 22: 285–292.

Meyerson, B.A., Ren, B., Herregodts, P., and Linderoth, B. (1995) Spinal cord stimulation in animal models of mononeuropathy: effects on the withdrawal response and the flexor reflex. Pain, 61: 229–243.

Michaelis, M. (2000) Coupling of sympathetic and somatosensory neurons following nerve injury: mechanisms and potential significance for the generation of pain. In: M. Devor, M.C. Rowbotham, and Z. Wiesemfeld-Hallin (Eds.), Progress in Pain Research and Management (pp. 645–656). IASP Press, Seattle.

Nashold, B.S., Somjen, G., and Friedman, H. (1972) Paresthesias and EEG potentials evoked by stimulation of the dorsal funiculi in man. Exp. Neurol., 36: 273–287.

Noordenbos, W. (1959) *Pain*. Elsevier, Amsterdam.

North, R. and Guarino, A. (1999) Spinal cord stimulation for failed back surgery syndrome: technical advances, patient selection and outcome. Neuromodulation, 2: 171–178.

North, R.B., Kidd, D.H., Zahurak, M., James, C.S., and Long, D.M. (1993) Spinal cord stimulation for chronic, intractable pain: experience over two decades. Neurosurgery, 32: 384–395.

Nyquist, J.K. and Greenhoof, J.H. (1973) Responses evoked from the thalamic centrum medianum by painful input: suppression by dorsal funiculus stimulation. Exp. Neurol., 9: 215–222.

Ochoa, J.L. and Yarnitsky, D. (1993) Mechanical hyperalgesias in neuropathic pain patients; dynamic and static subtypes. Ann. Neurol., 33: 465–472.

Ohnmeiss, D.D. and Rashbaum, R.F. (2001) Patient satisfaction with spinal cord stimulation for predominant complaints of chronic, intractable low back pain. Spine J., 1: 358–363.

Ossopov, H., Lai, J., Malan, T.P., and Porreca, F. (1999) Spinal and supraspinal mechanisms in neuropathic pain. Ann. N. Y. Acad. Sci., 909: 12–24.

Pan, H.-L., Chen, S.-R., and Eisenach, J.C. (1999) Intrathecal clonidine alleviates allodynia in neuropathic rats. Anesthesiology, 90: 509–514.

Pearl, G.S. and Anderson, K.V. (1977) Effect of high-frequency peripheral nerve and dorsal column stimulation on neuronal responses in feline nucleus reticularis gigantocellularis after nociceptive electrical stimulation. Exp. Neurol., 57: 307–321.

Price, D.D. (1991) The use of experimental pain in evaluating the effects of dorsal column stimulation on clinical pain. Pain, 45: 225–226.

Rees, H. and Roberts, M.H.T. (1989) Antinociceptive effects of dorsal column stimulation in the rat: involvement of the anterior pretectal nucleus. J. Physiol., 43: 375–388.

Ren, N., Linderoth, B., and Meyerson, B.A. (1996) Effects of spinal cord stimulation on the flexor reflex and involvement of supraspinal mechanisms: an experimental study in mononeuropathic rats. J. Neurosurg., 84: 244–249.

Roberts, M.H.T. and Rees, H. (1994) Physiological basis of spinal cord stimulation. Pain Rev., 1: 184–198.

Saadé, N.E., Tabet, M.S., Banna, N.R., Atweh, S.F., and Jabbur, S.J. (1985) Inhibition of nociceptive evoked activity in spinal neurons through a dorsal column-brainstem-spinal loop. Brain Res., 339: 115–158.

Saadé, N.E., Tabet, M.S., Soueidan, S.A., Bitar, M., Atweh, S.F., and Jabbur, S.V. (1986) Supraspinal modulation of nociception in awake rats by stimulation of the dorsal column nuclei. Brain Res., 369: 307–310.

Saadé, N.E., Atweh, S.F., Privat, A., and Jabbur, S.V. (1999) Inhibitory effects from various types of dorsal coulmn and raphe magnus stimulation on nociceptive withdrawal flexion reflexes. Brain Res., 846: 244–249.

Saadé, N.E., Baliki, S.F., El-Khoury, C., Hawwa, M., Atweh, S.F., Apkarian, A.V., and Jabbur, S.V. (2002) The role of dorsal columns in neuropathic behavior: evidence for plasticity and non-specificity. Neuroscience, 115: 403–413.

Schechtmann, G., Wallin, J., Meyerson, B.A., and Linderoth, B. (2003) Intrathecal clonidine suppresses tactile allodynia and potentiates spinal cord stimulation in neuropathic rats. (Submitted).

Sciacca, V., Tamorri, M., and Rocco, M. (1986) Modifications of transcutaneous oxygen tension in lower limb peripheral occlusive patients treated with spinal cord stimulation. Ital. J. Surg. Sci., 16: 279–282.

Seijo, F. (1994) Ischemic pain: nociceptive pain or deafferentation pain. In: J. Herreros, Y. Lazorthes, H. Boccalon, D. Galley, and G. Broggi (Eds.), *Spinal Cord Stimulation for Peripheral Vascular Disease: Advances and Controversies* (pp. 25–29). Editorial Libro del Ano, Madrid.

Seltzer, Z., Dubner, R., and Yoram, S. (1990) A novel behavioral model of neuropathic pain disorders produced in rats by partial sciatic nerve injury. Pain, 43: 205–218.

Shealy, C.N., Mortimer, J.T., and Reswick, J.B. (1967) Electrical inhibition of pain by stimulation of the dorsal columns: preliminary clinical report. Anesth. Analg., 46: 489–491.

Shimoyama, M., Shimoyama, N., and Hori, Y. (2000) Gabapentin affects glutaminergic excitatory neurotransmission in the rat dorsal horn. Pain, 85: 405–414.

Simpson, R.D., Robertson, C.S., and Goodman, J.C. (1993) Glycine: a potential mediator of electrically induced pain modification. Bio. Lett., 48: 193–207.

Sinclair, J.G., Fox, R.E., Mokha, S.S., and Iggo, A. (1980) The effect of naloxone on the inhibition of nociceptor driven neurones in the cat spinal cord. Q.J. Exp. Physiol. Cogn. Med. Sci., 65: 181–188.

Sotgiu, M., Biella, G., and Riva, L. (1995) Poststimulus afterdischarges of spinal WDR and NS units in rats with chronic nerve constriction. Neuroreport, 6: 1021–1024.

Stiller, C.-O., Cui, J.-G., O'Connor, W.T., Brodin, E., Meyerson, B.A., and Linderoth, B. (1996) Release of GABA in the dorsal horn and suppression of tactile allodynia by spinal cord stimulation in mononeuropathic rats. Neurosurgery, 39: 367–375.

Sun, H., Ren, K., Zhong, C.M., Ossipov, H., Malan, T.P., Lai, J., and Porreca, F. (2001) Nerve injury-induced tactile allodynia is mediated via ascending spinal dorsal column projections. Pain, 90, 105–111.

Tanaka, S., Barron, K.W., Chandler, M.J., Linderoth, B., and Foreman, R.D. (2003) Role of primary afferents in spinal cord stimulation-induced vasodilation: characterization of fiber types. Brain Res., 959: 191–198.

Taylor, C.P., Gee, N.S., Su, T.Z., Kocsis, J.D., and Welty, D.F. (1998) A summary of mechanistic hypothesis of gabapentin pharmacology. Epilepsy Res., 29: 233–249.

Tonelli, L., Setti, T., and Falasca, A. (1988) Investigation on cerebrospinal fluid opioid and neurotransmitters related to spinal cord stimulation. Appl. Neurophysiol., 51: 324–332.

Wallin, J., Cui, J.-G., Yakhnitsa, V., Schechtmann, G., Meyerson, B.A., and Linderoth, B. (2002) Gabapentin and pregabalin suppress tactile allodynia and potentiate spinal cord stimulation in a model of neuropathy. Eur. J. Pain, 6: 261–272.

Wallin, J., Fiskå, A., Tjölsen, A., Linderoth, B., and Hole, K. (2003) Spinal cord stimulation inhibits long-term potentiation of spinal wide dynamic range neurons. Brain Res., 973: 39–43.

White, J.C. and Sweet, W.H. (1969) *Pain and the Neurosurgeon* (pp. 888–904). Charles C Thomas, Springfield, Illinois, USA.

Willer, J. (1977) Comparative study of perceived pain and nociceptive flexion reflex in man. Pain, 3: 69–80.

Willis, W.D., Jr. (1985) *The Pain System: The Neural Basis of Nociceptive Transmission in the Mammalian Nervous System.* Karger, New York.

Woolf, C. and Doubell, T. (1994) The pathophysiology of chronic pain-increased sensitivity to low threshold A-beta fiber inputs. Curr. Opin. Neurobiol., 4: 525–534.

Yakhnitsa, V., Linderoth, B., and Meyerson, B.A. (1998) Modulation of dorsal horn neuronal activity by spinal cord stimulation in a rat model of neuropathy: the role of the dorsal funicles. Neurophysiology, 6: 424–427.

Yakhnitsa, V., Linderoth, B., and Meyerson, B.A. (1999) Effects of spinal cord stimulation on dorsal horn neuronal activity in a rat model of mononeuropathy. Pain, 79: 223–233.

Yakhnitsa, V., Linderoth, B., and Meyerson, B. (2003) The role of dorsal columns in the effect of spinal cord stimulation on dorsal horn hyperexcitability (in manuscript).

Zotterman, Y. (1939) The nervous mechanism of touch and pain. Acta Psychiat. Neurol., 14: 91–97.

Electrical Stimulation and the Relief of Pain
Pain Research and Clinical Management, Vol. 15
Edited by Brian A. Simpson

CHAPTER 12

Spinal cord and peripheral nerve stimulation: technical aspects

Richard B. North*

Departments of Neurosurgery, Anesthesiology and Critical Care Medicine, Johns Hopkins University School of Medicine, 600 N. Wolfe St., Meyer 8-181, Baltimore, MD 21287, USA

Abstract

Spinal cord and peripheral nerve stimulation are reversible 'neuro-augmentative' pain management techniques with low morbidity. Percutaneous placement of spinal epidural electrode arrays has facilitated minimally invasive therapeutic trials as well as permanent implants. The development of programmable, implanted stimulation devices, which allow non-invasive selection of anodes and cathodes from electrodes with multiple contacts, has significantly enhanced both technical and clinical results. This has added complexity to the adjustment process, but computerized methods of adjustment promise to address this, and to increase the longevity of implanted batteries.

Keywords: Spinal cord stimulation; Peripheral nerve stimulation; Electrical stimulation; Intractable pain

1. Introduction

In 1965 the publication of the 'gate theory' of pain provided a rationale for using electrical stimulation for the treatment of pain (Melzack and Wall, 1965). Conveniently, compact solid-state circuitry had been developed, and it had already been adapted for implantation in the hostile environment of the body for use in cardiac pacing; this was readily utilized for electrical stimulation of the nervous system. Ongoing advances in implantable electronics have been paralleled by improvements in our understanding of design requirements and underlying physiology. Implanted stimulation devices have become more useful and more reliable, leading to significantly better clinical results (North et al., 1991, 1993).

2. Mechanisms of pain relief by electrical stimulation

To the extent that the mechanisms of pain relief by electrical stimulation, in particular spinal cord stimulation (SCS), are understood, some are pertinent to the design and implantation of devices and therefore to this discussion of technical aspects of SCS. A growing body of research on neurochemical mediators, central mechanisms and psychophysics is beyond the scope of this discussion (Marchand et al., 1991; Linderoth and Meyerson, 2000).

According to the 'gate theory' the activity of cells in the dorsal horn of the spinal cord, mediating the central transmission of pain, is determined by the balance of large and small fibre

*Correspondence to: Richard B. North. Phone: +1 (410) 955-2438; Fax: +1 (410) 955-9112; E-mail: rnorth@jhmi.edu

activity in peripheral afferents. An excess of small fibre activity opens the 'gate', allowing central transmission of pain; an excess of large fibre activity closes the 'gate'. Conveniently, large fibres are depolarized by externally applied electrical fields more easily than small fibres, and so stimulation of a mixed peripheral nerve can recruit them selectively, closing the 'gate'.

Inconveniently, however, the threshold of motor fibres in a mixed peripheral nerve is very close to the sensory threshold, and so involuntary motor side effects may occur with stimulation; amplitude adjustment can be critical. In clinical practice, inconveniently, most pain syndromes involve the distribution of more than one peripheral nerve. The spinal cord contains large diameter primary afferents conveniently segregated from motor fibres, and located accessibly in the dorsal columns near the midline, away from the more ventral and lateral motor pathways. These afferents can be activated selectively ('dorsal column stimulation', or DCS) via dorsal midline electrodes, avoiding motor side effects. Action potentials are propagated not only orthodromically, via the lemniscal system, but also antidromically, through collaterals to the 'gates' in the dorsal horn and into afferent fibres in the periphery. Segmental activity, and therefore pain, can be influenced over a large area, in the distribution of multiple peripheral nerves. SCS addresses both of the major drawbacks of peripheral nerve stimulation (PNS) – spatial limitations and motor side effects.

From the beginning the 'gate theory' has been controversial (Nathan, 1976); there are pathological, painful conditions, some of them commonplace, which it does not explain. Large fibres can signal pain in hyperalgesic states, for example (Campbell et al., 1988). Perhaps in this circumstance relief of pain is achieved by a frequency-related conduction block, acting at branch points of primary afferents, where dorsal column fibres and dorsal horn collaterals diverge. Indeed, in clinical practice SCS patients have shown a significant preference for pulse repetition rates above a minimum of 25 per second (North et al.,

1993). This is consistent with the above hypothesis that frequency-related conduction block plays a role in pain relief by SCS. There are, of course, alternative mechanisms that may be frequency dependent; these might involve interneurons in the dorsal horn, sympathetic pathways, or other descending or ascending systems (Handwerker et al., 1975; Lindblom et al., 1977; Duggan and Foong, 1985; Linderoth et al., 1991). Whatever the mechanism, the requirement for a minimum pulse repetition rate is an important determinant of SCS design and adjustment.

The amplitude (voltage or amperage or, after multiplication by pulse width, charge per phase) of SCS is important to the design, and to adjustment in clinical practice. There have been many experimental studies of SCS mechanisms in anaesthetized animals and human subjects, in which the amplitude has simply been increased until some effect is observed on the dependent variable of interest. Amplitude must be scaled to clinically relevant levels, between that producing the first perception and that producing discomfort or motor activity (Law and Kirkpatrick, 1991).

Overlap of the patient's distribution of pain by stimulation-induced paraesthesias must be achieved at subjectively comfortable amplitudes, below discomfort threshold, to be clinically useful. Recent experimental models have recognized this and have been scaled appropriately (Meyerson et al., 1992).

Computerized finite element models of the electrical fields produced by SCS within the spinal canal and spinal cord have been developed and refined over the past two decades (Coburn and Sin, 1985; Holsheimer and Struijk, 1991). These models predict the distributions of current flow and voltage gradients; they have been validated by actual measurements in primate and cadaver spinal cord and by clinical observations (Sances et al., 1975). It is clear from these models that not only the dorsal columns, but also adjacent pathways and even dorsal roots, are subject to recruitment; hence the terminology 'spinal cord stimulation' (SCS) is preferable to 'dorsal column stimulation' (DCS).

Dorsal rootlets curve through the highly conductive cerebrospinal fluid (CSF) as they enter the spinal cord; fibres beginning their ascent in the dorsal columns are larger in diameter and they are relatively superficial within the first few segments of the fasciculus gracilis (Ohnishi et al., 1976; Dyck et al., 1985; Feirabend et al., 2002). All these anatomic factors reduce their threshold for depolarization by dorsal midline electrodes, and this accentuates local segmental effects. The thickness of the dorsal CSF space is maximal at the mid-thoracic levels and this accentuates the effect further (Holsheimer et al., 1994). Accordingly, during placement of SCS electrodes for the treatment of low back and leg pain, although advancing electrodes cephalad might be expected to broaden the area of paraesthesias, it may instead elicit excessive, unwanted local segmental effects at the amplitudes necessary to recruit the intended target areas (Law, 1983; Holsheimer, 1997). According to modelling studies, bipolar stimulation is more selective than monopolar stimulation for longitudinally oriented midline fibres; a contact separation of 1.4 times the thickness of the meninges and CSF, or 6–8 mm, is optimal (Holsheimer and Struijk, 1991). Clinical studies have confirmed the advantage of closely spaced bipoles with the cathode cephalad (Law, 1983). Clinical studies as well as models have shown advantages for adding anode(s) cephalad, creating a longitudinal tripole (North et al., 1991, 1992b; Holsheimer, 1997; Holsheimer and Wesselink 1997). Adding lateral anodes to create a transverse tripole should mitigate recruitment of lateral structures and, with a suitably designed pulse generator capable of directing current independently to right- and left-sided anodes, steering of the electrical field becomes possible (Holsheimer et al., 1998).

These models and clinical observations are best established for the most common clinical application of SCS, namely the failed back surgery syndrome, with low back and lower extremity pain. There have been detailed mapping studies of other applications, viz. cervical electrode placement, the results of which have been concordant (Barolat et al., 1993).

3. Implantable devices

3.1. SCS electrodes

SCS electrodes are available in two basic configurations. As shown in Fig. 1, there are catheter designs which can be inserted percutaneously, through a Tuohy needle, and there are insulated paddle or plate designs requiring open surgical placement via laminectomy. When SCS was introduced in the late 1960s, all the available electrodes required surgical exposure for placement in the epidural, endodural or subarachnoid space (Shealy et al., 1967; Nashold and Friedman, 1972; Sweet and Wepsic, 1974; Burton, 1975). As the technical objective of eliciting paraesthesias overlapping a patient's usual distribution of pain was appreciated, electrode placement under local

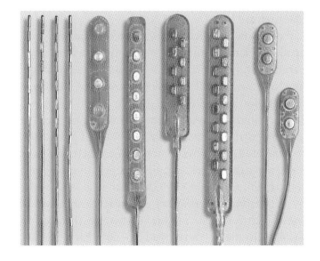

Fig. 1. Contemporary SCS electrode arrays are assemblies of multiple contacts. Catheter designs allow percutaneous placement through a Tuohy needle; insulated plate or paddle arrays require open surgical placement. These may be implanted in the spinal epidural space via a small laminectomy, or directly on a nerve to deliver peripheral nerve stimulation. (Courtesy Advanced Neuromodulation Systems, Inc., Plano, Texas.)

anaesthesia was necessary to be able to confirm this in real time. Open surgical placement was problematic, however, particularly if multiple longitudinal positions were to be tested. Furthermore, as pain relief did not necessarily occur even with technically successful electrode placement, the need for a minimally invasive approach became apparent.

Percutaneous methods for SCS electrode insertion were introduced in the 1970s to address this need (Hosobuchi et al., 1972; Erickson, 1975; Hoppenstein, 1975). The earliest electrode placements had been at high thoracic levels (Shealy et al., 1967; Nashold and Friedman, 1972) but this tended to cause excessive and unpleasant local segmental effects before recruitment of more caudal segments. Percutaneous electrode placement is not only minimally invasive but is also versatile; unlike laminectomy placement, it allows the electrode to be directed many segments away from the site of insertion. Under fluoroscopic guidance, it can be advanced and withdrawn and steered right and left, with test stimulation in the awake patient to establish optimal electrode placement.

Percutaneous electrodes were originally developed to screen patients for implantation of a permanent system, but they were adapted quickly for use as part of the permanent implant (Zumpano and Saunders, 1976; North et al., 1977). Single contact catheters were inserted in tandem for bipolar stimulation but this was often complicated by movement of one electrode with respect to the other, requiring operative revision (North et al., 1977, 1993). This was addressed by multicontact catheters – linear arrays which could be inserted as an assembly through a Tuohy needle – developed in the early 1980s. Concomitant improvements in electrode anchoring techniques addressed the problem of migration of the entire array. Complementing the development of multicontact arrays, programmable, multicontact pulse generators allowed selection of contacts as active anodes and cathodes noninvasively, after implantation. Within the bounds

set by the implanted array, this allows the stimulating anode and cathode positions to be reassigned post-operatively, with the patient in the position in which the device will be used, typically supine or upright. Implantation is constrained in time (as operating room time is expensive and lengthy operations incur added risk) and in space (as the position of the patient, viz. prone, may be irrelevant to everyday use).

Multicontact electrodes and programmable generators have resulted in a statistically significant improvement in technical and clinical results (North et al., 1991, 1993). Over a 20-year period, we recorded hardware failures and clinical failures and subjected them to Kaplan–Meier survival statistics. As shown in Figs. 2 and 3, contemporary programmable multicontact systems are significantly more reliable than single channel systems, by technical as well as clinical outcome measures. The need for surgical revision of electrode position is significantly lower, and clinical benefit is maintained significantly longer.

Comparative studies of electrode designs have been facilitated by the routine clinical practice of placing a temporary percutaneous quadripolar electrode, which is removed and discarded at the conclusion of the trial, followed by permanent implantation with a new electrode, which may be the same or a different design. Each patient may therefore serve as his or her own control. We have compared the performance of different SCS electrode designs in a series of studies using this methodology, along with randomized, blinded presentation of different stimulation parameters to patients, who adjust stimulation parameters to specific psychophysical thresholds using computerized equipment (North, 1998a,b). These studies have established the following:

(1) Insulated (plate) electrodes (requiring a small laminectomy) compare favourably with percutaneous electrodes, for the treatment of low back and lower extremity pain, in a study of linear arrays of four contacts with

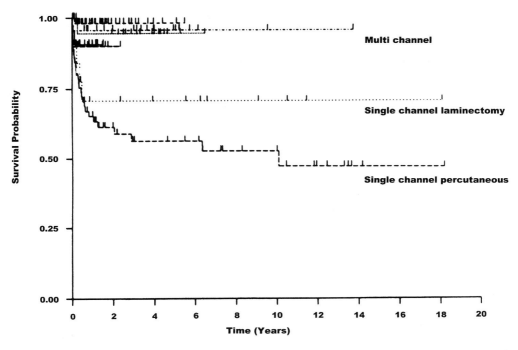

Fig. 2. Kaplan–Meier survival analysis for different electrode configurations used over two decades for SCS uses, as its statistical endpoint, a technical failure requiring return to the operating room for surgical revision of electrode position. Unless radiographically obvious, electrode migration can be difficult to distinguish from malposition such that stimulation paraesthesias do not satisfactorily overlap the patient's distribution of pain; for the purposes of this analysis, the two were equivalent. The uppermost curves represent contemporary multicontact percutaneous and laminectomy electrodes. These have been significantly more reliable than the bipolar, single-channel configurations plotted below. The lowermost curve, which shows eventual technical failure in a majority of patients, represents dual, independently inserted percutaneous electrodes which were vulnerable to migration as well as to malposition. The middle curve represents bipolar electrodes implanted by laminectomy. Neither of these single channel systems allowed non-invasive adjustment of anode and cathode positions. (Reproduced with permission from North et al. (1993).)

nearly identical contact area and spacing (North et al., 2002). The insulated electrode not only performed significantly better than the percutaneous electrode in the same patients by most technical measures, it also required half the power, doubling the predicted battery life. Clinical outcome was significantly better in the short term (1–2 years), but not long-term (3 years) (North, 1998b). Others have reported a superior clinical effectiveness of 'laminectomy' electrodes at a median 34 months (Villavicencio et al., 2000).

(2) 'Dual electrode' percutaneous arrays, consisting of two electrodes side by side, are inferior to a single electrode placed in the midline for the treatment of axial low back pain (North, 1998a). A prospective study comparing dual electrodes of two different spacings with single, midline electrodes, showed significant technical disadvantages for the dual electrodes. Previously reported case series have indicated some advantages for dual electrodes in this application; even if this is not the case, clinical benefit for axial low back pain has been reported consistently (Law and Kirkpatrick, 1991; Law, 1992; Rossi, 1996; Alo et al., 1998). A 16-contact insulated array, with two columns of contacts in parallel, has been used in a recent, successful multicentre trial of SCS for axial low back pain (Barolat et al., 2001, and see Chapter 6).

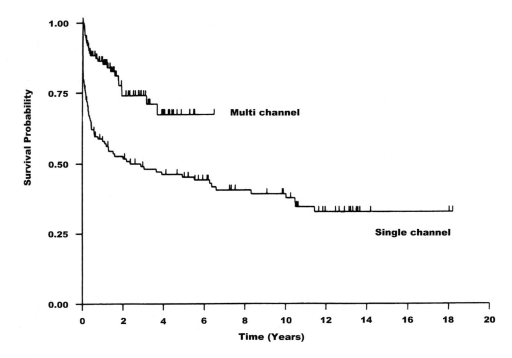

Fig. 3. Kaplan–Meier survival analysis from the same 20-year experience, using clinical failure (patient no longer using stimulator routinely) as the statistical endpoint. This included electro-mechanical failure of the device without replacement, and failure of the device to relieve pain (which could occur independently of technical failure). Programmable, 'multichannel' systems were significantly more reliable ($P < 0.001$). (Reproduced with permission from North et al. (1993).)

3.2. Peripheral nerve stimulation electrodes

Peripheral nerve stimulation (PNS), unlike SCS, was tested percutaneously in the earliest cases (Wall and Sweet, 1967). Over the past three decades, chronically implanted systems have generally used insulated arrays, placed surgically. Some have employed a cuff design, which encircles the involved nerve, but even when it is sized with some allowance for post-operative oedema the potential for constrictive injury remains. This has been avoided by the use of flat arrays of electrodes, which may be identical to SCS electrodes (Picaza et al., 1975; Campbell and Long, 1976; Law et al., 1980; Long et al., 1981; Racz et al., 1990). Most peripheral nerves involved in chronic pain syndromes have mixed sensory and motor function and so motor fibres may be recruited at amplitudes very close to that necessary to produce sensory effects. Peripheral nerves, fortunately, are less mobile than the spinal cord with respect to implanted electrodes and so postural effects are less pronounced. Some specialized electrode configurations and stimulus waveforms have been developed for functional applications, to achieve such effects as unidirectional propagation of action potentials (Van Den Honert and Mortimer, 1979), but these have not been employed in the management of pain.

Clinical application of peripheral nerve stimulation has been limited, compared with SCS, as clinical pain syndromes commonly involve the distribution of more than one nerve (Hassenbusch et al., 1996). Minimally invasive, percutaneous placement has also had limited application but endoscopic techniques are under development and there are some indications for which application to a nerve under direct vision is not required, e.g. suboccipital placement for occipital neuralgia and headache (Weiner, 2000).

3.3. Implanted pulse generators

Radiofrequency (RF) coupled, externally powered systems were the only systems available during the first decade of experience with implanted spinal cord and peripheral nerve stimulators; they remain in routine use. Implanted RF receivers function as amplitude modulated (AM) radio demodulators, rectifying and delivering the envelope of bursts of RF energy as stimulation pulses. They have no implanted batteries or other life-limiting components and thereby avoid the necessity for periodic replacement. They can be inconvenient to the patient, however, and it can be a source of skin irritation to wear an external antenna.

Internally powered 'implanted pulse generators' have been available for over 20 years. These devices have internal batteries and as this is more significant than the location of the pulse generator – which in a sense is implanted even with RF systems – the acronynm 'IPG' might refer properly to 'internally powered generators'. IPGs offer advantages of convenience, cosmetic, and in some cases patient compliance. Their limited battery longevity, however, necessitates periodic surgical replacement, with its attendant cost and morbidity, and therefore there may be compromises in stimulator settings and in usage by the patient, to maximize battery life. IPGs are sometimes referred to as 'totally implanted', but this is a misnomer; the patient must have an external device, such as a magnet or remote transmitter, to control the implant. Simple on–off control and limited amplitude adjustment may be accomplished with a magnet, with some systems; more elaborate external programming devices are necessary to adjust other parameters.

Battery longevity varies inversely as power requirements, which in turn vary directly with pulse amplitude, width, repetition rate (frequency), number of active contacts, and duty cycle (fraction of time used). For the most common application of SCS, the treatment of back and leg pain, typical thoracic electrode placements require high amplitude because of the thickness of the dorsal CSF layer, and therefore battery life can be unacceptably short. At the other extreme, PNS electrodes applied directly to a nerve require low amplitude, maximizing battery life. Individual patient power requirements and patterns of daily usage are evident during the temporary, percutaneous test phase and this can help to guide the choice of an IPG or an RF system.

Figure 4 shows representative implanted pulse generators, including IPGs as well as RF-coupled, externally powered devices.

4. Screening protocols

SCS is 'neuro-modulation' or 'neuro-augmentation', to be distinguished from other pain relieving interventions, such as anatomic procedures directed at a physical abnormality presumed to be causing pain, and ablative procedures which destroy portions of the nervous system to block pain transmission. Augmentative techniques are reversible, and they are amenable to pre-operative testing by a procedure (viz. temporary SCS electrode placement), which emulates the proposed treatment exactly. Anatomic procedures, on the other hand, are not amenable to trial (e.g. pre-operative bracing has limited prognostic value for the outcome of spinal fusion), and the outcome of ablative procedures is not consistently predicted by reversible local anaesthetic block. A temporary epidural electrode, placed percutaneously under local anaesthesia, may be used in a therapeutic trial to establish whether permanent SCS implantation is warranted. The temporary electrode placement also allows mapping of potential electrode positions, to determine the optimal placement of a permanent implant, as well as the choice of electrode design and generator.

Demonstration of pain relief with a temporary SCS or PNS electrode is not only useful clinically, it is required in some health care settings by third party payors before permanent implantation. This requirement may be met, at least technically, by test stimulation during implantation, proceeding

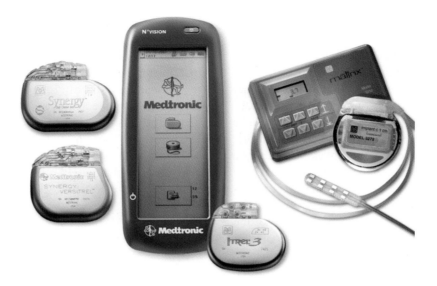

Fig. 4. Implanted generators used for spinal cord and peripheral nerve stimulation allow non-invasive programming, including selection of anode and cathode positions from an electrode array with multiple contacts. Some require or accept power from an externally worn device (right), via RF coupling to an antenna (not visible in this figure); others are powered by implanted primary cells (left). (Courtesy of Medtronic, Inc., Minneapolis, Minnesota.)

directly to internalization, and if the yield is sufficient an argument can be made that this is appropriate (Feler and Kaufman, 1992). A more prolonged trial with a temporary, percutaneous electrode has a number of advantages, however: (1) The pain-relieving effects of stimulation can be assessed outside the operating room (a) under everyday conditions of activity and posture and (b) on reduced pain medications, as appropriate. (2) If the temporary electrode simply exits percutaneously, through the needle tract, then (a) it can be placed in a fluoroscopy room rather than an operating room, minimizing expense and (b) it can be incrementally withdrawn at the bedside, allowing assessment of a greater number of contact positions. This allows the temporary array to be advanced to the most cephalad position, which gives promising results in the naive patient and then be adjusted as experience is gained. (3) As the permanent electrode will be placed independently, experience on the part of the patient and the physician with the temporary system assists with implantation of the permanent device.

A temporary electrode may be configured for later adaptation to a permanent implant. After percutaneous insertion, an incision can be made around the needle, the lead anchored and a percutaneous extension cable, intended for later removal, tunnelled subcutaneously, exiting percutaneously for connection to an external test generator. This saves the expense of the second electrode but it incurs several disadvantages: (1) The patient and physician are committed to two trips to the operating room, one for electrode placement, and another for internalization or, if the trial was unsuccessful, for removal. By comparison, a simple percutaneous lead may be removed at the bedside and only one trip to the operating room is required for those patients undergoing permanent implants. (2) Percutaneous lead extensions increase the risk of infection around the permanent system (Law, 1983; Koeze et al., 1987). This adds a certain urgency to concluding the trial and, given the necessity to return to the operating room in any event, a permanent generator may be implanted prematurely after an inconclusive trial. A temporary electrode destined for removal at the bedside involves no commitment to go to the operating room and therefore does not partially defeat the purpose of the trial. (3) Incisional pain associated with placement of a lead anchor and subcutaneous tunnelling may confound interpretation of the therapeutic trial.

Open surgical electrode placement may be required in some circumstances, e.g. prior spinal or peripheral nerve surgery may preclude percutaneous access. In general, open surgical placement has the technical advantage that it allows introduction of insulated electrodes (which prolong battery life and mitigate side effects, such as pain caused by unwanted recruitment of small fibres in the ligamentum flavum (North et al., 1997a, 2002). Plate electrodes inserted at a laminectomy can also be sutured to the dura, thereby contributing to their greater stability.

The criteria for proceeding from a temporary to a permanent implant have varied considerably. Some authors have required a percutaneous test phase for as long as 2 months (Meglio et al., 1989) while others have implanted in a single stage, with only intraoperative testing (Feler and Kaufman, 1992). Some have required as little as 30% reported pain relief (Bel and Bauer, 1991), while others have required as much as 70–75% (Leibrock et al., 1984; Meilman et al., 1989; De La Porte and Van De Kelft, 1993). If long-term 'success' is defined as a minimum reported percentage pain relief (commonly 50%), this will of course be increased by requiring an arbitrarily high reported percentage during the test phase. An extended trial likewise may be expected to increase the yield, by increasing the sampling period and by allowing more meaningful assessment of everyday activities and analgesic requirements. The author routinely requires a 3-day trial with a temporary electrode, extending it on an individual basis. A prolonged trial may incur not only increased risk of infection but also epidural scarring which may compromise the implantation of a permanent device.

5. Contraindications and complications

Tables I and II present contraindications to SCS, potential complications and adverse effects.

6. Computerized methods of stimulator adjustment

Programmable, multicontact generators and electrode arrays have significantly improved the technical as well as the clinical results of SCS. As the number of contacts on an array increases, the number of possible cathode and anode assignments grows disproportionately (50 for an array of 4, 6050 for an array of 8). This may be multiplied by pulse parameter choices (pulse width, rate and

TABLE I

Contraindications to SCS

Technical
    Demand cardiac pacemaker (requires monitoring EKG or changing pacemaker mode to fixed rate)
    Requirement for MRI
Medical
    Coagulopathy
    Sepsis
Psychological/behavioural
    Untreated, major comorbidity (e.g. depression)
    Serious drug-related, behavioural issues
    Secondary gain
    Inability to cooperate or control device

TABLE II

Potential complications and adverse effects of SCS

Specific to SCS
    Hardware failure
        Generator failure
        Electrode fatigue fracture
    Electrode migration/malposition
    Extraneous influences
        Electromagnetic fields e.g. Diathermy, Security systems
Generic spinal surgical/interventional
    Spinal cord or nerve injury
    CSF leak
    Infection
    Bleeding

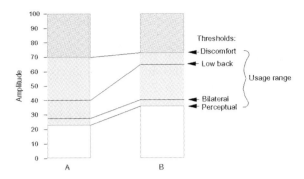

Fig. 5. The clinically relevant range of amplitudes for spinal cord and peripheral nerve stimulation is bounded by perceptual threshold as the minimum and discomfort (or motor) threshold as the maximum. The amplitude at which stimulation paraesthesias cover or overlap the area(s) of pain may be scaled to this range for comparison between settings (A and B). Lower scaled amplitudes are preferable.

amplitude). A range of amplitudes should be assessed for each useful setting, from first perception to discomfort, so that the amplitude at which paraesthesias overlap the distribution of pain can be scaled. This allows comparison between different configurations of electrodes and different pulse parameters, as shown in Fig. 5.

Adjustment of contemporary multicontact devices generates a large volume of data, best addressed by computerized methods (Law, 1987; North and Fowler, 1992; North et al., 1992a,b; Barolat et al., 1993). Data entry may be performed by a health care professional, working with the patient (Law, 1987; Barolat et al., 1993). Alternatively, the patient can interact directly with the computer (North and Fowler, 1992; North et al., 1992a,b, 1998, 2003). We have developed a system for this purpose, whereby the patient uses a graphic input device to control stimulus amplitude, draw areas of pain and stimulation paraesthesias, and enter ratings on a visual analog scale, as illustrated in Fig. 6.

Computerized methods have been applied to several populations of SCS patients, facilitating technical comparisons and development of rules and expert systems (Law, 1987; North et al., 1992a, 1997b, 2003; Barolat et al., 1993). Individual

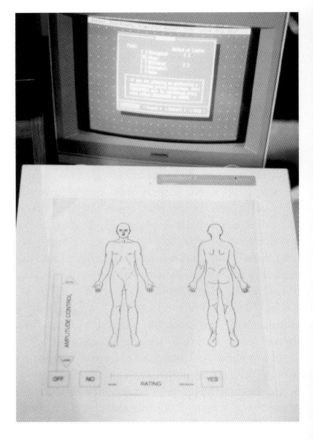

Fig. 6. A graphical user interface on a personal computer can be used by patients to control implanted stimulation devices easily and safely. 'Pain drawings', corresponding drawings of the location of stimulation paraesthesias, and associated 100 mm visual analog ratings may be entered directly by the patient. Quantitative measures of stimulator performance can be derived easily and automatically, to optimize settings for everyday clinical use and to maximize battery life (North et al., 1992a,b, 1998, 2003).

patients ultimately stand to benefit, not only with regard to therapeutic results, but also battery life and ultimately cost-effectiveness (North et al., 2003).

7. Conclusions

Future applications of SCS and PNS will foreseeably be enhanced by ongoing refinements in the design of electrodes and of supporting programmable implants, which are evolving from multicontact to true multichannel systems, functionally equivalent to multiple stimulators. Enhanced adjustment methods, including automated, patient-interactive control systems, will optimize the clinical benefit and overall utility of these systems. Optimizing power management will be important to minimizing the expense of surgical battery replacement, pending the development of improved (e.g. rechargeable) power sources.

References

Alo, K.M., Yland, M.J., Kramer, D.L., Charnov, J.H., and Redko, V. (1998) Computer assisted and patient interactive programming of dual Octrode spinal cord stimulation in the treatment of chronic pain. Neuromodulation, 1: 30–45.

Barolat, G., Massaro, F., He, J., Zeme, S., and Ketcik, B. (1993) Mapping of sensory responses to epidural stimulation of the intraspinal neural structures in man. J. Neurosurg., 78: 233–239.

Barolat, G., Oakley, J.C., Law, J.D., North, R.B., Ketcik, B., and Sharon, A. (2001) Epidural spinal cord stimulation with multiple electrode paddle leads is effective in treating intractable low back pain. Neuromodulation, 4: 59–66.

Bel, S. and Bauer, B.L. (1991) Dorsal column stimulation (DCS): cost to benefit analysis. Acta Neurochir. Suppl., 52: 121–123.

Burton, C. (1975) Dorsal column stimulation: optimization of application. Surg. Neurol., 4: 171–176.

Campbell, J.N. and Long, D.M. (1976) Peripheral nerve stimulation in the treatment of intractable pain. J. Neurosurg., 45: 692–699.

Campbell, J.N., Raja, S.N., Meyer, R.A., and Mackinnon, S.E. (1988) Myelinated afferents signal the hyperalgesia associated with nerve injury. Pain, 32: 89–94.

Coburn, B. and Sin, W. (1985) A theoretical study of epidural electrical stimulation of the spinal cord. Part I: Finite element analysis of stimulus fields. IEEE Trans. Biomed. Eng., 32: 971–977.

De La Porte, C. and Van De Kelft, E. (1993) Spinal cord stimulation in failed back surgery syndrome. Pain, 52: 55–61.

Duggan, A.W. and Foong, F.W. (1985) Bicuculline and spinal inhibition produced by dorsal column stimulation in the cat. Pain, 22: 249–259.

Dyck, P.J., Lais, A., Karnes, J., Sparks, M., and Dyck, P.J.B. (1985) Peripheral axotomy induces neurofilament decrease, atrophy, demyelination and degeneration of root and fasciculus gracilis fibers. Brain Res., 340: 19–36.

Erickson, D.L. (1975) Percutaneous trial of stimulation for patient selection for implantable stimulating devices. J. Neurosurg., 43: 440–444.

Feirabend, H.K.P., Choufoer, H., Ploeger, S., Holsheimer, J., and Van Gool, J.D. (2002) Morphometry of human superficial dorsal and dorsolateral column fibres: significance to spinal cord stimulation. Brain, 125: 1137–1149.

Feler, C. and Kaufman, S. (1992) Spinal cord stimulation: one stage?. Acta Neurochir., 117: 91.

Handwerker, H.O., Iggo, A., and Zimmerman, M. (1975) Segmental and supraspinal actions on dorsal horn neurons responding to noxious and non-noxious skin stimuli. Pain, 1: 147–165.

Hassenbusch, S.J., Stanton-Hicks, M., Schoppa, D., Walsh, J.G., and Covington, E.C. (1996) Long-term results of peripheral nerve stimulation for reflex sympathetic dystrophy. J. Neurosurg., 84: 415–423.

Holsheimer, J. (1997) Effectiveness of spinal cord stimulation in the management of chronic pain: analysis of technical drawbacks and solutions. Neurosurgery, 40: 990–999.

Holsheimer, J. and Struijk, J.J. (1991) How do geometric factors influence epidural spinal cord stimulation? A quantitative analysis by computer modeling. Stereotact. Funct. Neurosurg., 56: 234–249.

Holsheimer, J. and Wesselink, W. (1997) Optimum electrode geometry for spinal cord stimulation: The narrow bipole and tripole. Med. Biol. Eng. Comput., 35: 493–497.

Holsheimer, J., Den Boer, J.A., Struijk, J.J., and Rozeboom, A.R. (1994) MR assessment of the normal position of the spinal cord in the spinal canal. Am. J. Neuroradiol., 15: 951–959.

Holsheimer, J., Nuttin, B., King, G.W., Wesselink, W.A., Gybels, J.M., and De Sutter, P. (1998) Clinical evaluation of paresthesia steering with a new system for spinal cord stimulation. Neurosurgery, 42: 541–547.

Hoppenstein, R. (1975) Electrical stimulation of the ventral and dorsal columns of the spinal cord for relief of chronic intractable pain: preliminary report. Surg. Neurol., 4: 187–194.

Hosobuchi, Y., Adams, J.E., and Weinstein, P.R. (1972) Preliminary percutaneous dorsal column stimulation prior to permanent implantation. J. Neurosurg., 37: 242–245.

Koeze, T.H., Williams, A.C., and Reiman, S. (1987) Spinal cord stimulation and the relief of chronic pain. J. Neurol. Neurosurg. Psychiatry, 50: 1424–1429.

Law, J. (1983) Spinal stimulation: statistical superiority of monophasic stimulation of narrowly separated, longitudinal bipoles having rostral cathodes. Appl. Neurophys., 46: 129–137.

Law, J.D. (1987) Targeting a spinal stimulator to treat the "failed back surgery syndrome". Appl. Neurophys., 50: 437–438.

Law, J.D. (1992) Spinal stimulation in the "failed back surgery syndrome": comparison of technical criteria for palliating pain in the leg vs. in the low back. Acta Neurochir., 117: 95.

Law, J.D. and Kirkpatrick, A.F. (1991) Pain management update: spinal cord stimulation. Am. J. Pain Manage., 2: 34–42.

Law, J.D., Swett, J., and Kirsch, W.M. (1980) Retrospective analysis of 22 patients with chronic pain treated by peripheral nerve stimulation. J. Neurosurg., 45: 692–699.

Leibrock, L., Meilman, P., Cuka, D., and Green, C. (1984) Spinal cord stimulation in the treatment of chronic low back and lower extremity pain syndromes. Nebr. Med. J., 69(6): 180–183.

Lindblom, U., Tapper, N., and Wiesenfeld, Z. (1977) The effect of dorsal column stimulation on the nociceptive response of dorsal horn cells and its relevance for pain suppression. Pain, 4: 133–144.

Linderoth, B. and Meyerson, B.A. (2000) Spinal cord stimulation. I. Mechanisms of action. In: K. Burchiel (Ed.), *Pain Surgery*. Thieme, New York.

Linderoth, B., Gunasekera, L., and Meyerson, B.A. (1991) Effects of sympathectomy on skin and muscle microcirculation during dorsal column stimulation: animal studies. Neurosurgery, 29: 874–879.

Long, D.M., Erickson, D., Campbell, J., and North, R. (1981) Electrical stimulation of the spinal cord and peripheral nerves for pain control. Appl. Neurophysiol., 44: 207–217.

Marchand, S., Bushnell, M.C., Molina-Negro, P., Martinez, S.N., and Duncan, G.H. (1991) The effects of dorsal column stimulation on measures of clinical and experimental pain in man. Pain, 45: 249–257.

Meglio, M., Cioni, B., and Rossi, Gf (1989) Spinal cord stimulation in management of chronic pain. A 9-year experience. J. Neurosurg., 70: 519–524.

Meilman, P.W., Leibrock, L.G., and Leong, F.T.L. (1989) Outcome of implanted spinal cord stimulation in the treatment of chronic pain: arachnoiditis versus single nerve root injury and mononeuropathy. Clin. J. Pain, 5: 189–193.

Melzack, P. and Wall, P.D. (1965) Pain mechanisms: a new theory. Science, 150(3699): 971–978.

Meyerson, B.A., Herregodts, P., and Linderoth, B. (1992) Enhanced flexor reflex in the mononeuropathic rat is attenuated by spinal cord stimulation. Acta Neurochir., 117: 88.

Nashold, B.S., Jr. and Friedman, H. (1972) Dorsal column stimulation for control of pain, preliminary report on 30 patients. J. Neurosurg., 36: 590–597.

Nathan, P.W. (1976) The gate-control theory of pain: a critical review. Brain, 99: 123–158.

North, R.B., 1998a, Spinal cord stimulation for axial low back pain: single versus dual percutaneous electrodes, International Neuromodulation Society Abstracts, Lucerne, Switzerland, p. 212.

North, R.B., 1998b, Quantitative studies of spinal cord stimulation electrode designs, International Neuromodulation Society Abstracts, Lucerne, Switzerland, p. 212.

North, R.B. and Fowler, K.R. (1992) Computer-controlled, patient-interactive neurological stimulation system. Acta Neurochir., 117: 90–91.

North, R.B., Fischell, T.A., and Long, D.M. (1977) Chronic stimulation via percutaneously inserted epidural electrodes. Neurosurgery, 1: 215–218.

North, R.B., Ewend, M.G., Lawton, M.T., and Piantadosi, S. (1991) Spinal cord stimulation for chronic, intractable pain: superiority of 'multichannel' devices. Pain, 44: 119–130.

North, R.B., Fowler, K.R., Nigrin, D.A., and Szymanski, R.E. (1992a) Patient-interactive, computer-controlled neurological stimulation system: clinical efficacy in spinal cord stimulation. J. Neurosurg., 76: 689–695.

North, R.B., Fowler, K.R., Nigrin, D.A., Szymanski, R.E., and Piantadosi, S. (1992b) Automated 'pain drawing' analysis by computer-controlled, patient-interactive neurological stimulation system. Pain, 50: 51–57.

North, R.B., Kidd, D.H., Zahurak, M., James, C.S., and Long, D.M. (1993) Spinal cord stimulation for chronic, intractable pain: two decades' experience. Neurosurgery, 32: 384–395.

North, R.B., Lanning, A., Hessels, R., Cutchis, P.N. (1997a) Spinal cord stimulation with percutaneous and plate electrodes: side effects and quantitative comparisons. Neurosurg. Focus, 2(1): Article 3.

North, R.B., McNamee, P., Wu, L., Piantadosi, S. (1997b) Artificial neural networks: application to electrical stimulation of the human nervous system for intractable pain. Neurosurg. Focus, 2(1): Article 1.

North, R.B., Sieracki, J.M., Fowler, K.R., Alvarez, B., and Cutchis, P.N. (1998) Patient-interactive, microprocessor-controlled neurological stimulation system. Neuromodulation, 1(4): 185–193.

North, R.B., Kidd, D.H., Olin, J., and Sieracki, J.M. (2002) Spinal cord stimulation electrode design: a prospective, randomized, controlled trial comparing percutaneous and laminectomy electrodes. Part I: Technical outcomes. Neurosurgery, 51: 381–389.

North, R.B., Calkins, S.K., Campbell, D.S., Sieracki, J.M., Piantadosi, S., Daly, M.J., Dey, P.B., and Barolat, G. (2003) Automated, patient-interactive spinal cord stimulator adjustment: a randomized controlled trial. Neurosurgery, 52: 572–580.

Ohnishi, A., O'Brien, P.C., Okazaki, H., and Dyck, P.J. (1976) Morphometry of myelinated fibers of fasciculus gracilis of man. J. Neurol. Sci., 27: 163–172.

Picaza, J.A., Cannon, B.W., Hunter, S.E., Boyd, A.S., Guma, J., and Maurer, D. (1975) Pain suppression by peripheral nerve stimulation. Surg. Neurol., 4: 105–114.

Racz, G.B., Lewis, R., Heavner, J.E., and Scott, J. (1990) Peripheral nerve stimulator implant for treatment of causalgia. In: M. Stanton-Hicks (Ed.), *Pain and the Sympathetic Nervous System* (pp. 225–239). Kluwer Academic Publishers, Boston.

Rossi, U., 1996, Technical advances in neuromodulation: state of the art hardware technology in neurostimulation, Abstracts of the 3rd International Congress, International Neuromodulation Society, Orlando p. 11.

Sances, A., Swiontek, T.J., Larson, S.J., Cusick, J.F., Meyer, G.A., Millar, E.A., Hemmy, D.C., and Myklebust, J.

(1975) Innovations in neurologic implant systems. Med. Instrum., 9(5): 213–216.

Shealy, C.N., Mortimer, J.T., and Reswick, J.B. (1967) Electrical inhibition of pain by stimulation of the dorsal columns: preliminary clinical report. Anesth. Analg., 46: 489–491.

Sweet, W. and Wepsic, J. (1974) Stimulation of the posterior columns of the spinal cord for pain control. Clin. Neurosurg., 21: 278–310.

Van Den Honert, C. and Mortimer, J. (1979) Generation of unidirectionally propagated action potentials in a peripheral nerve by brief stimuli. Science, 206: 1311–1312.

Villavicencio, A.T., Leveque, J.-C., Rubin, L., Bulsara, K., and Gorecki, J.P. (2000) Laminectomy versus percutaneous electrode placement for spinal cord stimulation. Neurosurgery, 46: 399–406.

Wall, P.D. and Sweet, W.H. (1967) Temporary abolition of pain in man. Science, 155: 108–109.

Weiner, R.L. (2000) The future of peripheral neurostimulation. Neurol. Res., 22: 299–304.

Zumpano, B.J. and Saunders, R.L. (1976) Percutaneous epidural dorsal column stimulation. J. Neurosurg., 45: 459–460.

Electrical Stimulation and the Relief of Pain
Pain Research and Clinical Management, Vol. 15
Edited by Brian A. Simpson

CHAPTER 13

Motor cortex stimulation

Jean-Paul Nguyen,[a,*] Jean Pascal Lefaucheur,[b] and Yves Keravel[a]

[a]*Department of Neurosurgery, Hôpital Henri Mondor, 51 Avenue du Maréchal de Lattre de Tassigny,
94010 Créteil, France*
[b]*Department of Neurophysiology, Hôpital Henri Mondor, 51 Avenue du Maréchal de Lattre de Tassigny,
94010 Créteil, France*

Abstract

Chronic motor cortex stimulation is a rapidly developing treatment modality essentially indicated for the treatment of chronic deafferentation pain refractory to medical treatment and which cannot be treated by other stimulation techniques. The surgical technique has been improved, and is now more precise, as a result of neuronavigation and easier application of computed tomography (CT) or magnetic resonance imaging (MRI) reconstruction techniques. This technical progress has shown that, in the very great majority of cases, the somatotopical organization of the motor cortex must be taken into account when defining the site of stimulation. A review of the literature shows that the success rate of this procedure ranges from 44 to 88% depending on the indications. The indications must therefore be very carefully selected. At present, the best indications are deafferentation facial pain and central pain, but the success rate can also vary considerably even within these selected indications. The presence of major deafferentation appears to be a factor of poor prognosis for facial pain, while the presence of a severe motor deficit could constitute a cause of failure of treatment of central pain. The indications for MCS for brachial plexus, spinal cord or peripheral nerve injury pain are currently under evaluation.

Ongoing research will probably improve the clinical results and provide a better understanding of the mechanisms of action. Transcranial magnetic stimulation may be predictive of the analgesic effect of implanted stimulation and could therefore constitute a method of selection of candidates for MCS. This technique may also allow the development of indications other than treatment of deafferentation pain, especially abnormal movements and psychiatric disorders. Functional MRI already appears to be essential when the intensity of the neurological disorder suggests a possible somatotopical reorganization of the motor cortex. Positron emission tomography (PET) scanning has shown that MCS mainly acts by activating pathways descending to the thalamus, brainstem and spinal cord, which play a well-known role in inhibition of nociceptive stimuli. In addition to these structures, MCS also activates the cingulate gyrus and insula, which are involved in affective perception of pain. The respective roles of these two mechanisms have not yet been clearly defined. The specific structures activated by MCS also need to be defined: which layer of the cortex; cell bodies or axons; pathways tangential or perpendicular to the cortical surface? Answers to these questions would probably allow more precise definition of stimulation parameters, which are currently only empirical.

Keywords: Motor cortex stimulation; Chronic pain; Deafferentation pain; Neurosurgery; Electrophysiological mapping

*Correspondence to: Dr. J.-P. Nguyen. Phone: + 33 49 81 22 03; Fax: + 33 49 81 22 02; E-mail: mondor@micronet.fr or jean-paul.nguyen@hmm.ap-hop-paris.fr

1. Introduction

Deafferentation pain secondary to a cerebral lesion (so-called central pain) or to a trigeminal nerve lesion (neuropathic facial pain) are generally difficult to treat. Drug treatments are usually not very effective and classical stimulation techniques are unsuitable or ineffective. Stimulation of the ventrolateral nucleus of the thalamus, designed to improve neuropathic facial pain, has been disappointing. Pain secondary to a thalamic lesion (so-called thalamic pain) is also generally refractory to thalamic stimulation.

For these various reasons, the cortex stimulation technique, proposed in 1991 by Tsubokawa (Tsubokawa et al., 1991), constituted a very promising alternative. Tsubokawa observed that central lesions in animals could induce the development of abnormal neuronal hyperactivity in the thalamus, and that this hyperactivity could be reduced by chronic stimulation of the sensorimotor cortex. The results of a first series of patients with thalamic pain confirmed the efficacy of chronic cortex stimulation on this type of pain (Tsubokawa et al., 1993). In this series, 67% of patients obtained marked and lasting improvement, a much higher success rate than that obtained with thalamic stimulation. Surprisingly, stimulation of the motor cortex was found to be more effective than stimulation of the sensory cortex, which sometimes even induced exacerbation of pain.

In 1993, Meyerson confirmed that motor cortex stimulation (MCS) was effective against deafferentation pain (Meyerson et al., 1993). Meyerson's series mainly comprised patients with neuropathic facial pain. All of these patients were improved, but MCS was not effective in two patients with central pain, in contrast with the results reported by Tsubokawa. This discordance can probably be explained by the fact that the surgical technique, at that time, was relatively imprecise and poorly reproducible, as the motor cortex was identified preoperatively by the position of the coronal suture and scalp recording of somatosensory evoked potentials. The electrode placement technique could also increase the imprecision of the procedure, as it consisted of introducing a 4-plate electrode (Resume™, Medtronic, Minneapolis) into the epidural space via a standard burr hole. The quality of electrode positioning therefore essentially depended on the position of the burr hole (Nguyen et al., 1997). As the position of the electrode often had to be changed during the operation, this technique was associated with a risk of epidural haematoma. With time, the technique has become more precise with a lower risk of complications. In parallel with improvement of the technique, the results of other teams have shown that the indications for MCS could be extended to other types of pain (Nguyen et al., 1999; Franzini et al., 2000; Saitoh et al., 2000; Katayama et al., 2001; Roux et al., 2001b).

In this review, we will successively describe the various steps leading to improvement of the surgical procedure, the current main indications and the various hypotheses concerning the mechanism of the analgesic action of chronic MCS.

2. Technique

2.1. Preoperative mapping of the motor cortex

Clinicopathological and electrophysiological studies have established, a long time ago, that the primary motor cortex (Brodman's area; Brodman, 1925) is situated in the anterior part of the central fissure and the part of the cortex immediately anterior to this fissure. Penfield's studies also demonstrated the somatotopical representation of the lower limbs, upper limbs and face that are represented on the superior, middle and inferior parts of the precentral gyrus, respectively (Penfield and Rasmussen, 1950). The motor cortex can therefore be mapped indirectly by determining the anatomical position of the central fissure (Fig. 1). This fissure is visible on computed tomography (CT) scanning and even more clearly visualized on

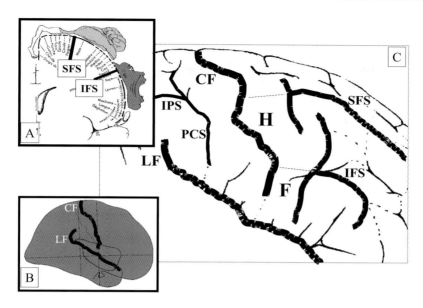

Fig. 1. Anatomical landmarks of the central region and correlations with functional zones of the motor cortex: (A) Penfield's homunculus. The functional zones of the motor cortex (face (F image C), hand (H image C) and lower part of the body) are defined schematically by the position of the superior frontal sulcus (SFS) and inferior frontal sulcus (IFS). (B) General view of the central region showing the position of the central fissure (CF) and lateral fissure (LF). (C) Detail of the central region showing the position of the SFS, which is connected to the superior precentral sulcus, the IFS, which is connected to the inferior precentral sulcus, and the post-central sulcus (PCS), which is connected to the intraparietal sulcus (IPS).

magnetic resonance imaging (MRI). However, classical axial, frontal and sagittal views are unsuitable to identify the various zones (superior, middle and inferior) of the central and precentral region. Progress in the field of digital image processing now allows identification of these various zones. These various structures can be easily identified on images obtained after curved reconstruction following the curvature of the cortical surface (Lee et al., 1998). Visualization of the inferior and superior frontal sulci and the longitudinal cerebral fissure and lateral fissure allows objective delineation of the three main functional zones of the precentral gyrus. Images corresponding to the cortical surface are generally difficult to interpret, as the folds of the gyri often create the appearance of intermediate sulci that interfere with identification of the main sulci and fissures. However, these structures are generally very easily identified on deeper reconstructions (Fig. 2). In our experience, images situated 5 mm

below the surface of the cortex are the easiest to interpret. The ideal site of stimulation, based on our knowledge of the somatotopical representation of this region, can be easily determined on these images.

Theoretically, to treat neuropathic facial pain, MCS should be applied to the lower part of the precentral gyrus corresponding to the representation of the face on the motor homunculus. According to the studies by Penfield (Penfield and Rasmussen, 1950), Woolsey (Woolsey et al., 1979) and McCarthy (McCarthy et al., 1993), this zone is limited inferiorly by the frontoparietal operculum and lateral fissure and superiorly by a horizontal line corresponding to a posterior continuation of the inferior frontal sulcus. The zone of stimulation for treatment of deafferentation pain affecting the upper limb is situated between the levels of the inferior and superior frontal sulci. The motor cortex situated between the levels of the superior frontal sulcus and

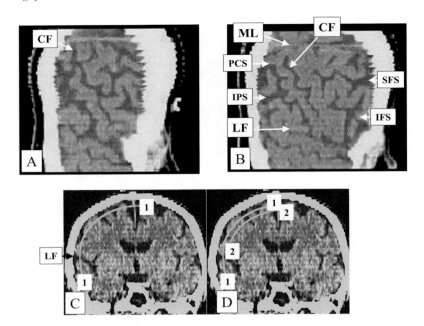

Fig. 2. Curved reconstructions following the plane of the cerebral surface: (A) Superficial reconstruction according to curve 1 (image C). The central fissure (CF) is difficult to identify as it receives connections from adjacent sulci. (B) Reconstruction according to a deeper curve (2 image D). The central fissure (CF), lateral fissure (LF), post-central sulcus (PCS), intraparietal sulcus (IPS), superior frontal sulcus (SFS) and inferior frontal sulcus (IFS) are easily identified. ML: Midline.

longitudinal cerebral fissure corresponds to the representation of the trunk and proximal part of the lower limbs. The distal part of the lower limbs is classically represented essentially in the internal surface of the hemisphere. However, Woolsey showed that, in some cases, this representation could extend to the superior part of the hemisphere, even as far as the superior frontal sulcus.

These various functional zones are easily identified by neuronavigation systems, but, at present, these systems are unable to perform curved reconstructions. However, oblique reconstructions, relatively parallel to the cortical surface, can be very easily obtained. The various structures visualized by curved reconstructions (performed preoperatively) can be identified on these oblique reconstructions (Fig. 3), which can be used to define the same target. The neuronavigation system allows the centre of the craniotomy to be placed very precisely over the target (Fig. 4).

Other examinations can also be helpful for preoperative target planning: functional MRI (fMRI) and especially transcranial magnetic stimulation (TMS). fMRI provides good visualization of the sensorimotor cortex and its spatial resolution is sufficient to establish somatotopical maps (Rao et al., 1995). The results of fMRI are well correlated with the results of direct cortical stimulation and intraoperative somatosensory evoked potentials (SEP) (Roux et al., 2001b). Some teams regularly use fMRI for preoperative motor cortex target planning (Sol et al., 2001). TMS can also be used to identify the motor cortex (Migita et al., 1995).

2.2. Craniotomy

Several authors have demonstrated the advantages of craniotomy over a burr hole (Peyron et al., 1995; Ebel et al., 1996; Nguyen et al., 1999). By allowing suspension of the dura mater, a true

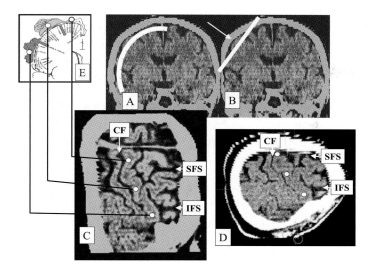

Fig. 3. Superficial curved and oblique reconstructions: (A) Superficial curved reconstruction represented on image C, visualizing the central fissure (CF), superior frontal sulcus (SFS) and inferior frontal sulcus (IFS). White circles correspond to functional zones of the face, hand and lower part of the body, represented on image E. (B) Superficial oblique reconstruction represented on image D. This type of reconstruction can be used with all neuronavigation systems (so-called 'surgeon's eye' or 'tool view' function indicated by the white arrow on image (B). The potential location of functional areas of the motor cortex is represented by white circles. In this particular case, the target (open circle) was placed just anteriorly to the central fissure, between the functional zones of the face and the hand.

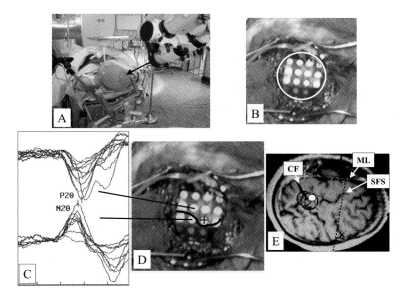

Fig. 4. Craniotomy and recording of SEP: (A) The neuronavigation system ensures that the craniotomy (white circle on image B) is correctly centred over the target selected by imaging (black arrow). (B) A 16-plate electrode is placed on the dura mater. (C) SEP are recorded by the 16-plate electrode after stimulation of the median nerve at the wrist. (D) The position of the electrodes at which the P20 (precentral) and N20 (post-central) waves are recorded corresponds to the theoretical position of the central fissure (black line). The good correspondence with the anatomical targeting (white circle on image E) can be immediately verified on the imaging (in this case MRI) by pointing (laser beam or cursor of neuronavigation system) on one of the plates (black cross) situated just anteriorly to the central fissure (CF image E). ML: midline, SFS: superior frontal sulcus.

craniotomy limits the risk of postoperative epidural haematoma. A craniotomy 4–5 cm in diameter allows sufficient exploration of the central region to identify the appropriate area of the motor cortex to be stimulated. A larger access also allows a multi-plate electrode to be placed on the dura mater to optimize intraoperative electrophysiological testing. We use a 16-plate diagnostic electrode array (Cormedica, Vaulx-Milieu, France) allowing recording of SEP as well as intraoperative MCS (Fig. 4).

2.3. Intraoperative electrophysiological testing

The first step of electrophysiological testing consists of confirming the position of the central sulcus detected by the neuronavigation system by recording SEP. Theoretically, the polarity of the potentials recorded 20 ms after stimulation of the median nerve at the wrist is reversed across the central sulcus (N20/P20 phase shift). The zone of N20 potential recording is situated anteriorly to this sulcus and globally corresponds to the part of the motor cortex corresponding to representation of the hand. Potentials recorded after stimulation of the posterior tibial nerve or labial commissure are difficult to interpret and are consequently rarely used to identify the central sulcus. Fig. 4 shows the N20 and P20 waves recorded by the 16-plate diagnostic electrode applied to the dura mater. The good correlation between radiological and electrophysiological data can be easily verified in real time by using the pointer system or laser guidance beam of the neuronavigation system. In our experience, a very good correlation has always been obtained between SEP data and the anatomical position of the central fissure indicated by the neuronavigation system. In the case of severe deafferentation, SEP may be difficult or even impossible to record. The absence of preoperative SEP does not necessarily mean that they will be absent intraoperatively, as SEP recording from electrodes placed on the dura mater is more sensitive than scalp recording.

The second step consists of confirming the position of the motor cortex by stimulation. The objective of this step is to stimulate the contacts of the grid placed over the motor cortex to trigger muscle jerks in the zone corresponding to the pain (Fig. 5). In the case of upper limb pain, those contacts providing the highest N20 potentials will be stimulated. For pain of the face and lower half of the body, contacts situated below or above this zone will be stimulated. The following stimulation parameters are generally used: pulse width: 1 ms; frequency: 16–20 Hz; intensity: 5–10 mA. The stimulation amplitude mainly varies according to the depth of general anaesthesia and the distance between the dura mater and the cerebral cortex.

2.4. Implantation technique

The site of the Resume™ 4-plate electrode (Fig. 5) for chronic stimulation depends on the results of the electrophysiological tests (SEP and stimulation). The electrode is positioned perpendicularly in the direction of the central sulcus to ensure that at least one of the contacts is situated over the motor cortex, whose width varies considerably from one part of the central region to another (Figs. 6 and 7). This positioning also allows verification of the potential analgesic efficacy of stimulation of the sensory cortex or premotor cortex (Fig. 7). This electrode is sutured to the dura mater with two sutures.

The electrode is connected to a lead wire which is tunnelled out onto the skin to test the efficacy of stimulation for several days. When the efficacy of stimulation has been confirmed, this temporary lead wire is replaced by a completely internalized lead wire connected to a pulse generator implanted subcutaneously (Itrel 3™ or Synergy™, Medtronic, Minneapolis), generally in the supraclavicular region.

2.5. Stimulation parameters

Mean stimulation parameters based on our experience are as follows: frequency: 40 Hz

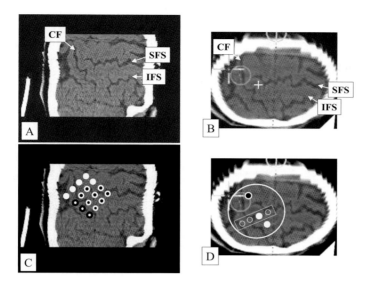

Fig. 5. Example of treatment of deafferentation pain of the upper limb: (A) Superficial curved reconstruction clearly showing the central fissure (CF), superior frontal sulcus (SFS) and inferior frontal sulcus (IFS). (B) Superficial oblique reconstruction showing the same landmarks. The target (indicated by a white cross) has been placed at the midpoint between the termination of the superior frontal sulcus and the central fissure. (C) Representation of the position of the 16-plate electrode. The electrodes at which P20 waves were recorded (SEP by stimulation of the median nerve) are represented by black circles with a white outline. The electrodes at which N20 waves were recorded are represented by white circles with a black outline. No potentials were recorded at the electrodes represented by white circles. (D) Positions of the craniotomy and the electrodes at which stimulation was followed by muscle contractions of the hand (white circles) and foot (black circle with a white outline). The 4-plate chronic stimulation electrode (Resume^{TM}, Medtronic, Minneapolis) is represented by a white rectangle. This electrode has been placed perpendicularly to the central fissure (see comments in the text).

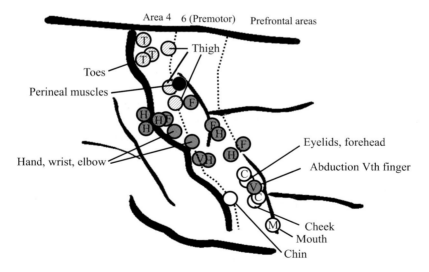

Fig. 6. Correlations between anatomical targeting and motor effects (19 patients): The various circles represent the position of the electrodes at which stimulation induced muscle contractions. White circles: region of the face. Grey circles: region of the upper limb. Black circle: pelvic region. Hatched circle: region of the lower limb. Vertical dotted lines indicate the theoretical position of the motor, premotor and prefrontal cortex. M: Mouth, C: Cheek, H: Hand, F: Fingers, V: Little finger, T: Toes.

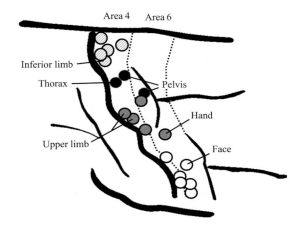

Fig. 7. Correlations between anatomical targeting and analgesic effects (19 patients obtaining an excellent or good analgesic result): Same legends as for the previous figure. An analgesic effect on intercostal deafferentation pain was obtained by chronic stimulation of a zone situated between the level of the superior frontal sulcus and the midline. Several effective stimulation sites are situated in the premotor region.

(range: 25–55); pulse width: 82.4 μs (range: 60–180); amplitude: 2.1 V (range: 1.3–4). Bipolar stimulation is used in most cases with the negative pole overlying the motor cortex and the positive pole over the sensory cortex. Some teams have obtained good results by using higher stimulation voltages, approximately corresponding to 70–80% of motor threshold values (Tsubokawa et al., 1991; Meyerson et al., 1993; Mogilner and Rezai, 2001). Continuous stimulation can be used but our experience with spinal cord stimulation has encouraged us to use a cycling mode, which is preferable. This prolongs the battery life and it also seems to offer a more stable response in the long term. The duration of the cycling phases depends on the duration of the post-stimulation effect. We use either 3 h on and 3 h off or 12 h on and 12 h off.

3. Indications and results

A review of the literature reveals two main indications: central pain and trigeminal neuropathic pain (Tsubokawa et al., 1991, 1993; Hosobuchi, 1993; Meyerson et al., 1993; Canavero, 1995; Herregodts et al., 1995; Migita et al., 1995; Peyron et al., 1995; Ebel et al., 1996; Nguyen et al., 1997, 1998, 1999; Rainov et al., 1997; Yamamoto et al., 1997; Katayama et al., 1998, 2001; Canavero et al., 1999; Garcia-Larrea et al., 1999; Mertens et al., 1999; Carroll et al., 2000; Franzini et al., 2000; Saitoh et al., 2000, 2001; Mogilner and Rezai, 2001; Pirotte et al., 2001; Roux et al., 2001a,b; Sol et al., 2001).

3.1. Central pain

Central pain, especially pain related to a thalamic lesion, theoretically constitutes the best indication for MCS. Moreover, Tsubokawa developed this treatment modality specifically in order to treat this type of pain (Tsubokawa et al., 1991).

In most cases published in the literature, the pain is secondary to haemorrhagic or ischaemic stroke: 11 cases for Tsubokawa (Tsubokawa et al., 1993), 11 cases for Nguyen (Nguyen et al., 1999), three cases for Katayama (three cases of Wallenberg syndrome; Katayama et al., 1998) and two cases for Migita (Migita et al., 1995). Central pain can also be secondary to other causes, e.g. head injury or thalamic abscess (Nguyen et al., 1999). The review of the literature indicates that 159 cases of central pain secondary to stroke have been published to date. It is difficult to analyse the results of these cases, as the assessment criteria are not always the same. When only very good results are considered (> 50% improvement on the Visual Analog Scale: VAS) the success rate is 52% (82/159 patients).

These results need to be modulated, however, as they do not take into account those patients who obtained a satisfactory improvement without achieving a 50% improvement on the VAS. For example, in our series of 18 cases of central pain (Nguyen, 2002), seven (38.9%) obtained very marked improvement (> 60% improvement on the VAS), eight (44.5%) obtained an improvement considered to be satisfactory (40–60%

improvement on the VAS) and three (16.6%) were not improved. The mean clinical follow-up was 46 months. More than 80% of the patients declared themselves to be satisfied with the operation.

3.2. Trigeminal neuropathic pain

Trigeminal neuropathic pain represents the second main indication. In the majority of cases in our series, the pain was secondary to thermocoagulation of the trigeminal ganglion (54.5%). In 36.3% of cases, the pain was secondary to surgery to the maxillary sinus, posterior fossa or cavernous sinus (Nguyen et al., 1999). Forty-five cases of neuropathic facial pain have been reported in the literature. A very good improvement (> 50% improvement on the VAS) was obtained in 33 patients (73%), but these results also need to be modulated. In our series of 22 patients, 13 (59%) obtained very marked improvement, five (22.8%) obtained satisfactory improvement and four were not improved (Nguyen, 2002).

3.3. Other indications

The other indications concern deafferentation pain of the upper limbs, lower limbs or trunk. This type of pain can theoretically be improved by cervical or thoracic spinal cord stimulation; MCS is in general only considered following failure of these techniques.

Several authors have demonstrated the efficacy of MCS in the treatment of *phantom limb pain*. However, fairly discordant results have been reported. Overall (19 cases published in the literature), very good results were obtained in about 53% of patients. The results were less favourable in Katayama's series (Katayama et al., 2001), as only 20% patients were improved. According to this author, thalamic stimulation (nucleus ventralis caudalis) was more effective (60% good results). Somatotopical reorganization could account for these disappointing results of MCS. fMRI would theoretically be able to identify

these changes and may explain the much better results obtained by Sol and colleagues (2001).

Pain related to *brachial plexus injury* can also be treated with MCS. Eighteen cases have been published in the literature. The results are relatively disappointing, as only 44% of patients were improved. As in phantom limb pain, fMRI could be useful to detect somatotopical modifications, which may be considerable in the case of complete sensorimotor deficit. In this case, the absence of SEPs and of a motor effect of cortical stimulation make target mapping considerably more difficult.

Similar problems are encountered in patients with pain related to complete *paraplegia* or *quadriplegia*. Curiously, the published results appear to be much better (seven out of eight patients improved). In all of these cases, treatment was designed to relieve pain below the lesion. Unilateral MCS has been shown to be effective even in the case of bilateral pain (Nguyen et al., 1999).

Only five cases of pain related to a *peripheral nerve lesion* have been published. Four of these five patients were markedly improved. Some of these patients presented with nerve root or nerve trunk pain related to multi-operated neurofibromas in the context of Von Recklinghausen disease (Nguyen et al., 1999; Smith et al., 2001). One case of intercostal herpes zoster responded favourably to MCS (Nguyen et al., 1999).

3.4. Case selection

Regardless of the method of evaluation used, the results obtained in the treatment of neuropathic facial pain are clearly better than those obtained in the treatment of central pain. Katayama's group (1998) have shown that patients with central pain and a marked motor deficit have a significantly less favourable response to MCS than other patients. In our series, the mean improvement on the VAS was $38.1 \pm 8\%$ in patients with motor weakness and $46.5 \pm 9\%$ in patients with no evidence of motor weakness. A similar difference was reported by Katayama, but the difference between the two groups was not significant ($P = 0.53$). Similarly, severe sensory deafferentation can also be considered to be a factor of poor prognosis. In our series, the mean improvement on the VAS was $39.5 \pm 8\%$ in patients with a marked sensory deficit and allodynia and $47.8 \pm 8\%$ in the other patients; this difference was not statistically significant ($P = 0.52$).

Repetitive transcranial magnetic stimulation (rTMS) of the motor cortex has been shown to be a very useful tool to predict the effect of stimulation by implanted electrodes (Lefaucheur et al., 2001a). We studied the effect of preoperative rTMS in seven patients with central pain (Nguyen, 2001): three patients obtained a major analgesic effect, while this stimulation had no effect in the other four patients. All patients were subsequently operated: the three patients who were improved by rTMS were all improved by subsequent MCS (mean improvement on the VAS: $72 \pm 14\%$) and the four patients not improved by rTMS were not improved postoperatively (mean improvement on the VAS: $32.2 \pm 11\%$). Although the difference was not significant ($P = 0.07$), these results confirm those reported in the literature (Lefaucheur et al., 2001b; Drouot et al., 2002).

3.5. Adverse and side effects

Globally, 11.4% of published cases experienced an adverse effect (Tsubokawa et al., 1991, 1993; Hosobuchi, 1993; Meyerson et al., 1993; Canavero, 1995; Herregodts et al., 1995; Migita et al., 1995; Peyron et al., 1995; Ebel et al., 1996; Nguyen et al., 1997, 1998, 1999; Rainov et al., 1997; Yamamoto et al., 1997; Katayama et al., 1998, 2001; Canavero et al., 1999; Garcia-Larrea et al., 1999; Mertens et al., 1999; Carroll et al., 2000; Franzini et al., 2000; Saitoh et al., 2000, 2001; Mogilner and Rezai, 2001; Pirotte et al., 2001; Roux et al., 2001a,b; Sol et al., 2001). The most serious represent 3.6% of all cases: epi- or subdural haematoma (2.2%), epileptic seizures (0.7%) and speech disorders (0.7%). The larger

craniotomy should improve the epi- or subdural haematoma risk (Nguyen et al., 1999). The low incidence of epileptic seizures during chronic stimulation shows that stimulation of the cortex through the dura with reasonable intensity is safe (Bezard et al., 1999). Skin ulceration and infection was encountered in 0.7 and 2.2% of published cases. Side effects induced by stimulation consisted of paraesthesia and dysaesthesia (2.2%) and pain at the site of implanted electrode (0.7%).

4. Mechanism of action

The mechanism of action of MCS has not been fully elucidated. In his first publications, Tsubokawa proposed the hypothesis that MCS antidromically activated neurons of the sensory cortex (Tsubokawa et al., 1993), allowing descending impulses to activate structures inhibiting the abnormal thalamic hyperactivity which occurred secondary to the deafferentation phenomenon. However, several results tended to refute this hypothesis. The clinical improvement after MCS of some patients with infarction of the post-central region and the absence of modification of cerebral blood flow in the post-central region on position emission tomography (PET) scanning during MCS (Garcia-Larrea et al., 1999), argued against the potential role of neurons of sensory areas.

In contrast, these studies showed that the most marked changes in regional blood flow in response to MCS mainly concerned the nucleus ventralis lateralis and the nucleus ventralis anterior of the thalamus. These structures are directly connected to the motor cortex and direct activation of these nuclei can explain the effects of MCS on motor disorders: improvement of spasticity (Garcia-Larrea et al., 1999) or tremor (Nguyen et al., 1998). The role of these structures in the analgesic effect is more difficult to explain. MCS also induces changes in blood flow in other structures more directly involved in pain mechanisms, especially the midline thalamic nuclei, anterior cingulate gyrus, insula, and the upper part of the brainstem (Garcia-Larrea et al., 1999). The role of the anterior cingulate gyrus and insula in pain mechanisms and their relations with the midline thalamic nuclei have been clearly established. Connections between these cortical regions and anterior thalamic nuclei have also been demonstrated (Garcia-Larrea et al., 1999). The direct action of the pyramidal tract on the posterior horn of the spinal cord may also play a major role in the analgesic effects of MCS (Coulter et al., 1974).

It is now fairly well established that the analgesic effect of MCS depends on the zone of motor cortex stimulated. It is therefore essential to take the somatotopical organization of the cortex into account; as our studies (Nguyen et al., 1999) have demonstrated, the sites of stimulation effective against pain correspond to the sites at which intraoperative stimulation triggers motor responses (Figs. 6 and 7). MCS clearly stimulates the motor cortex as a whole; not only the primary motor area (area 4) but also the premotor area (area 6). The results of MCS on phantom limb pain showed that somatotopical reorganization must also be taken into account and these can be demonstrated by fMRI and/or rTMS. Activation of inhibitory descending structures (especially anterior thalamic nuclei) may only be effective when the somatotopical organization of the motor cortex is taken into account.

The specific structures activated by MCS need to be defined: which layer of the cortex? cell bodies or axons? pathways tangential or perpendicular to the cortical surface? Answers to these questions would probably allow more precise definition of stimulation parameters, which are currently only empirical. The difficulty of adjusting stimulation parameters is mainly due to the latency of the analgesic effect, as the effect of an adjustment can often only be determined on the following day or even several days later. In rare cases, the analgesic effect has been obtained during the minutes following the start of stimulation. In these patients, the best effect was obtained with a relatively low stimulation amplitude, about 2 mA

(2 V for an impedance of 1000 Ω) at a frequency of about 40 Hz with a pulse width of 60 ms.

5. Conclusions

Motor cortex stimulation, introduced and recommended by Tsubokawa, is a promising treatment modality for deafferentation pain. It is essentially indicated for the treatment of pain that cannot be controlled by spinal cord stimulation: central pain and neuropathic facial pain. Optimal selection of the best indications must be based on a technique that precisely identifies the zone to be stimulated. A relatively large craniotomy and the use of a neuronavigation system appear to be essential. Other indications need to be confirmed, especially paraplegic pain, phantom limb pain, and plexus injury pain. The more systematic use of functional MRI and repetitive TMS will probably contribute to extension of the indications of MCS. We also obviously need to improve our understanding of the mechanisms of action of MCS.

Acknowledgments

The authors would like to thank Thierry Poiraud for his assistance in the review of the literature.

References

Bezard, E., Boraud, T., Nguyen, J.P., Velasco, F., Keravel, Y., and Gross, C. (1999) Cortical stimulation and epileptic seizure: a study of the potential risk in primates. Neurosurgery, 45: 346–350.

Brodman K. (1925) In: Barth JA (Ed.), Vergleichende Lokalisationslehre der Grosshirnrinde in Prinzipien darges-tellt auf Grund des Zellenbaues. Leipzig.

Canavero, S. (1995) Cortical stimulation for central pain. J. Neurosurg., 83: 1117.

Canavero, S., Bonicalzi, V., Castellano, G., Perozzo, P., and Massa-Micon, B. (1999) Painful supernumerary phantom arm following motor cortex stimulation for central post-stroke pain. J. Neurosurg., 91: 121–123.

Carroll, D., Joint, C., Maartens, N., Schlugman, D., Stein, J., and Aziz, T.Z. (2000) Motor cortex stimulation for chronic neuropathic pain: a preliminary study of 10 cases. Pain, 84: 431–437.

Coulter, J.D., Maunz, R.A., and Willis, W.D. (1974) Effects of stimulation of sensorimotor cortex on primate spinothalamic neurons. Brain Res., 64: 351–356.

Drouot, X., Nguyen, J.P., Peschanski, M., and Lefaucheur, J.P. (2002) The antalgic efficacy of chronic motor cortex stimulation is related to sensory changes in the painful zone. Brain, 125: 1660–1664.

Ebel, H., Rust, D., Tronnier, V., Böker, D., and Kunze, S. (1996) Chronic precentral stimulation in trigeminal neuropathic pain. Acta Neurochir., 138: 1300–1306.

Franzini, A., Ferroli, P., Servello, D., and Broggi, G. (2000) Reversal of thalamic hand syndrome by long-term motor cortex stimulation. J. Neurosurg., 93: 873–875.

Garcia-Larrea, L., Peyron, R., Mertens, P., Gregoire, M.C., Lavenne, F., Le Bars, D., Convers, P., Maugière, F., Sindou, M., Laurent, B. (1999) Electrical stimulation of motor cortex for pain control: a combined PET-scan and electrophysiological study. Pain, 83: 259–273.

Herregodts, P., Stadnik, T., De Ridder, F., and D'Haens, J. (1995) Cortical stimulation for central neuropathic pain: 3-D surface MRI for easy determination of the motor cortex. Acta Neurochir. Suppl., 64: 132–135.

Hosobuchi, Y. (1993) *Motor Cortex Stimulation for Control of Central Deafferentation Pain. Electrical and Magnetic Stimulation of the Brain and Spinal Cord* (pp. 215–217). Raven Press, New York.

Katayama, Y., Fukaya, C., and Yamamoto, T. (1998) Poststroke pain control by chronic motor cortex stimulation: neurological characteristics predicting a favorable response. J. Neurosurg., 89: 585–591.

Katayama, Y., Yamamoto, T., Kobayashi, K., Kasai, M., Oshima, H., and Fukaya, C. (2001) Motor cortex stimulation for phantom limb pain: a comprehensive therapy with spinal cord and thalamic stimulation. Stereotact. Funct. Neurosurg., 77: 159–161.

Lee, U., Bastos, A.C., Alonso-Vanegas, M.A., Morris, R., and Olivier, A. (1998) Topographic analysis of the gyral patterns of the central area. Stereotact. Funct. Neurosurg., 70: 38–51.

Lefaucheur, J.P., Drouot, X., Keravel, Y., and Nguyen, J.P. (2001a) Pain relief induced by repetitive transcranial magnetic stimulation of precentral cortex. Neuroreport, 12: 1–3.

Lefaucheur, J.P., Drouot, X., and Nguyen, J.P. (2001b) Interventional neurophysiology for pain control: duration of pain relief following repetitive transcranial magnetic stimulation of the motor cortex. Neurophysiol. Clin., 31: 247–252.

McCarthy, G., Allison, T., and Spencer, D.D. (1993) Localization of the face area of human sensorimotor cortex by intracranial recording of somatosensory evoked potentials. J. Neurosurg., 79: 874–884.

Mertens, P., Nuti, C., Sindou, M., Guenot, M., Peyron, R., Garcia-Larrea, L., and Laurent, B. (1999) Precentral cortex stimulation for the treatment of central neuropathic pain. Stereotact. Funct. Neurosurg., 73: 122–125.

Meyerson, B.A., Lindblom, U., Lind, G., and Herregodts, P. (1993) Motor cortex stimulation as treatment of trigeminal neuropathic pain. Acta Neurochir. Suppl., 58: 150–153.

Migita, K., Tohru, U., Kazunori, A., and Shuji, M. (1995) Transcranial magnetic coil stimulation in patients with central pain. Technique and application. Neurosurgery, 36: 1037–1040.

Mogilner A.Y., Rezai A.R. (2001) Epidural motor cortex stimulation with functional imaging guidance. Neurosurg. Focus 11: Article 4.

Nguyen J.P. (2001) Motor cortex and transcranial magnetic stimulation. Neuromodulation symposium, Cleveland, June.

Nguyen J.P. (2002) Motor cortex stimulation. 10th World Congress on Pain, San Diego.

Nguyen, J.P., Keravel, Y., Feve, A., Uchiyama, T., Cesaro, P., Le Guerinel, C., and Pollin, B. (1997) Treatment of deafferentation pain by chronic stimulation of the motor cortex: report of a series of 20 cases. Acta Neurochir. Suppl., 68: 54–60.

Nguyen, J.P., Pollin, B., Feve, A., Geny, C., and Cesaro, P. (1998) Improvement of action tremor by chronic cortical stimulation. Mov. Disord., 13: 84–88.

Nguyen, J.P., Lefaucheur, J.P., Decq, P., Uchiyama, T., Carpentier, A., Fontaine, D., Brugières, P., Pollin, B., Feve, A., Rostaing, S., Cesaro, P., Keravel, Y. (1999) Chronic motor cortex stimulation in the treatment of central and neuropathic pain. Correlations between clinical, electrophysiological and anatomical data. Pain, 82: 245–251.

Penfield, W. and Rasmussen, T. (1950) *The Cerebral Cortex of Man. A Clinical Study of Localization of Function.* Macmillan, New York.

Peyron, R., Garcia-Larrea, L., Deiber, M.P., Cinotti, L., Convers, P., Sindou, M., Maugière, F., and Laurent, B. (1995) Electrical stimulation of precentral cortical area in the treatment of central pain: electrophysiological and PET study. Pain, 62: 275–286.

Pirotte B., Voordecker P., Joffroy F., Massager N., Wilker D., Baleriaux D., Levivier M., Brotchi J. (2001) The Zeiss-MKM system for frameless image-guides approach in epidural motor cortex stimulation for central neuropathic pain. Neurosurg. Focus, 11: Article 3.

Rainov, N.G., Fels, C., Heidecke, V., and Burkert, W. (1997) Epidural electrical stimulation of the motor cortex in patients with facial neuralgia. Clin. Neurol. Neurosurg., 99: 205–209.

Rao, S.M., Binder, J.R., Hammeke, T.A., Bandettini, P.A., Bobholz, J.A., Frost, J.A., Myklebust, B.M., Jacobson, R.D., and Hyde, J.S. (1995) Somatotopic mapping of the human primary motor cortex with functional magnetic resonance imaging. Neurology, 45: 919–924.

Roux, F.E., Ibarrola, D., Lazorthes, Y., and Berry, I. (2001a) Chronic motor cortex stimulation for phantom limb pain: a functional Magnetic Resonance Imaging study: technical case report. Neurosurgery, 48: 681–688.

Roux, F.E., Ibarrola, D., Tremoulet, M., Lazorthes, Y., Henry, P., Sol, J.C., and Berry, I. (2001b) Methodological and technical issues for integrating functional Magnetic Resonance Imaging data in a neuronavigation system. Neurosurgery, 49: 1145–1157.

Saitoh, Y., Shibata, M., Hirano, S.I., Hirata, M., Mashimo, T., and Yoshimine, T. (2000) Motor cortex stimulation for central and peripheral deafferentation pain. J. Neurosurg., 92: 150–155.

Saitoh Y., Hirano S.I., Kato A., Kishima H., Hirata M., Yamamoto K., Yoshimine T. (2001) Motor cortex stimulation for deafferentation pain. Neurosurg. Focus 11: Article 1.

Smith, H., Joint, C., Schlugman, D., Nandi, D., Stein, J.F., Aziz, T.Z. (2001) Motor cortex stimulation for neuropathic pain. Neurosurg. Focus, 11: Article 2.

Sol, J.C., Casaux, J., Roux, F.E., Lotterie, J.A., Bousquet, P., Verdié, J.C., Mascott, C., and Lazorthes, Y. (2001) Chronic motor cortex stimulation for phantom limb pain: correlations between pain relief and functional imaging studies. Stereotact. Funct. Neurosurg., 77: 172–176.

Tsubokawa, T., Katayama, Y., Yamamoto, T., Hirayama, T., and Koyama, S. (1991) Chronic motor cortex stimulation for the treatment of central pain. Acta Neurochir. Suppl., 52: 137–139.

Tsubokawa, T., Katayama, Y., Yamamoto, T., Hirayama, T., and Koyama, S. (1993) Chronic motor cortex stimulation in patients with thalamic pain. J. Neurosurg., 78: 393–401.

Woolsey, C.N., Erickson, T.C., and Gilson, W.E. (1979) Localization in somatic sensory and motor areas of human cerebral cortex as determined by direct recording of evoked potentials and electrical stimulation. J. Neurosurg., 51: 476–506.

Yamamoto, T., Katayama, Y., Hirayama, T., and Tsubokawa, T. (1997) Pharmacological classification of central post-stroke pain: comparison with the results of chronic motor cortex stimulation therapy. Pain, 72: 5–12.

Electrical Stimulation and the Relief of Pain
Pain Research and Clinical Management, Vol. 15
Edited by Brian A. Simpson

CHAPTER 14

Deep brain stimulation

Volker M. Tronnier*

*Department of Neurological Surgery, University Hospital, Ruprecht-Karls-University Heidelberg,
Im Neuenheimer Feld 400, D-69120 Heidelberg, Germany*

Abstract

Electrical deep brain stimulation (DBS) is a valuable tool for the treatment of chronic pain states which did not respond to less invasive more conservative treatment techniques. Careful patient selection, choice of the correct indication, accurate target localization and identification with neurophysiological techniques as well as a blinded test evaluation are the key requirements for a good outcome. Despite optimal treatment conditions, however, there are several pain syndromes which do not respond to this kind of treatment. Central pain syndromes, especially the thalamic pain syndrome or post-stroke pain, are not relieved by DBS. This might be due to the limited understanding of central reorganization and neuroplastic changes of the pain-transmitting pathways and pain-modulation centres after brain and spinal cord lesions. Considering a neuronal network of pain-processing modules at the subcortical and cortical levels, new imaging studies will hopefully lead to the identification of new targets for therapeutic neuromodulation.

Keywords: Brain stimulation; Nucleus ventroposterolateralis (VPL); Periaqueductal grey (PAG); Periventricular grey (PVG); Microrecordings; Somatosensory evoked potentials (SEPs); Neuropathic pain; Nociceptive pain

1. Introduction

Besides the 'classical' method of placing lesions in pain-conducting pathways (Spiegel and Wycis, 1953), the idea of 'positive enforcement' by electrical stimulation of certain brain areas was transferred from the rodent to the human brain in the mid 1950s. Heath (Heath, 1954) and Pool (Pool et al., 1956) reported pain relief obtained in patients with significant psychopathology by stimulating the septal nuclei including the diagonal band of Broca anterolateral to the fornical columns. These areas are considered to be mainly involved in behavioural activities. Heath and Mickle (1960) later also reported pain relief in six

patients with intractable pain due to malignancy and rheumatoid arthritis. Ervin described pain relief in a patient with facial pain due to malignancy by stimulating the caudate nucleus (Ervin et al., 1966). Gol (1967), however, reported only limited success in chronic pain patients with stimulation of both the caudate nucleus and the septal region.

At about the same time Mazars (Mazars et al., 1960) described the stimulation of the pain-conducting neospinothalamic pathway at its termination in the lateral somatosensory thalamus (VPL – nucleus ventroposterolateralis). Together with the stimulation of the periaqueductal/periventricular grey region these targets resemble

*Correspondence to: Prof. Dr. Volker Tronnier. Phone: +49 (6221) 566301; Fax: +49 (6221) 565534
E-mail: volker_tronnier@med.uni-heidelberg.de

the classical targets for deep brain stimulation (DBS) today.

2. Classical targets

2.1. Somatosensory thalamus (VPL and VPM) and internal capsule

Stimulation of the somatosensory pathways was introduced by Mazars, producing stimulation-induced paraesthesias with simultaneous long-lasting pain relief in patients with deafferentation pain (Mazars et al., 1960). Stimulation of the posterior limb of the internal capsule also evoked paraesthesias and was used for permanent implantation of electrodes by some surgeons (Adams et al., 1974; Fields and Adams, 1974). Since then several series have been published (Table I, pp. 224–226) with a considerable number of patients and varying results (Bechtereva et al., 1972; Hosobuchi et al., 1973; Mazars, 1976; Turnbull et al., 1980; Dieckmann and Witzmann, 1982; Siegfried, 1982; Tsubokawa et al., 1985; Young et al., 1985). However, there was a consensus that pain due to deafferentation responds better than nociceptive pain or pain due to 'excessive afferentation' (Mazars, 1975) to lateral somatosensory thalamus or internal capsule stimulation.

2.1.1. Rationale for stimulation of the somatosensory thalamus and the internal capsule

The somatosensory thalamus (VPL – nucleus ventroposterolateralis and VPM – nucleus ventro-posteromedialis) is the major terminal of the neospinothalamic tract, and it is proposed that neurons in these structures signal either acute pain or generate symptoms of central pain syndromes due to alterations in their activity. Increased neuronal-bursting activity has been found in pain due to deafferentation or central pain syndromes (Kenshalo et al., 1980; Chung et al., 1986; Lenz et al., 1987, 1993a,b, 1994a,b, 1995; Gorecki et al., 1989; Hirayama et al., 1989; Lenz, 1992; Yamashiro

et al., 1997). This increased neuronal firing parallels the clinical findings in central pain syndromes with lesions in the pain-signalling pathways and the occurrence of spontaneous and evoked pain to noxious (hyperalgesia) and innocuous (allodynia) stimuli (Cassinari and Pagni, 1969). It has been proposed that after deafferentation a somatotopic reorganization in the somatosensory thalamus takes place and that a mismatch between receptive fields (RFs) and projection fields evoked by microstimulation exists (Lenz et al., 1994c). The spinothalamic tract (STT) projects to VPM and VPL and ends in clusters intermingled with lemniscal fibres organized somatotopically in rods. Other terminations of the STT are the medial thalamic nuclei (centralis lateralis, submedius) and the posterior group including the posterior nucleus, the anterior pulvinar, the nucleus limitans, the magnocellular medial geniculate and supragenicu-late nuclei (Mantyh, 1983; Apkarian and Hodge, 1989; Ralston and Ralston, 1992). At least in the medial and intralaminar nuclei, spontaneous hyperactivity due to deafferentation was also demonstrated (Rinaldi et al., 1991a; Liz-Planells et al., 1992; Jeanmonod et al., 1993) and nociceptive neurons were described (Ishijima et al., 1975). New binding studies with calbindin and parvalbumin have not confirmed the existence of a special nucleus (Vmpo – ventromedialis posterior) exclusively yielding terminations of nociceptive and thermoceptive fibres (Craig et al., 1994; Blomquist et al., 2000; Jones et al., 2001).

Further evidence for the effect of VPL stimulation comes from animal studies. Stimulation of VPL inhibits STT neurons in the dorsal horn of monkeys (Gerhart et al., 1981, 1983). Somatosensory thalamic stimulation in rat has been shown to inhibit neuronal activity in the centromedianum–parafascicular (CM–PF) complex (Benabid et al., 1983; Cesaro et al., 1986). Internal capsule stimulation in cat inhibits nociceptive-evoked VPM cells (Nishimoto et al., 1984). Finally, VPL stimulation is able to reduce mechanical allodynia in an animal chronic pain model which uses a partial nerve injury (Gybels et al., 1993).

2.2. *PAG and PVG stimulation*

The periaqueductal grey (PAG) is considered to be a target for chronic stimulation since the observations by Reynolds (1969). The electrodes were placed close to the aqueduct at the mesencephalic level in rats and stimulation permitted laparotomy with no anaesthetic. In humans, stimulation of the ventral PAG revealed an opioid-mediated mechanism because its pain-suppressing effect is reversed by naloxone. In contrast stimulation of the dorsal PAG is not opioid-mediated. Stimulation of the dorsal PAG suppresses pain only while the current is delivered; there is no lasting effect after cessation of stimulation. This stimulation is not very well tolerated by the patients as it induces fear, anxiety and sometimes excitation. High-intensity stimulation in ventral and dorsal PAG causes vertical gaze paralysis, lateral gaze paralysis and oscillopsia, and because of these side effects the target was shifted to the periventricular grey (PVG) in humans for chronic stimulation.

2.2.1. Rationale for stimulation of the PAG/PVG area

The mechanism of pain modulation with PAG/PVG stimulation is mainly related to an opioid-dependent pathway, although also non-opioid-dependent mechanisms are discussed (Young and Chambi, 1987; Rinaldi et al., 1991b). From animal research the phenomenon of 'stimulation-produced analgesia' (SPA) was coined by Reynolds (1969). Stimulation of the PAG completely suppressed acute nociceptive stimuli. Further animal studies revealed that SPA was at least partially reversed by the opiate antagonist naloxone and that a cross-tolerance between exogenously given opiates and PAG stimulation exists (Mayer and Hayes, 1975; Basbaum and Fields, 1978). Elevation of endogenous opioids, such as β-endorphin and met-enkephalin, has been found in patients after PAG and PVG stimulation but not after VPL stimulation (Akil et al., 1978a,b; Hosobuchi et al., 1979; Young et al., 1993). Although the application of contrast medium

during ventriculography was blamed for the elevation of endogenous opioids (Dionne et al., 1984; Fessler et al., 1984), later studies without contrast medium confirmed the earlier findings (Young et al., 1993). SPA was proven to be effective in acute and chronic pain states in humans (Adams, 1976; Hosobuchi et al., 1977; Richardson and Akil, 1977a,b; Meyerson et al., 1979). The neural substrates of this endogenous analgesia pathway include the PVG, parts of the PAG, the nucleus raphe magnus and the magnocellular part of the nucleus reticularis gigantocellularis (Basbaum and Fields, 1978; Hosobuchi, 1988). Stimulation of this pathway is able to inhibit STT neurons in the dorsal horn of the spinal cord (Yezierski et al., 1982; Gerhart et al., 1984; Sandkühler et al., 1987) mainly via serotoninergic descending inhibition. On the other hand, sectioning of this pathway in the dorsolateral funiculus in the rat has been shown to increase the response to noxious stimuli (Li et al., 1998). The implantation of a macroelectrode in humans causes a simultaneous stimulation of the nucleus parafascicularis (PF) and parts of the nucleus centromedianum (CM) due to current spread. This accounts probably also for a non-opioid-dependent pathway (Andersen and Dafny, 1983; Peschansky and Besson, 1984). Our group was able to demonstrate that stimulation of the PVG area could inhibit neuronal activity in VPL neurons in humans (Rinaldi et al., 1991a). Also medial thalamic nuclei activity was suppressed by central grey-matter stimulation in cat (Gura et al., 1991).

3. Other targets

3.1. *CM–PF complex*

As mentioned in the previous section, while implanting a chronic DBS electrode in the PVG region, usually a concomitant activation of the PF and CM occurs. The medial and intralaminar nuclei were a target for DBS quite early (Thoden et al., 1979; Boivie and Meyerson, 1982). Boivie and Meyerson provided autopsy data showing that the active pole of the stimulating electrodes were located at the PF/PVG border. According to the atlas of Schaltenbrand and Wahren (1977) most of our electrodes were located with their active poles at the transition of PVG and nucleus endymalis although pain relief was sometimes yielded with the proximal electrodes located in the dorsomedial nucleus (Nucleus medialis fasciculosus of Hassler). The medial and intralaminar nuclei are also targets for terminations of the STT (usually bilaterally), and it has been shown that spontaneous hyperactivity also occurs in these nuclei (Rinaldi et al., 1991b).

Spinal-cord stimulation attenuates the activity in CM (Modesti and Waszak, 1975) as stimulation of the dorsal raphe nucleus attenuates activity in PF (Reyes-Vazquez et al., 1989). Ray and Burton (1980) implanted chronic-stimulating electrodes in the CM–PF complex in 28 patients with a successful pain reduction (> 50%) in 76% of their patients with a mean follow-up of several months. Andy (1980) used CM–PF stimulation in four patients with painful dyskinesias and reported a faster pain relief than improvement of the motor disorder. However, he stimulated three of the four patients with high-frequency (125 Hz) stimulation, which makes the results difficult to explain considering that usually lower frequencies (50–75 Hz) are used for DBS in chronic pain patients. In a subsequent publication (Andy, 1983), he added five patients with pure chronic pain describing good to excellent pain relief in all with the typical stimulation parameters (200 μs pulse width, 50 Hz, intensities up to 5 V). Although a follow-up is not given, one can read from the case reports that the follow-up was shorter than 12 months in four of five patients. An opioid-dependent mechanism in CM–PF cannot be ruled out because morphine injected in PF changed acute pain behaviour in rats (Reyes-Vazquez et al., 1989; Harte et al., 2000).

The role of the CM–PF complex in pain transmission is not yet fully understood. Although these nuclei are known as a part of the ascending reticulo-thalamo-cortical activating system (Moruzzi and Magoun, 1949; Paré et al., 1988), they also receive strong inputs from the motor and premotor cortex as well as the basal ganglia. Their main output projections are not directed to sensory cortical areas but to the striatum (Fenelon et al., 1991; Sadikot et al., 1992). A recent study, however, describes the modulation of tonically active striatal neurons by sensory events (auditory, visual and somatosensory) mediated through the CM–PF complex, although painful stimuli were not tested specifically (Matsumoto et al., 2001). It is possible that the pain-reducing mechanism is via current spread to afferent fibres to the nucleus centralis lateralis (CL), which is known to be a sensory nucleus involved in pain transmission (Mehler et al., 1960; Jones and Burton, 1974).

3.2. Septal area

Based on the early results by Heath and Pool, some authors continued to use septal stimulation for the relief of chronic pain. Schvarcz (1985) implanted chronic electrodes in the septal area of 10 patients additionally to conventional (PAG and VPL) targets. The follow-up time ranged between 1 and 42 months. No side effects were reported. Stimulation-induced effects were a sensation of warmth, well-being and relaxation. Six patients experienced pain relief greater than 50%, although it was not mentioned whether this was due to septal stimulation alone or combined stimulation. Similar results were reported by Richardson (1982), stimulating five patients in the superior and five patients in the inferior septal area.

3.3. Hypothalamus

Posteromedial hypothalamotomy was originally developed by Sano as a treatment for aggressive behavioural disorders (Sano et al., 1970). Later this technique was applied for intractable pain by Fairman and Mayanagi (Fairman, 1976; Mayanagi et al., 1982). Stimulation created an increase in β-endorphins. Additionally, sympathomimetic responses (increase in blood pressure and heart rate) were elicited. Most of the cases were lesioned after initial stimulation. However, one case with a chronic-implanted electrode was described. The hypothalamus has not been considered by many neurosurgeons as a target for chronically implanted electrodes in the past.

3.4. Koelliker-Fuse region

Stimulation of the dorsolateral midbrain tegmentum is rarely performed although the fundamental basis, supported by anatomical studies, is probably a direct stimulation of descending inhibitory pathways. Katayama described electrical stimulation of the parabrachial area in cats and in two patients with morphine-insensitive pain (Katayama et al., 1984a,b, 1985). Although there are discrepancies in the nomenclature between different species, the Koelliker-Fuse nucleus (KF) is closely associated with the parabrachial area. Electrical stimulation of this nucleus in cats was described by Hodge et al. (1986). This group was able to demonstrate inhibition of dorsal horn cells with KF stimulation. This effect could be antagonized by reserpine, implicating a catecholamine-mediated mechanism. Young stimulated this area in humans and found pain relief in three of six patients (Young et al., 1992). On the other hand, stimulation of the pedunculopontine nucleus created panic attacks in the patients.

4. Deep brain stimulation and microrecordings

The main question remains: Is the bursting pattern recorded in patients with chronic pain using microelectrode-recording techniques in medial and lateral thalamus really related to pain or just to deafferentation? Hyperpolarisation of thalamic neurons causes bursting discharges known as low-threshold spikes (LTSs). The deinactivation of rapidly inactivating calcium channels result in an inward calcium current which leads to an activation of sodium-dependent action potentials (Llinás and Jahnsen, 1982; Pedroarena and Llinás, 1997; Steriade et al., 1997). The LTS-induced bursting exhibits a characteristic firing pattern comprising progressively increasing interspike intervals (ISIs) in each burst. The first ISI shows a progressive shortening with an increased number of spikes. This type of bursting was also demonstrated in patients asleep during surgery and in non-pain patients (Zirh et al., 1998; Jeanmonod et al., 2001). A recent study also questioned the correlation between thalamic-bursting activity and chronic pain, demonstrating bursting patterns in awake pain and non-pain patients with a similar burst index (number of bursts per encountered neurons) in both patient groups (Radhakrishnan et al., 1999).

In contrast our group has found an increased number of bursting neurons in different thalamic nuclei after rhizotomies in rat as compared to a control group (sham-operated). The animals developed self-mutilating behaviour 2–3 weeks after the deafferentation. At the same time the number of RFs decreased, which confirmed earlier animal experiments (Lombard et al., 1979; Albe-Fessard and Lombard, 1983) and the human data of Lenz (Figs. 1 and 2). Yamashiro has shown in a rat study similar to ours that iontophoretically

Localization	Postrhizotomy			Control		
	Bursting	Non-bursting	Total	Bursting	Non-bursting	Total
Lateral	75 (56.4%)	58 (43.6%)	133	16 (32.6%)	33 (67.4%)	49
Medial	21 (65.6%)	11 (34.4%)	32	6 (20%)	24 (80%)	30

Fig. 1. After rhizotomy the number of neurons exhibiting a bursting firing pattern increases in rat. Recordings were from the nucleus medialis dorsalis, centre median, centralis lateralis and reunion (medial thalamic group), and from the nucleus ventroposterolateralis and posteromedialis as well as the nucleus reticularis thalami (lateral group).

Receptive field (RF)	Postrhizotomy		Control	
	Lateral	Medial	Lateral	Medial
Pain	34 (25.5%)	12 (37.5%)	13 (26.6%)	3 (10%)
Tactile stimuli	26 (19.5%)	–	18 (36.7%)	–
No RF	73 (55%)	20 (62.5%)	18 (36.7%)	27 (90%)
Total	133	32	49	30

Fig. 2. Deafferentation causes a reduction of neurons with RFs in the lateral thalamus of rats. The neurons in the medial thalamus responding to nociceptive stimuli increase after deafferentation.

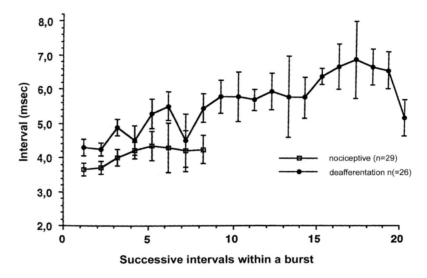

Fig. 3. Patients with pure deafferentation pain reveal bursts with more spikes/burst and longer ISIs within a burst as compared to patients with pure nociceptive pain.

applied glutamate increased the bursting while gamma-aminobutyric acid (GABA) and an N-methyl-D-aspartate (NMDA) antagonist reduced the spontaneous bursting activity (Yamashiro et al., 1997). We also compared the number of ISIs in patients with deafferentation pain and nociceptive pain and found a marked difference in the number and length of ISIs between these patient groups (Fig. 3; Liz-Planells et al., 1992).

Putting these data together we can conclude that bursting, especially the LTS-induced bursting, is not related to pain solely but appears in different states of wakefulness and also in non-pain patients. However, deafferentation increases the bursting (burst index and number of ISIs), and chronic deafferentation pain generates a

'thalamocortical dysrhythmia' (Jeanmonod et al., 2001). The downregulation of GABA-A receptors after deafferentation in the nociceptive pathways might be one of the mechanisms causing the above-described disinhibition in thalamocortical relay neurons. After dorsal rhizotomies in monkeys, not only has a downregulation of GABA-A receptors been found but also an upregulation of calbindin immunostaining (as a sign of increased innervation of intact spinothalamic afferents) and downregulation of parvalbumin immunostaining (as a function of decreased lemniscal input; Rausell et al., 1992). Among other influences the application of GABA has been found to decrease the RF size in VPL neurons of cats while the GABA antagonist bicuculline increases the RFs

(Hicks et al., 1986). This is another hint of the involvement of GABA in chronic pain states and fits into Lenz' hypothesis that the RFs are increased in areas adjacent to a deafferentation site in VPL. Since microstimulation or macrostimulation is able to produce pain in the area exhibiting abnormal spontaneous and evoked activity (Hassler and Riechert, 1959; Lenz et al., 1993b), this suggests that these neurons are involved in the generation of pain or are an expression of pain.

5. DBS and evoked potentials

Evoked potentials have been used since the beginning of functional stereotactic neurosurgery to improve the positioning of either stimulating or lesioning electrodes. Usually macroelectrodes or semimacroelectrodes are used for determination of the exact position of the electrodes in the human motor and sensory thalamus but also in related structures such as the subthalamic nucleus. Somatic signals arrive in the VPL or VPM via the medial lemniscus. A mapping of the thalamic somatotopy is possible with evoked potentials from different body areas (Albe-Fessard et al., 1986; Yamashiro et al., 1989). While upper and lower extremity stimulation usually evokes activity in the contralateral VPL, stimulation of the face, the inside of the mouth, tongue and lips creates bilateral evoked potentials at the thalamic and cortical level. Today mapping with evoked potentials (waves) is substituted by microelectrode recordings of evoked sensations (single or multi-unit responses). We used short latency evoked potentials in 20 patients with implanted deep brain electrodes to find the best contact combinations in PVG and lateral somatosensory thalamus. Evoked responses in the contralateral VPL showed typical P9 and P11 deflections. P13/14 was often masked by a large P15 deflection with a N16 negative component. In the medial thalamus contralateral stimulation produced a P9, P11 and a P13/14a lemniscal response; additionally a P15 farfield

potential was demonstrated. Brainstem and lemniscal potentials decreased with rapid (12 Hz) stimulation. Ipsilateral median nerve evoked potentials revealed a weak P15 in the ipsilateral VPL and a more prominent P15 in the medial thalamus suggesting farfield effects (Fig. 4).

6. DBS and functional imaging

Functional imaging is an exciting method of studying pain processing and modulation at subcortical and cortical levels. Most of the studies deal with experimental pain in human volunteers. However, several studies have been performed in patients with chronic pain but very few studies have examined the effect of implanted deep brain electrodes (Duncan et al., 1998; Davis et al., 2000; Kupers et al., 2000; Peyron et al., 2000). Based on these limited patient studies and our own results, one can only conclude that different areas involved in pain processing and modulation are activated by DBS. Stimulation of the lateral somatosensory thalamus not only activates areas of the lateral neospinothalamic pathway but also areas of the limbic cortex (anterior cingulate, insula, hippocampus) considered to be involved in the affective components of pain and 'pain memory' (Fig. 5). This leads to the conclusion that at diencephalic and cortical levels no segregation of two different pain-mediating pathways exists but one rather has to consider a neuronal network of central pain processing and modulation (Wiech, 2001).

7. Patient selection

Chronic pain can be divided into nociceptive and non-nociceptive pain. *Nociceptive pain* occurs due to chronic activation or overactivation of peripheral nociceptors. The pain-conducting pathways, peripheral as well as central, are intact. Examples are pain due to degenerative bone and joint disease or malignant invasion of soft tissue or of joints and bones. This type of pain very often responds

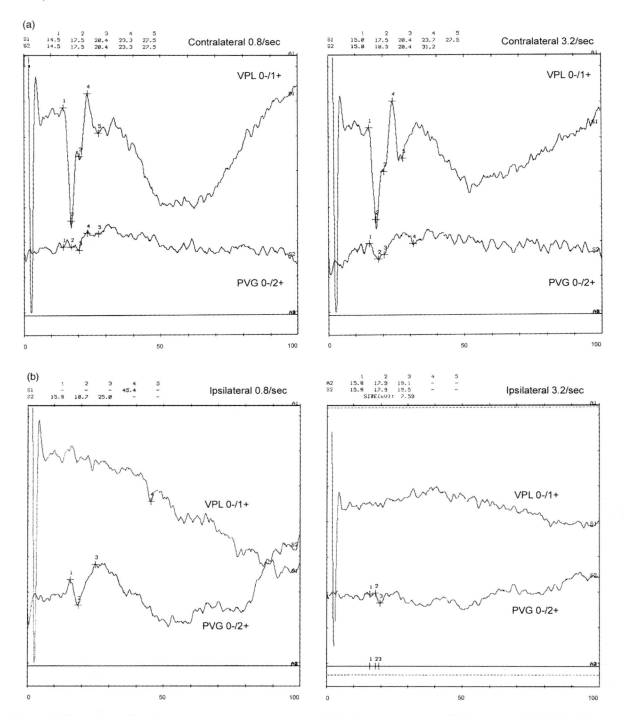

Fig. 4. (a) Two traces of median nerve evoked potentials recorded in the somatosensory (VPL) and medial (PVG) thalamus contralateral to the stimulation via the implanted electrodes at 0.8 and 3.2 Hz stimulation frequencies. Marked responses are seen in VPL; however, small responses could be observed in medial thalamus. (b) Two traces recorded in the thalamus ipsilateral to median nerve stimulation. Note the decreased response in ipsilateral PVG with faster stimulation.

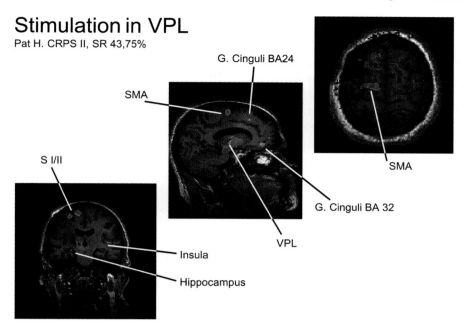

Stimulation in VPL
Pat H. CRPS II, SR 43,75%

G. Cinguli BA24

SMA

SMA

S I/II

G. Cinguli BA 32

VPL

Insula

Hippocampus

Fig. 5. 0^{15}-PET (positron-emission tomography) in a patient with a lesion of the tibial nerve and several operative revisions (CRPS II – complex regional pain syndrome). Suprathreshold stimulation in VPL revealed activation, not only in SI and SII but also in the cingulate gyrus, the insula and the hippocampus.

well to opiates. Therefore, PVG stimulation is generally used to treat different forms of nociceptive pain.

Non-nociceptive pain occurs in response to lesions of the peripheral or central nervous system and is referred to as *neuropathic pain*. Although the term deafferentation pain describes very well the pathophysiology and is obvious in certain pain states such as plexus avulsion, it is not widely accepted in the non-neurosurgical literature. Therefore, we will use the terms *neuropathic pain of peripheral origin* (CRPS II – complex regional pain syndrome type II, previously called causalgia, phantom pain and post-herpetic neuralgia – PHN), which activates peripheral and central pain mechanisms and *central pain* activating only central pain mechanisms. Due to surgical considerations we differentiate further between central pain of spinal cord origin and central post-stroke pain. Neuropathic pain and central pain are considered to respond better to stimulation of the somatosensory thalamus, the internal capsule

or even the motor cortex. However, a large group of patients responding quite well to DBS, those with failed back surgery syndrome (FBSS), have mixed nociceptive (back) and neuropathic (radicular) pain components.

Deep brain stimulation is a treatment option in patients not responding to less invasive or more conventional therapeutic measures. A neural substrate for the origin of the pain should be obvious. Patients with diffuse pain states without a feasible reason for the pain should be excluded. Also pain states in the rectal, genital or perineal region do not respond to DBS according to our experience. One reason might be the small representation of those midline areas in the brain.

Medical treatment should be exhausted in patients considered for brain stimulation, either due to inefficacy or due to intolerable side effects. However, a careful patient history should be taken to rule out inefficient dosages or side effects due to missing comedication. In particular, patients with neuropathic pain should be treated for a sufficient period of time with tricyclic antidepressants (i.e. amitriptyline), anticonvulsants (i.e. carbamazepine and gabapentin) and other medications (i.e. mexiletine, baclofen). Pain of peripheral origin should be treated first with spinal cord or peripheral nerve stimulation if appropriate. A morphine test (Hosobuchi, 1986, 1990) is not considered to be helpful before implantation (Young and Chambi, 1987; Young and Rinaldi, 1994). On the contrary, we try to withdraw all narcotics before implantation.

Patients should be treated in a multidisciplinary pain clinic before being referred to a neurosurgeon for DBS. Psychiatric and psychological testing should be carried out before considering a patient for implantation. In our department all patients undergo a psychological interview and are screened with the questionnaire of the German chapter of the IASP including a visual analogue scale (Scott and Huskisson, 1976), a verbal rating scale, the pain disability index (PDI) (Tait et al., 1990), the SF 36 Health Survey (Ware and Sherbourne, 1992), a modified MMPI (Melzack and Katz, 1992), a pain-experience measure (SES) (Geissner et al., 1992), the Beck Depression Inventory (Beck et al., 1961) and others including a pain diary. Depression is considered to be a consequence of the chronic pain state and not a contraindication for implanting electrodes (Fishbain et al., 1997). All patients receive two electrodes (PVG and somatosensory thalamus, Fig. 6), which are tested separately and in combination in a double-blinded fashion. After determination of the threshold of experiencing any stimulation-induced effects (paraesthesias in somatosensory thalamus; floating, dizziness, panic in PVG) testing is carried out with subthreshold stimulation, half of the intensity of subthreshold stimulation and placebo stimulation (intensity set to zero). The patient, as well as the evaluating nurse who takes the VAS, is not aware of the stimulator setting. Internalization of the extension cable and of the stimulating device is carried out if the pain reduction is at least 50% and the daily activities are markedly increased. One or two

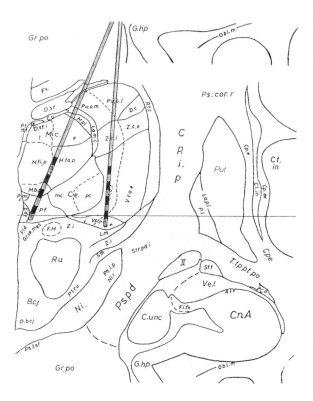

Fig. 6. Modified coronal slice of the Schaltenbrand–Wahren atlas with localisation of the electrodes in the somatosensory thalamus [VPL – nucleus ventralis caudalis, pars parvocellularis (Vcpc) according to Hasslers' nomenclature] and the PVG (nucleus endymalis, nucleus parafascicularis – PF).

Itrel 3^{TM} (Medtronic Inc.) pulse generators are used for single or dual stimulation; the two-channel pulse generator Synergy^{TM} (Medtronic Inc.) is not suitable for DBS for pain because independent frequency settings are not available. Prior to internalisation a magnetic resonance imaging (MRI) scan (3D T1-weighted sequences) is carried out to confirm the electrode positions (Fig. 7).

8. Operative technique

In our unit the procedure is carried out as follows: Electrode implantation is performed under local anaesthesia with intravenous analgosedation during frame placement (ramifentanil and propofol). This analgosedation is stopped during the imaging

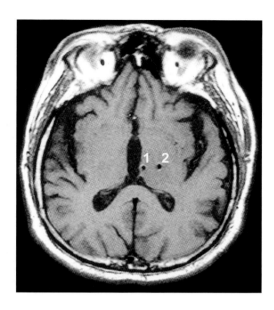

Fig. 7. Postoperative MRI, demonstrating one electrode (1) close to the ventricular wall (PVG) and the other electrode (2) in the lateral thalamus (VPL) in a patient with phantom pain.

procedure. The stereotactic frame (Zamorano-Dujovny, Fischer-Leibinger, Freiburg, Germany) is aligned parallel to the orbitomeatal line in order to be as parallel as possible to the intercommissural line. Since 1990 we have relied solely on MR imaging for target localization. In patients with cardiac pacemakers CT localization is used. In our opinion there is no necessity for ventriculography anymore (Young and Rinaldi, 1997). When using MRI, however, certain precautions, such as phantom measurements with the different components of the stereotactic system, are necessary to rule out distortions. Frameless stereotaxy is not useful for electrode placements in functional neurosurgery (Tronnier et al., 1996). After visualization and calculation of the coordinates of the posterior commissure (PC), the target coordinates are determined.

The coordinates for the lateral somatosensory thalamus are as follows: $Y = 3$ to 5 mm anterior to the PC; $Z = 0$ to -2 mm under the intercommissural line; $X = 10$ to 12 mm lateral to the midline for facial pain, 12 to 15 mm for pain in the upper extremity, 15 to 18 mm for pain in the lower extremity (corrections have to be made according to the width of the third ventricle)

The coordinates for PVG are: $Y = 2$ to 3 mm anterior to PC; $Z = 2$ above to 2 mm below the intercommissural line; $X = 2$ mm lateral to the wall of the third ventricle.

A 14-mm precoronal burr hole is created 2 cm lateral to the midline to fix either the burr hole cap provided by Medtronic (Medtronic Inc., Minneapolis, MA, USA) or the burr hole cap by IGN (Image Guided Neurologics, Melbourne, FL, USA), which has the advantage that the electrodes are not pushed into the brain below the intended target when the electrodes are secured. Both electrodes are placed through the same burr hole.

Target refinement is performed using microelectrode recording (Figs. 8 and 9), and micro- and macrostimulation. Microrecordings have been performed for many years with custom made bipolar concentric tungsten electrodes, now commercially available with diameters of 0.5 and 0.9 mm (Inomed, Teningen, Germany). Meanwhile, several companies offer solutions for microrecordings comprising manually- or motor-driven microdrives and recording software. The impedance of the microelectrodes varies between 0.5 and 2 MΩ at 1000 kHz.

In patients with large areas of deafferentation (e.g. paraplegia), cells in the representation of the anaesthetic body part have no thalamic RFs (Lenz et al., 1994c). In other patients we found a distortion of the receptive and projection fields (i.e. face instead of the amputated arm at 16 mm lateral) as described by Lenz (Lenz et al., 1998). Microstimulation can be carried out up to 100 µA without damaging the electrode tip. With the concentric electrode we use, macrostimulation is possible up to a distance of 0.5 mm from the microelectrode tip.

Stimulation in the PVG creates a feeling of warmth, floating and dizziness at threshold stimulation with frequencies of 50 Hz and a pulse width of 210 µs. At higher intensities the patients reported anxiety or even panic. Below the intercommissural line diplopia, gaze deviation or

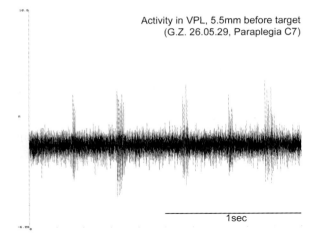

Activity in VPL, 5.5mm before target
(G.Z. 26.05.29, Paraplegia C7)

1sec

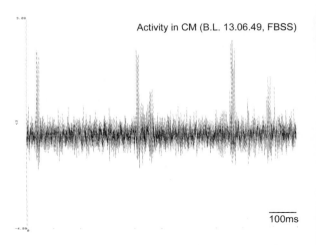

Activity in CM (B.L. 13.06.49, FBSS)

100ms

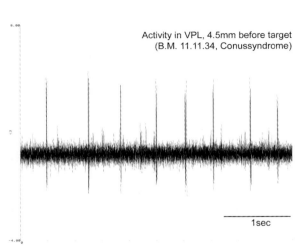

Activity in VPL, 4.5mm before target
(B.M. 11.11.34, Conussyndrome)

1sec

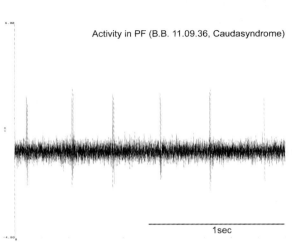

Activity in PF (B.B. 11.09.36, Caudasyndrome)

1sec

Fig. 8. Microrecordings in VPL in two patients with neuropathic pain revealing bursting activity at 2–3 Hz.

Fig. 9. Microrecordings in CM (a) in a patient with FBSS and PF (b) in a patient with neuropathic pain.

gaze paralysis can be elicited. Further posterior, paraesthesias in the contralateral body without somatotopy are sometimes reported, caused by current spread to the medial lemniscus. Reproducible elevations of the blood pressure and heart rate at threshold stimulation are a very helpful guide in PVG stimulation (Young and Rinaldi, 1994). Interestingly, these effects fade with chronic stimulation. In some cases pain can be evoked by stimulation, similar to the pain experienced originally by the patient; however, this occurs more often in the lateral thalamus.

Stimulation of the lateral thalamus elicits paraesthesias in different body areas according to the laterality of the electrode placement. We can confirm the results of Lenz and others, that there is a mismatch of receptive field and projection field, especially in patients with phantom pain or central pain syndromes. In patients with thalamic pain or paraplegia only very few cells have RFs at all. Suprathreshold stimulation is often reported as painful, especially by patients with thalamic pain. In one of our patients with phantom pain, just placing the macroelectrode caused immense pain in his phantom. Dystonic movements of the extremities are caused by stimulation of the internal capsule. In those cases the electrode has to be moved more medially.

After the electrodes have been placed in the suspected correct targets, they are fixed in the burr hole either with a silastic cap (under X-ray control) or with a burr hole fixation system (Fig. 10). In cases where the latter device (IGN, Melbourne, FL, USA) is used, a second small groove is made in the outer ring with a microdrill to keep the second electrode in place. Both electrodes are connected to external extension leads for consecutive testing. These extension wires are externalised in the temporal area in front of the ears away from the placement of definitive extensions in order to minimise the risk of infection.

Patients undergo a test trial period of about 7 days under antibiotic cover. A double-blinded test stimulation is carried out as described earlier. At least 50% pain reduction is mandatory for the decision for permanent implantation (internalization). No narcotics are taken during the test trial. Non-steroidal anti-inflammatory drugs, tricyclic antidepressants and clonidine (especially after withdrawal of narcotics) are allowed during the testing period. Finally, the decision of whether to remove one or the other, or both, electrodes or to proceed to the internalization of the system is discussed with the patient and his or her relatives.

Typical stimulation parameters are as follows:

Lateral thalamus (VPL)	frequency 75 Hz pulse width 210 μs amplitude 0.3–3.0 V continuous stimulation
PVG	frequency 50 Hz pulse width 210 μs amplitude 1.0–3.0 V intermittent stimulation (e.g. 3–6 times per day for 0.5–2 hr)

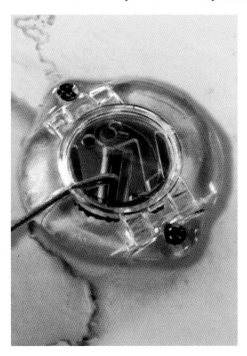

Fig. 10. New device to fix the electrode at the burr hole level without the risk of final dislocation (Navigus™ system, Image Guided Neurologics, Melbourne, FL, USA).

9. Results

Reviewing the literature confirms the criticisms described by Duncan and others in a review article in the journal 'Pain' in 1991 (Duncan et al., 1991). According to the criteria of evidence-based medicine, most publications on DBS are level 5, i.e. historic case-control studies. Only a few studies used an independent third-party examiner for evaluation of the results. There are, in general, no standardised selection and evaluation criteria in those studies. In particular, no blinded stimulation was carried out and finally a 'pharmacologically dose–response relationship' was postulated. This review article led the FDA (Food and Drug Administration) to restrict DBS for chronic pain to the status of an investigational procedure. Since then no further publications have appeared. A summary of most of the published studies is given in Tables I and II.

Our own results in 56 patients are presented with respect to the different pain etiologies (Tables III, IV, V, VI, VII, VIII, IX and X).

TABLE I

Summary of published patient series with somatosensory thalamic stimulation or combined stimulation

Author	Year	Target	Pain	Follow-up	Outcome	Measurement of pain	Evidence level
Hosobuchi et al.	1973	VPM (5)	anaesthesia dolorosa	up to 24 months	4/5 good	verbal	5
Hosobuchi et al.	1975	Internal capsule (8)	thalamic pain (4) paraplegia (1) medullary lesion (2) postcordotomy	?	3 good good failure failure		5
Adams et al.	1977	Internal capsule (10)	thalamic pain	6–40 months (22 months)	8/10 good	excellent = pain free	5
		lateral thalamus (1)			2/10 = 0	w/o medication; good = pain reduction; 0 = no effect	
		lateral thalamus (7)	anaesthesia dolorosa	4–60 months (27 months)	3/7 excellent		
		PVG (3)			3/7 good 1/7 = 0		
		Internal capsule (5)	phantom pain	12–24 months (17 months)	1/5 excellent	failure (one electrode migration, one infection)	
		lateral thalamus (1) PVG (3)			1/5 good 3/5 = 0		
		Internal capsule (2) lateral thalamus (1)	paraplegia postherpetic	14–48 months 13 months	1 good 1 excellent		
Mundinger	1977	lemniscus medial (4)	postherpetic (3) neuropathic trigeminal	21 months	excellent (2), fair (1) good	verbal, fair = < 50% pain relief intermittent analgesics good = pain relief up to 70% excellent = pain relief > 70%	5
Turnbull et al.	1980	lateral thalamus (14)	lumbar arachnoiditis (8) causalgia (2) plexus avulsion (1) central pain (1)	1–47 months	5 pain free 2 partially relieved 2 pain free partially relieved pain free	verbal	5

Author	Year	Target	Indication	Follow-up	Results	Evaluation	
Dieckmann et al.	1982	lateral thalamus or PVG	plexus avulsion, phantom pain, anaesthesia dolorosa, thalamic pain, paraplegia, postherpetic pain	6 months–4.5 years	3 good, 2 moderate (5 slight pain reduction), 2 good, 5 slight, 3=0, 4 slight, 3=0, 5 slight, 3 slight, 1=0, 1 good, 1 moderate, 1=0		5
Plotkin	1982	lateral thalamus	anaesthesia dolorosa (5), thalamic pain (1), paraplegia (2), phantom pain (2)	3 years	3 pain free, failure, failure, 1 pain free	verbal, preoperatively morphine test	5
Roldan	1982	VPM (2)	anaesthesia dolorosa	5–11 months	pain free	verbal	5
Siegfried	1982	VPM (10)	postherpetic	8–17 months	5 excellent, 3 good, 2 failure	verbal, use of narcotics relative evaluation	5
Tsubokawa et al.	1982	VPL (6)	carcinoma (2), central pain (4)	1 year	excellent (3), good (2)	poststimscore/prestimscore × 100	5
Hosobuchi	1983	lateral thalamus + PAG	failed back surgery	1–3 years	11/11 good with thalamus, 9/11 good with PAG	?	5
Broggi et al.	1984	VPL/VPM (9)	postherpetic (5), thalamic pain (2), trigeminal neuropathia, plexus avulsion	18 months	7/9 excellent	VAS; excellent = 80–90% pain reduction	5
Namba et al.	1985	IC posteromedial (11)	thalamic pain	?	3 excellent, 2 good, 2 fair, 3 poor	?	5
Hosobuchi et al.	1986	lateral thalamus (76)	thalamic pain (13), anaesthesia dolorosa (12), postherpetic (5)	2–14 years	6 successful, 4 successful, 2 successful	successful = pain reduction + no narcotics	5

(Continued.)

TABLE I
Continued

Author	Year	Target	Pain	Follow-up	Outcome	Measurement of pain	Evidence level
			plexus avulsion (6)		2 successful		
			postcordotomy dys. (9)		8 successful		
			lumbar radiculopathy (21)		19 successful		
			paraplegia (8)		2 successful		
Levy et al.	1987	lateral thalamus (48)	thalamic pain (25)	80 months	24% long-term success	verbal, questionnaire third party	4
			peripheral neuropathy (16)		50% long-term success		
			anaesthesia dolorosa (12)		18% long-term success		
			paraplegia (11)		0% long-term success		
			postcordotomy dys. (5)		40% long-term success		
			phantom pain (5)		20% long-term success		
Siegfried	1987	lateral thalamus (89)	postherpetic (V^1) pain (21)	< 2 years	67% excellent, 14% good	VAS, use of narcotics pain profile, ADL	4
			anaesthesia dolorosa (18)		39% excellent, 44% good		
			thalamic pain (14)		42% excellent, 29% good		
			plexus avulsion (11)		36% excellent, 36% good		
			phantom/stump (10)		50% excellent, 20% good		
			paraplegia (4)		50% excellent, 50% good		
Tsubokawa et al.	1987	lateral thalamus (24)	peripheral neuropathy (6)	?	4 excellent, 2 good	verbal, excellent = > 80% pain reduction; good = 60–80%; fair < 60%	5
			central pain (8)		2 excellent, 3 good, 3 fair		
			carcinoma pain (10)		3 excellent, 1 good, 6 fair		
Kumar et al.	1990	lateral thalamus (10)	thalamic pain (3)	6–70 months	no long-term success		5
			phantom pain (2)		no long-term success		
Gybels et al.	1993	VPL/VPM, internal capsule	thalamic pain (5)	4 years	1 good	?	5
			anaesthesia dolorosa (6)		2 good		
			root avulsion (7)		3 good		
			phantom pain (4)		1 good		
			spinal cord lesion (5)		2 good		
			postherpetic (5)		0 good		

TABLE II
Summary of published patient series with stimulation in periaqueductal/periventricular grey or medial thalamus (CM–PF)

Author	Year	Target	Type of pain	Follow-up	Outcome	Pain measurement	Evidence level
Mundinger	1977	CM	paraplegia (1) root avulsion (3)	21 months	fair good (2), fair (1)	verbal, fair = <50% relief good = 50–70% relief	5
		PVG	phantom pain (1)		good		
Richardson and Akil	1977	PVG	postdiscectomy (5)		2 excellent, 1 good	4-point scale based on pain relief, side effects	5
			carcinoma (2) plexus avulsion (1)	?	2 good excellent	long-term results (more than 2 years) quantitative sensory testing	
Richardson and Akil	1977	PVG	postdiscectomy (10)	1–46 months	6 excellent, 4 = 0	excellent = >50% pain relief	5
			carcinoma (4) paraplegia (3) thalamic pain (2) scoliosis (2)	18 months	3 excellent, 1 fair 1 excellent, 1 fair 1 excellent, 1 = 0 2 excellent	fair = <50% pain relief	
Andy	1980	CM–PF	pain with movement disorders (4)	3 months–6 years	pain relief in all cases	verbal response	5
Plotkin	1982	PVG (48)	postdiscectomy (35)	3 years	80% success	verbal response, preoperative morphine test	5
Andy	1983	CM–PF	CRPS II (2) thalamic pain (2) migraine (1)	?	1 good, 1 excellent 1 good, 1 excellent good	4-point scale	5

(continued)

TABLE II
Continued

Author	Year	Target	Type of pain	Follow-up	Outcome	Pain measurement	Evidence level
Young et al.	1985	PAG/PVG (26) +combinations	postdiscectomy (16)	2–60 months	9 excellent, 5 partially	verbal, morphine test	5
			carcinoma (7)		3 excellent, 3 partially		
			paraplegia (6)		1 excellent, 3 partially		
			anaesthesia dolorosa (4)		2 partially, 2 poor		
			root avulsion (4)		2 partially, 2 poor		
			postherpetic (2)		2 partially		
Hosobuchi et al.	1986	PAG (65)	carcinoma (7)	2–14 years	5 successful	successful = pain relief + no narcotics; preoperative morphine test	5
			failed back (49)		39 successful		
			nociceptive pain (9)		6 successful		
Hosobuchi	1987	dorsal PAG	head/neck–carcinoma (7)	?	2 good, 5 failure	verbal	5
Levy et al.	1987	PVG (57)	failed back (51)	80 months	32% long-term success	verbal, questionnaire, disinterested third party	4
			carcinoma (6)		33% long-term success		
Kumar et al.	1990	PVG (38)	failed back (34)	6–118 months	73% long-term success	success = good–excellent pain relief + no narcotics preoperative psychological testing	5

The best long-term results were seen in patients with the so-called 'failed back surgery syndrome' (Table III). Despite the option of other techniques, e.g. spinal cord stimulation (SCS) and intrathecal opioids, we have performed DBS in those patients with combined low back and radicular pain. According to our experience, SCS relieves only the radicular component of the patients' pain, while intrathecal opioids better relieve the low back component. Considering the long-term side effects of intrathecal opioids, we believe that DBS is an alternative treatment option for those patients who did not respond to more conservative, less invasive procedures. PVG stimulation is recommended for the low back pain, while VPL stimulation improves the radicular neuropathic pain component. These favourable results in this patient group have been confirmed by other authors (Young, 1996). Less favourable are the results in patients with central pain syndromes. In the case of central pain due to spinal cord lesions, patients with complete deafferentation and diffuse infralesional pain respond less. Usually the electrode in

TABLE III

Results of the combined stimulation for the treatment of the 'failed back surgery syndrome' ($n = 13$, mean follow-up: 3.5 years)

Patient	Age/sex	Implantation	Internalization	Follow-up	Pain relief
DG	48/m	VPL/PVG	PVG	5 years	75–100%
CF	66/m	VPL/PVG	–	–	0
JG	61/m	VPL/PVG	VPL/PVG	6 months	0
JG	48/f	VPL/PVG	VPL	3 years	75–100%
BD	67/f	VPL/PVG	PVG	6 years	25–50%
GR	67/m	VPL/PVG	VPL/PVG	4 years	75–100%
PQ	44/m	VPL/PVG	VPL/PVG	4 years	50–75%
DR	58/m	VPL/PVG	–	–	0
GR	36/m	VPL/PVG	VPL/PVG	2 years	50–75%
VR	72/f	VPL/PVG	VPL/PVG	2 years	50–75%
LS	42/f	VPL/PVG	VPL/PVG	2 years	50–75%
JS	71/m	VPL/PVG	VPL/PVG	2 years	50–75%
BM*	37/f	VPL/PVG	PVG	8 years	75–100%

*Radicular pain is treated with SCS.

TABLE V

Results of the combined stimulation for the treatment of phantom pain (mean follow-up: 2.8 years)

Patient	Age/sex	Implantation	Internalization	Follow-up	Pain relief
MM	71/f	VPL/PVG	VPL/PVG	6 months	0
MS	67/m	VPL/PVG	VPL/PVG	6.5 years	75–100%
FV	41/m	VPL/PVG	PVG	1.5 years	25–50%
HB*	39/m	VPL/PVG	–	–	0

*Despite pain reduction of > 50% and cessation of narcotic intake, the patient wanted explantation of the electrodes.

TABLE IV

Results of the combined stimulation for the treatment of 'central pain' due to spinal cord injury ($n = 12$, mean follow-up: 3.5 years)

Patient	Age/sex	Pain origin	Implantation	Internalization	Follow-up	Pain relief
GB	60/m	Brown-Sequard	VPL/PVG	–	0	0
JM	55/f	Myelopathy	VPL/PVG	VPL/PVG	3 years	25–50%
DK	35/m	Tetraplegia	VPL/PVG	VPL/PVG	5 years	0–25%
UJ*	51/m	Post-Drez	VPL/PVG	VPL/PVG	6 months	75–100%
HA	64/m	Paraplegia	VPL/PVG	–	0	0
GZ	67/m	Paraplegia	VPL/PVG	–	0	0
FK	58/m	Paraplegia	VPL/PVG	–	0	0
BM	62/f	Conus syndrome	VPL/PVG	–	0	0
FK	66/m	Syringomyelia	VPL/PVG	–	0	0
RJ	42/m	Plexus avulsion	VPL/PVG	PVG	4 years	0–25%
ES**	55/m	Paraplegia	VPL/PVG	VPL	2.5 years	0–25%
KG	67/f	Myelopathy	VPL/PVG	–	0	0

*Committed suicide.
**Was treated later with intraventricular morphine, committed suicide.

TABLE VI

Results of the combined stimulation for the treatment of dysaesthesia dolorosa (mean follow–up: 3 years)

Patient	Age/sex	Implantation	Internali-zation	Follow-up	Pain relief
PS	36/m	VPM/PVG	VPM/PVG	3 years	75–100%
HL	64/m	VPM/PVG	VPM/PVG	6 months	0
RS	68/f	VPM/PVG	VPM/PVG	4.5 years	25–50%
MW	45/f	VPM/PVG	VPM/PVG	5 years	75–100%
JL	26/f	VPM/PVG	VPM/PVG	2 years	50–75%
HM*	71/m	VPM/PVG	–		0

*Bilateral distal pain in upper gums and lips.

TABLE VII

Results of the combined stimulation for the treatment of CRPS II (mean follow-up: 4.1 years)

Patient	Age/sex	Implanta-tion	Internali-zation	Follow-up	Pain relief
SD	51/m	VPL/PVG	–	0	0
CP	50/f	VPL/PVG	VPL/PVG	4 years	75–100%
OB	59/m	VPL/PVG	VPL/PVG	2 years	50–75%
HH	35/m	VPL/PVG	VPL/PVG	8 years	75–100%
CL	41/f	VPL/PVG	–	0	0
FP	53/m	VPL/PVG	VPL/PVG	5.5 years	50–75%

TABLE VIII

Results of the combined stimulation for the treatment of central pain (thalamic pain syndrome)

Patient	Age/sex	Implanta-tion	Internali-zation	Follow-up	Pain relief
RP	55/f	VPL/PVG	PVG	1 year	50–75%
HK	53/m	VPL/PVG	PVG	2.5 year	25–50%
GH	64/m	VPL/PVG	–	–	0
RW	44/m	VPL/PVG	–	–	0
GR	70/m	VPL/PVG	–	–	0
SC	55/f	VPL/PVG	–	–	0
DH	64/m	VPL/PVG	–	–	0
HH	50/m	VPL/PVG	–	–	0
SB	68/m	VPL/PVG	–	–	0
KW	61/m	VPL/PVG	–	–	0
HH	61/f	VPL/PVG	–	–	0

TABLE IX

Results of the combined stimulation for the treatment of PHN

Patient	Age/sex	Implanta-tion	Internali-zation	Follow-up	Pain relief
RI	71/m	VPL/PVG	VPL/PVG	5.5 years	50–75%
EF	80/m	VPM	–		0

the lateral somatosensory thalamus was implanted on the side contralateral to the worst pain. In patients with bilateral pain of equal intensity, the non-dominant side was chosen (Table IV).

Phantom pain, a primary peripheral neuropathic pain with secondary central changes, is considered a rather good indication because of the well-circumscribed pain (Table V). However, we and others have had mixed results. Another fairly good indication is trigeminal neuropathic pain and/or dysaesthesia dolorosa (Table VI). In these patients our results with Gasserian stimulation are disappointing mainly due to side effects and complications (motor activation and electrode migration). An alternative, however, might be stimulation of the motor cortex (see Chapter 13).

Patients with peripheral neuropathic pain (CRPS II) respond very well to DBS (Table VII). Again, we usually have to deal with a rather circumscribed area of pain. Most of our patients had been treated earlier with SCS, but had complications (electrode migration, spinal cord compression by plate electrodes) or needed very high current intensities which made impulse generator replacements necessary at very short intervals.

Our results in patients with the thalamic pain syndrome (post-stroke pain) were very frustrating. Although we observed some beneficial effects regarding the allodynia with PVG stimulation, this did not increase the patients' quality of life because of the persisting chronic burning pain component and intermittent lancinating pain attacks. Suprathreshold as well as subthreshold stimulation in VPL usually increased the pain (Table VIII). Unfortunately, most of those patients also did not respond to motor cortex stimulation either.

Owing to the limited numbers of patients, we cannot draw any conclusions from patients with pure nociceptive pain or patients with PHN. Our

TABLE X

Results of combined stimulation for the treatment of nociceptive pain

Patient	Age/sex	Pain origin	Implantation	Internalisation	Follow-up	Pain relief
HF	60/m	Coccydynia	VPL/PVG	–	–	0
VF	62/f	Polyarthritis	VPL/PVG	PVG	1 year	50–75%

impression with the latter group, however, that patients with long-lasting PHN and complete deafferentation are poor responders due to central changes within the spinal cord or at even more central sites (Tables IX and X).

10. Complications

The most serious complications in functional stereotactic neurosurgery are intracranial haemorrhages. The incidence in major series ranged between 1.9% and 4.1%. Following improvements in electrode design, the risk of haemorrhage has decreased considerably. Nevertheless, permanent neurological complications occur in about 2%. In some cases just the insertion of the electrodes can cause neurological deficits (e.g. diplopia in PAG) without visible haemorrhage on postoperative imaging.

Some patients develop compulsive stimulation behaviour with stimulation in the lateral somatosensory thalamus. In our series this happened in two patients with the lowest electrode contacts probably stimulating hypothalamic fibres. A similar case was described by Portenoy (Portenoy et al., 1986) with VPL stimulation.

The risk of infection ranges between 3% and 12%. In our series infection occurred in one patient who had a purulent otitis media and diabetes (2%). Prophylactic oral antibiotics are routinely administered during the trial stimulation. The connector between the electrode and the extension cable should be placed over the parietal skull and not behind the ear. The latter position increases the risk of disconnection and of fracture of the connecting cables (an analogous problem is well known in shunt surgery). New extension cables with smaller connectors were recently developed and these reduce the risk of scalp erosion. A persisting problem concerns the burr hole cap provided by the manufacturer of DBS devices. The fixation with a silicon cap can push the electrode 2 or 3 mm deeper into the brain. Intraoperative X-ray and final stimulation with control of the stimulation parameters are essential. A new burr hole-fixating device (IGN, Melbourne, FL, USA; Fig. 10) has solved this problem very elegantly but it is expensive.

11. Conclusion

Deep brain stimulation is a therapeutic option for patients where more conservative and less invasive measures have failed. Careful patient selection, including blinded evaluation trials, is essential for yielding long-term success. DBS should be just one module in a multidisciplinary pain-treatment regimen, including medical treatment (e.g. tricyclics or gabapentin for neuropathic pain), physical therapy, psychological and psychiatric support to increase the patients' activity and their own responsibility to fight the chronic pain problem.

References

Adams, J.E. (1976) Naloxone reversal of analgesia produced by brain stimulation in human. Pain, 2: 161–166.

Adams, J.E., Hosobuchi, Y., and Fields, H.L. (1974) Stimulation of internal capsule for relief of chronic pain. J. Neurosurg., 41: 740–744.

Akil, H., Richardson, D.E., Barchas, J.D., and Li, C.H. (1978a) Appearance of beta-endorphin-like immunoreactivity in human ventricular cerebrospinal fluid upon analgesic electrical stimulation. Proc. Natl. Acad. Sci., 75: 5170–5172.

Akil, H., Richardson, D.E., Hughes, J., and Barchas, J.D. (1978b) Enkephalin-like material elevated in ventricular cerebrospinal fluid of pain patients after analgesic focal stimulation. Science, 201: 463–465.

Albe-Fessard, D. and Lombard, M.C. (1983) Use of animal model to evaluate the origin and protection against deafferentation pain. Adv. Pain Res. Ther., 5: 691–700.

Albe-Fessard, D., Tasker, R., Yamashiro, K., Chodakiewitz, J., and Dostrovsky, J. (1986) Comparison in man of short latency averaged evoked potentials recorded in thalamic and scalp hand zones of representation. Electroencephalogr. Clin. Neurophysiol., 65: 405–415.

Andersen, E. and Dafny, N. (1983) An ascending serotoninergic pain modulation pathway from the dorsal raphe nucleus to the parafascularis nucleus of the thalamus. Brain Res., 269: 57–67.

Andy, O.J. (1980) Parafascicular-Center median nuclei stimulation for intractable pain and dyskinesia (painful dyskinesia). Appl. Neurophysiol., 43: 133–144.

Andy, O.J. (1983) Thalamic stimulation for chronic pain. Appl. Neurophysiol., 46: 116–123.

Apkarian, A.V. and Hodge, C.J., Jr. (1989) Primate spinothalamic pathways. III. Thalamic terminations of the dorsolateral and ventral spinothalamic pathways. J. Comp. Neurol., 288: 493–511.

Basbaum, A.I. and Fields, H.L. (1978) Endogenous pain control mechanism: review and hypothesis. Ann. Neurol., 4: 451–462.

Bechtereva, N.P., Bondcharuk, A.N., Smirnov, V.M., and Melyucheva, L.A. (1972) Curative electric stimulation of deep-lying brain structures. Vopr. Neirokhir., 1: 7–12.

Beck, A.T., Ward, C.H., Mendelson, M., Mock, J., and Erbaugh, J. (1961) An inventory for measuring depression. Arch. Gen. Psychiatry, 4: 561–571.

Benabid, A.L., Henriksen, S.J., McGinty, J.F., and Bloom, F.E. (1983) Thalamic nucleus ventroposterolateralis inhibits nucleus parafascicularis response to noxious stimuli through a non opioid pathway. Brain Res., 280: 217–231.

Blomquist, A., Zhang, E.T., and Craig, A.D. (2000) Cytoarchitectonic and immunohistochemical characterization of a specific pain and temperature relay, the posterior portion of the ventral medial nucleus in the human thalamus. Brain, 123: 601–619.

Boivie, J. and Meyerson, B.A. (1982) Correlative anatomical and clinical study of pain suppression by deep brain stimulation. Pain, 13: 113–126.

Cassinari, V. and Pagni, P. (1969) *Central Pain: A Neurosurgical Survey*. Harvard University Press, Cambridge, MA.

Cesaro, P., Amsallem, B., Pollin, B., Nguyen-Legros, J., and Moretti, J.L. (1986) Organization of the median and intralaminar nuclei of the thalamus: hypotheses on their role in the onset of certain central pain. Rev. Neurol., 142: 297–302.

Chung, J.M., Lee, K.H., Surmeier, D.J., Sorkin, L.S., Kim, J., and Willis, W.D. (1986) Response characteristics of neurons in the ventral posterior lateral nucleus of the monkey thalamus. J. Neurophysiol., 56: 370–390.

Craig, A.D., Bushnell, M.C., Zhang, E.T., and Blomqvist, A. (1994) A thalamic nucleus specific for pain and temperature sensation. Nature, 372: 770–773.

Davis, K.D., Taub, E., Duffner, F., Lozano, A.M., Tasker, R.R., Houle, S., and Dostrovsky, J.O. (2000) Activation of the anterior cingulate cortex by thalamic stimulation in patients with chronic pain: a positron emission tomography study. J. Neurosurg., 92: 64–69.

Dieckmann, G. and Witzmann, A. (1982) Initial and long-term results of deep brain stimulation for chronic intractable pain. Appl. Neurophysiol., 45: 167–172.

Dionne, R.A., Mueller, G.P., Young, R.F., Greenberg, R.P., Hargreaves, K.M., Gracely, R.H., and Dubner, R. (1984) Contrast medium causes the apparent increase in beta-endorphin levels in human cerebrospinal fluid following brain stimulation. Pain, 20: 313–321.

Duncan, G.H., Bushnell, M.C., and Marchand, S. (1991) Deep brain stimulation: a review of basic research and clinical studies. Pain, 45: 49–59.

Duncan, G.H., Kupers, R.C., Marchand, S., Villemure, J.G., Gybels, J., and Bushnell, M.C. (1998) Stimulation of human thalamus for pain relief. Possible modulatory circuits revealed by positron emission tomography. J. Neurophysiol., 80: 3326–3330.

Ervin, F.R., Brown, C.E., and Mark, V.H. (1966) Striatal influence on facial pain. Confinia Neurol., 27: 75–86.

Fairman, D. (1976) Neurophysiological basis for the hypothalamic lesion and stimulation by chronic implanted electrodes for the relief of intractable pain in cancer. Adv. Pain Res. Ther., 1: 843–847.

Fenelon, G., Francois, C., Percheron, G., and Yelnik, J. (1991) Topographic distribution of neurons of the central complex (centremédian-parafascicular complex) and of other thalamic neurons projecting to the striatum in macaques. Neuroscience, 45: 495–510.

Fessler, R.G., Brown, F.D., Rachlin, J.R., Mullan, S., and Fang, V.S. (1984) Elevated beta-endorphin in cerebrospinal fluid after electrical brain stimulation: artifact of contrast infusion? Science, 224: 1017–1019.

Fields, H.L. and Adams, J.E. (1974) Pain after cortical injury relieved by electrical stimulation of the internal capsule. Brain, 97: 169–178.

Fishbain, D.A., Cutler, R.B., Rosomoff, H., and Steele-Rosomoff, R. (1997) Chronic pain-associated depression: antecedent or consequence of chronic pain? Clin. J. Pain, 13: 116–137.

Geissner, E., Dalbert, C., and Schulte, A. (1992) Die Messung der Schmerzempfindung. In: E. Geissner and G. Jungnitsch (Eds.), *Psychologie des Schmerzes* (pp. 79). Psychologie Verlags Union, Weinheim.

Gerhart, K.D., Yezierski, R.P., Fang, Z.R., and Willis, W.D. (1983) Inhibition of spinothalamic tract neurons by stimulation in ventral posterior lateral (VPL) thalamic nuclei. J. Neurophysiol., 49: 406–423.

Gerhart, K.D., Yezierski, R.P., Wilcox, T.K., Grossman, A.E., and Willis, W.D. (1981) Inhibition of primate spinothalamic tract neurons by stimulation in ipsilateral or contralateral ventral posterior lateral (VPLC) thalamic nucleus. Brain Res., 229: 514–519.

Gerhart, K.D., Yezierski, R.P., Wilcox, T.K., and Willis, W.D. (1984) Inhibition of primate spinothalamic tract neurons by stimulation in periaqueductal gray or adjacent midbrain reticular formation. J. Neurophysiol., 51: 450–466.

Gol, A. (1967) Relief of pain by electrical stimulation of the septal area. J. Neurosci., 5: 115–120.

Gorecki, J., Hirayama, T., Dostrovsky, J.O., Tasker, R.R., and Lenz, F.A. (1989) Thalamic stimulation and recording in patients with deafferentation and central pain. Stereotact. Funct. Neurosurg., 52: 219–226.

Gura, E.V., Garkavenko, V.V., and Limansky, Y.M. (1991) Influences of central gray matter stimulation on thalamic neuron responses to high and low threshold stimulation of trigeminal nerve structures. Neuroscience, 41: 681–693.

Gybels, J., Kupers, R., and Nuttin, B. (1993) What can the neurosurgeon offer in peripheral neuropathic pain!? Acta Neurochir., Suppl. 58: 136–140.

Harte, S.E., Lagman, A.L., and Borszcz, G.S. (2000) Antinociceptive effects of morphine injected into the nucleus parafascicularis thalami of the rat. Brain Res., 874: 78–86.

Hassler, R. and Riechert, T. (1959) Klinische und anatomische Befunde bei stereotaktischen Schmerzoperationen im Thalamus. Arch. Psychiatr. Nervenkr., 200: 93–122.

Heath, R. (1954) *Studies in Schizophrenia: A Multidisciplinary Approach to Mind-Brain Relationships.* Harvard University Press, Cambridge, MA.

Heath, R.G. and Mickle, W.A. (1960) Evaluation of 7 years' experience with depth electrode studies in human patients. In: E.R. Ramey and D.S. O'Doherty (Eds.), Electrical Studies on the Unanesthetized Brain (pp. 214–247). P. Hoeber, New York.

Hicks, T.P., Metherate, R., Landry, P., and Dykes, R.W. (1986) Bicuculline-induced alterations of response properties in functionally identified ventroposterior thalamic neurones. Exp. Brain Res., 63: 248–264.

Hirayama, T., Dostrovsky, J.O., Gorecki, J., Tasker, R.R., and Lenz, F.A. (1989) Recordings of abnormal activity in patients with deafferentation and central pain. Stereotact. Funct. Neurosurg., 52: 120–126.

Hodge, C.J., Jr., Apkarian, A.V., and Stevens, R.T. (1986) Inhibition of dorsal horn cell responses by stimulation of the Koelliker-Fuse nucleus. J. Neurosurg., 65: 825–833.

Hosobuchi, Y. (1986) Subcortical electrical stimulation for control of intractable pain in humans. J. Neurosurg., 64: 543–553.

Hosobuchi, Y. (1988) Current issues regarding subcortical electrical stimulation for pain control in humans. Prog. Brain Res., 77: 189–192.

Hosobuchi, Y. (1990) Intracerebral stimulation for the relief of chronic pain. In: J.R. Youmans (Ed.), Neurological Surgery (pp. 4128–4143). W.B. Saunders, Philadelphia.

Hosobuchi, Y., Adams, J.E., and Rutkin, B. (1973) Chronic thalamic stimulation for the control of facial anesthesia dolorosa. Arch. Neurol., 29: 158–161.

Hosobuchi, Y., Adams, J.E., and Linchitz, R. (1977) Pain relief by electrical stimulation of the central gray matter in human and its reversal by naloxone. Science, 197: 183–186.

Hosobuchi, Y., Rossier, J., and Bloom, F.E. (1979) Stimulation of human periaqueductal gray for pain relief increases immunoreactive beta-endorphin in ventricular fluid. Science, 203: 279–281.

Ishijima, B., Yoshimasu, N., Fukushima, T., Hori, T., Sekino, H., and Sano, K. (1975) Nociceptive neurons in the human thalamus. Confinia Neurol., 37: 99–106.

Jeanmonod, D., Magnin, M., and Morel, A. (1993) Thalamus and neurogenic pain: physiological, anatomical and clinical data. Neuroreport, 4: 475–478.

Jeanmonod, D., Magnin, M., Morel, A., Siegemund, M., Cancro, R., Lanz, M., Llinás, R.R., Ribary, U., Kronberg, E., Schulman, J., Zonenshayn, M. (2001) Thalamocortical dysrhythmia II. Clinical and surgical aspects. Thalamus Relat. Syst., 1: 245–254.

Jones, E.G. and Burton, H. (1974) Cytoarchitecture and somatic sensory connectivity of thalamic nuclei other than the ventrobasal complex in the cat. J. Comp. Neurol., 154: 173–245.

Jones, E.G., Lensky, K.M., and Chan, V.H. (2001) Delineation of thalamic nuclei immunoreactive for calcium-binding proteins in and around the posterior pole of the ventral posterior complex. Thalamus Relat. Syst., 1: 213–224.

Katayama, Y., DeWitt, D.S., Becker, D.P., and Hayes, R.L. (1984a) Behavioral evidence for a cholinoceptive pontine inhibitory area: descending control of spinal motor output and sensory input. Brain Res., 296: 241–262.

Katayama, Y., Watkins, L.R., Becker, D.P., and Hayes, R.L. (1984b) Non opiate analgesia by carbachol injection into the pontine parabrachial region of the cat. Brain Res., 296: 263–283.

Katayama, Y., Tsubokawa, T., Hirayama, T., and Yamamoto, T. (1985) Pain relief following stimulation of the pontomesencephalic parabrachial region in human. Brain sites for non-opiate-mediated pain control. Appl. Neurophysiol., 48: 195–200.

Kenshalo, D.R., Giesler, G.J., Leonard, R.B., and Willis, W.D. (1980) Responses of neurons in primate ventral posterior lateral nucleus to noxious stimuli. J. Neurophysiol., 43: 1594–1614.

Kupers, R.C., Gybels, J.M., and Gjedde, A. (2000) Positron emission tomography study of a chronic pain patient successfully treated with somatosensory thalamic stimulation. Pain, 87: 295–302.

Lenz, F.A. (1992) The ventral posterior nucleus of thalamus is involved in the generation of central pain syndromes. APS J., 1: 42–51.

Lenz, F.A., Tasker, R.R., Dostrowsky, J.O., Kwan, H.C., Gorecki, J., Hirayama, T., and Murphy, J.T. (1987) Abnormal single-unit activity recorded in the somatosensory thalamus of a quadriplegic patient with central pain. Pain, 31: 225–236.

Lenz, F.A., Seike, M., Lin, Y.C., Baker, F.H., Rowland, L.H., Gracely, R.H., and Richardson, R.T. (1993a) Neurons in the area of human thalamic nucleus ventralis caudalis respond to painful heat stimuli. Brain Res., 623: 235–240.

Lenz, F.A., Seike, M., Richardson, R.T., Lin, Y.C., Baker, F.H., Khoja, I., Jaeger, C.J., and Gracely, R.H. (1993b) Thermal and pain sensations evoked by microstimulation in the area of human ventrocaudal nucleus. J. Neurophysiol., 70: 200–212.

Lenz, F.A., Gracely, R.H., and Hope, E.J. (1994a) The sensation of angina can be evoked by stimulation of the human thalamus. Pain, 59: 119–125.

Lenz, F.A., Gracely, R.H., Rowland, L.H., and Dougherty, P.M. (1994b) A population of cells in the human thalamic principal sensory nucleus respond to painful mechanical stimuli. Neurosci. Lett., 180: 46–50.

Lenz, F.A., Kwan, H.C., Martin, R., Tasker, R., Richardson, T., and Dostrovsky, J.O. (1994c) Characteristics of somatotopic organization and spontaneous neuronal activity in the region of the thalamic principal sensory nucleus in patients with spinal cord transsection. J. Neurophysiol., 72: 1570–1587.

Lenz, F.A., Gracely, R.H., Romanoski, A.J., Hope, E.J., Rowland, L.H., and Dougherty, P.M. (1995) Stimulation in the human somatosensory thalamus can produce both the affective and sensory dimensions of previously experienced pain. Nat. Med., 1: 910–913.

Lenz, F.A., Zirh, T.A., Garonzik, I.M., and Dougherty, P.M. (1998) Neuronal activity in the region of the principle sensory nucleus of the human thalamus (ventralis caudalis) in patients with pain following amputations. Neuroscience, 86: 1065–1081.

Li, H.S., Monhemius, R., Simpson, B.A., and Roberts, M.H.T. (1998) Supraspinal inhibition of nociceptive dorsal horn neurones in the anaesthetized rat: tonic or dynamic?. J. Physiol., 506.2: 459–469.

Liz-Planells, M., Tronnier, V., and Rinaldi, P.C. (1992) Neural activity of medial and lateral thalamus in a deafferentation model. Soc. Neurosci. Abstr., 18: 288.

Llinás, R.R. and Jahnsen, H. (1982) Electrophysiology of mammalian thalamic neurons in vitro. Nature, 297: 406–408.

Lombard, M.C., Nashold, B.S., and Pelissier, T. (1979) Thalamic recordings in rats with hyperalgesia. Adv. Pain Res. Ther., 3: 767–772.

Mantyh, P.W. (1983) The spinothalamic tract in primate: a reexamination using wheatgerm agglutinin conjugated with horse radish peroxidase. Neuroscience, 9: 847–863.

Matsumoto, N., Minamimoto, T., Graybiel, A.M., and Kimura, M. (2001) Neurons in the thalamic CM-PF complex supply striatal neurons with information about behaviorally significant sensory events. J. Neurophysiol., 85: 960–976.

Mayanagi, Y., Sano, K., Suzuki, I., Kanazawa, I., Aoyagi, I., and Miyachi, Y. (1982) Stimulation and coagulation of the posteromedial hypothalamus for intractable pain, with reference to β-endorphins. Appl. Neurophysiol., 45: 136–142.

Mayer, D.J. and Hayes, R.L. (1975) Stimulation produced analgesia: development of tolerance and cross-tolerance to morphine. Science, 188: 941–943.

Mazars, G., Ruge, R., and Mazars, Y. (1960) Résultats de la stimulation du faisceau spino-thalamique et leur incidence sur la pathophysiologie de la douleur. Rev. Neurol., 103: 136–138.

Mazars, G.J. (1975) Intermittent stimulation of nucleus ventralis posterolateralis for intractable pain. Surg. Neurol., 4: 93–96.

Mazars, G.J. (1976) Etat actual de la chirurgie de la douleur. Neurochirurgie, Suppl. 22: 95–98.

Mehler, W.R., Feferman, M.E., and Nauta, W.J.H. (1960) Ascending axon degeneration following anterolateral cordotomy. An experimental study in the monkey. Brain, 83: 718–751.

Melzack, R. and Katz, J. (1992) The McGill Pain Questionnaire: appraisal and current status. In: D.C. Turk and R. Melzack (Eds.), Handbook of Pain Assessment (pp. 152–168). Guildford Press, New York.

Meyerson, B.A., Boethius, J., and Carlsson, A.M. (1979) Alleviation of malignant pain by electrical stimulation in the periventricular-periaqueducal region. Pain relief as related to stimulation sites. In: J.J. Bonica, J.C. Liebeskind, and D. Albe-Fessard (Eds.), Advances in Pain Research and Therapy (pp. 525–533). Raven Press, New York.

Modesti, L.M. and Waszak, M. (1975) Firing pattern of cells in human thalamus during dorsal column stimulation. Appl. Neurophysiol., 38: 251–258.

Moruzzi, G. and Magoun, H.W. (1949) Brain stem reticular formation and the activation of the EEG. Electroencephalogr. Clin. Neurophysiol., 1: 455–473.

Nishimoto, A., Namba, S., Nakao, Y., Matsumoto, Y., and Ohmoto, T. (1984) Inhibition of nociceptive neurons by internal capsule stimulation. Appl. Neurophysiol., 47: 117–127.

Paré, D., Smith, Y., Parent, A., and Steriade, M. (1988) Projections of brainstem core cholinergic and non-cholinergic neurons of cat to intralaminar and reticular thalamic nuclei. Neuroscience, 25: 69–86.

Pedroarena, C. and Llinás, R.R. (1997) Dendritic calcium conductances generate high-frequency oscillation in thalamocortical neurons. Proc. Natl. Acad. Sci., 94: 724–728.

Peschansky, M. and Besson, J.M. (1984) Diencephalic connections of the raphe nuclei of the rat brainstem: an anatomical study with reference to the somatosensory system. J. Comp. Neurol., 224: 509–534.

Peyron, R., Laurent, B., and Garcia-Larrea, L. (2000) Functional imaging of brain responses to pain. A review and meta-analysis. Neurophysiol. Clin., 30: 263–288.

Plotkin, R. (1982) Results in 60 cases of deep brain stimulation for chronic intractable pain. Appl. Neurophysiol., 45: 173–178.

Pool, J.L., Clark, W.D., Hudson, P., and Lombardo, M. (1956) *Hypothalamus-Hypophyseal Interrelationships.* Charles Thomas, Springfield.

Portenoy, R.K., Jarden, J.O., Sidtis, J.J., Lipton, R.B., Foley, K.M., and Rottenberg, D.M. (1986) Compulsive thalamic self-stimulation: a case with metabolic, electrophysiologic and behavioral correlates. Pain, 27: 277–290.

Radhakrishnan, V., Tsoukatos, J., Davis, K.D., Tasker, R.R., Lozano, A.M., and Dostrovsky, J.O. (1999) A comparison of the burst activity of lateral thalamic neurons in chronic pain and non pain patients. Pain, 80: 567–575.

Ralston, H.J., III and Ralston, D. (1992) The primate dorsal spinothalamic tract: evidence for a specific termination in the posterior nuclei (Po/SG) of the thalamus. Pain, 48: 107–118.

Rausell, E., Cusick, C.G., Taub, E., and Jones, E.G. (1992) Chronic deafferentation in monkeys differentially affects nociceptive and nonnociceptive pathways distinguished by specific calcium binding proteins and down-regulates γ-aminobutyric acid type A receptors at thalamic levels. Proc. Natl. Acad. Sci., 89: 2571–2575.

Ray, C.D. and Burton, C.V. (1980) Deep brain stimulation for severe chronic pain. Acta Neurochir., Suppl. 30: 289–293.

Reyes-Vazquez, C., Qiao, J.T., and Dafny, N. (1989) Nociceptive responses in nucleus parafascicularis thalami are modulated by dorsal raphe stimulation and microiontophoretic application of morphine and serotonin. Brain Res. Bull., 23: 405–411.

Reynolds, D.V. (1969) Surgery in the rat during electrical analgesia induced by focal brain stimulation. Science, 164: 444–445.

Richardson, D.E. (1982) Analgesia produced by stimulation of various sites in the human beta-endorphin system. Appl. Neurophysiol., 45: 116–122.

Richardson, D.E. and Akil, H. (1977a) Pain reduction by electrical brain stimulation in man. I. Acute administration in periaqueductal and periventricular sites. J. Neurosurg., 47: 178–183.

Richardson, D.E. and Akil, H. (1977b) Pain reduction by electrical stimulation in man: II. Chronic selfadministration in the periventricular grey matter. J. Neurosurg., 47: 184–194.

Rinaldi, P.C., Young, R.F., and Tronnier, V.M. (1991a) Bursting activity of thalamic neurons from chronic pain patients is modified by electrical stimulation in PVG. Soc. Neurosci. Abstr., 17: 1560.

Rinaldi, P.C., Young, R.F., Albe-Fessard, D., and Chodakiewitz, J. (1991b) Spontaneous neuronal hyperactivity in the medial and intralaminar thalamic nuclei of patients with deafferentation pain. J. Neurosurg., 74: 415–421.

Sadikot, A.F., Parent, A., and Francois, C. (1992) Efferent connections of the centromedian and parafascicular thalamic nuclei in the squirrel monkey: a PHA-L study of subcortical projections. J. Comp. Neurol., 315: 137–159.

Sandkühler, J., Fu, Q.G., and Zimmermann, M. (1987) Spinal pathways mediating tonic or stimulation-produced descending inhibition from the periaqueductal gray or nucleus raphe magnus are separate in cat. J. Neurophysiol., 58: 327–341.

Sano, K., Mayanagi, Y., Sekino, H., Ogashiwa, M., and Ishijima, B. (1970) Results of stimulation and destruction of the posterior hypothalamus in man. J. Neurosurg., 33: 689–707.

Schaltenbrand, G. and Wahren, W. (1977) *Atlas for Stereotaxy of the Human Brain.* 2nd ed. Thieme, New York.

Schvarcz, J.R. (1985) Chronic stimulation of the septal area for the relief of intractable pain. Appl. Neurophysiol., 48: 191–194.

Scott, J. and Huskisson, E.C. (1976) Graphic representations of pain. Pain, 2: 175–184.

Siegfried, J. (1982) Monopolar electrical stimulation of nucleus ventroposteromedialis thalami for postherpetic pain. Appl. Neurophysiol., 45: 179–184.

Spiegel, E.A. and Wycis, H.T. (1953) Mesencephalotomy in treatment of 'intractable' facial pain. Arch. Neurol. Psychiatry, 69: 1–13.

Steriade, M., Jones, E.G., and McCormick, D.A. (1997) *Thalamus.* Elsevier, Amsterdam.

Tait, R.C., Chibnall, J.T., and Krause, S. (1990) The pain disability index: psychometric properties. Pain, 40: 171–182.

Thoden, U., Doerr, M., Dieckmann, G., and Krainick, J.U. (1979) Medial thalamic permanent electrodes for pain control in man: an electrophysiological and clinical study. Electroencephalogr. Clin. Neurophysiol., 47: 582–591.

Tronnier, V.M., Wirtz, C.R., Knauth, M., Bonsanto, M.M., Hassfeld, S., Albert, F.K., and Kunze, S. (1996) Intraoperative computer-assisted neuronavigation in functional neurosurgery. Stereotact. Funct. Neurosurg., 66: 65–68.

Tsubokawa, T., Katayama, Y., Yamamoto, T., and Hirayama, T. (1985) Deafferentiation pain and stimulation of the thalamic sensory relay nucleus: clinical and experimental study. Appl. Neurophysiol., 48: 166–171.

Turnbull, I.M., Shulman, R., and Woodhurst, B. (1980) Thalamic stimulation for neuropathic pain. J. Neurosurg., 52: 486–493.

Ware, J.E. and Sherbourne, C.D. (1992) The MOS 36-item short form of health survey (SF-36). I. Conceptual framework and item selection. Med. Care, 6: 473.

Wiech, K. (2001) Neuronale Netzwerke und Schmerzverarbeitung. Ergebnisse bildgebender Verfahren. Anästhesist, 50: 2–12.

Yamashiro, K., Tasker, R.R., Iwayama, K., Mori, K., Albe-Fessard, D., Dostrovsky, J.O., and Chodakiewitz, J.W. (1989) Evoked potentials from the human thalamus: correlation with microstimulation and single-unit recording. Stereotact. Funct. Neurosurg., 52: 127–135.

Yamashiro, K., Tomiyama, N., Ishida, A., Terada, Y., Mukawa, J., Yoshii, Y., Tasker, R.R., and Albe-Fessard, D. (1997) Characteristics of neurons with high-frequency discharge in the central nervous system and their relationship to chronic pain. Stereotact. Funct. Neurosurg., 68: 149–154.

Yezierski, R.P., Wilcox, T.K., and Willis, W.D. (1982) The effects of serotonin antagonists on the inhibition of primate spinothalamic tract cells produced by stimulation of the nucleus raphe magnus or periaqueductal gray. J. Pharmacol. Exp. Ther., 220: 266–277.

Young, R.F. (1996) Deep brain stimulation for failed back syndrome. In: P.L. Gildenberg and R.R. Tasker (Eds.), Textbook of Stereotactic and Functional Neurosurgery (pp. 1621–1625). McGraw-Hill, New York.

Young, R.F. and Chambi, I. (1987) Pain relief by electrical stimulation of the periaqueductal and periventricular grey matter. J. Neurosurg., 66: 364–377.

Young, R.F. and Rinaldi, P.C. (1994) Brain stimulation. In: P.D. Wall (Ed.), Textbook of Pain (pp. 1225–1232). Churchill Livingstone, London.

Young, R.F. and Rinaldi, P.C. (1997) Brain stimulation in pain. In: R.M. Levy and R.B. North (Eds.), Neurosurgical Management of Pain. Springer Verlag, New York.

Young, R.F., Kroening, R., Fulton, W., Feldman, R.A., and Chambi, I. (1985) Electrical stimulation of the brain in treatment of chronic pain. J. Neurosurg., 62: 389–396.

Young, R.F., Tronnier, V.M., and Rinaldi, P.C. (1992) Chronic stimulation of the Koelliker-Fuse nucleus region for relief of intractable pain in humans. J. Neurosurg., 76: 979–985.

Young, R.F., Bach, F.W., Van Norman, A.S., and Yaksh, T.L. (1993) Release of beta-endorphin and met-enkephalin into cerebrospinal fluid during deep brain stimulation for chronic pain. Effects of stimulation locus and site of sampling. J. Neurosurg., 79: 816–825.

Zirh, T.A., Lenz, F.A., Reich, S.G., and Dougherty, P.M. (1998) Patterns of bursting occurring in thalamic cells during Parkinsonian tremor. Neuroscience, 83: 107–121.

Electrical Stimulation and the Relief of Pain
Pain Research and Clinical Management, Vol. 15
Edited by Brian A. Simpson

CHAPTER 15

Selection of patients and assessment of outcome

Brian A. Simpson*

Department of Neurosurgery, University Hospital of Wales, Heath Park, Cardiff CF14 4XW, UK

Abstract

The outcome from therapeutic neurostimulation depends heavily upon case selection, but although an enormous experience has accrued over the past 35 years the selection of patients remains problematical. The clinical diagnosis and the use of trial stimulation provide the mainstays of selection but the success rate in neuropathic pain remains no better than approximately two out of three, overall. Our relatively poor understanding of some of the neuropathic conditions being treated, e.g. complex regional pain syndrome (CRPS), probably contributes to the failure rate. Trial stimulation is widely regarded as an essential prerequisite but, at least in the context of spinal cord stimulation (SCS), it has definite limitations which are discussed. The role of psychological factors is also considered. A higher success rate is achieved for ischaemic pain, predominantly via SCS, aided by greater diagnostic specificity and the availability of physiological parameters to guide selection.

In neuropathic pain syndromes there is uncertainty about what is meant by 'success'. The long-term nature of the conditions and of the treatment needs to be taken into greater account, as does the resistance of the pain to other treatments. The simple application of visual analogue and numerical rating pain scales, though widespread, is flawed and inadequate; the need for more complex assessments including functional aspects, quality of life (QoL) measures, etc. is increasingly recognised. The '50% pain relief' notation is conventional and convenient but has no intrinsic meaning, and the pitfalls and limitations of its use are discussed. There is a need to study failures, including late failures. The latter constitute a complex phenomenon; some may not be failures at all. In ischaemic conditions assessment of outcome is again rather more straightforward. More neurostimulation cost-effectiveness data are needed, and many more prospective, controlled trials but incorporating better ways of assessing individual cases.

Keywords: Diagnosis; Trial stimulation; Psychological factors; Percentage pain relief; Pain scales; Functional assessment; Pain memory; Cost-effectiveness; Controlled trials

"In order to identify target groups, to conduct research, to prescribe treatment, to evaluate treatment efficacy, and for policy and decision-making, it is essential that some consensually validated criteria are used to describe groups of individuals who share a common set of relevant attributes."

(Turk and Rudy, 1992)

1. Selection of patients

It is now well established that the main indications for the use of implanted neurostimulators for pain control fall broadly into the two categories of ischaemic pain and neuropathic pain (although some nociceptive pain other than ischaemic pain responds to deep brain stimulation). The outcome

*Correspondence to: Brian A. Simpson. Phone: +44 (29) 20742708; Fax: +44 (29) 20742560;
E-mail: brian.simpson@cardiffandvale.wales.nhs.uk

of this form of treatment depends heavily upon case selection. This may be more straightforward in ischaemic pain, both cardiac and peripheral, where it is aided by radiological and physiological parameters (e.g. transcutaneous oxygen tension measurement – $TcpO_2$ – in critical limb ischaemia; see Chapter 9). In non-ischaemic neuropathic pain syndromes, however, the position regarding selection remains far from clear and it is therefore with these that this chapter will primarily be concerned.

1.1. Diagnosis

As with any medical or surgical treatment, the first consideration is the diagnosis. Pain is a symptom, a perception; it is not a diagnosis. When it is due to otherwise inoperable coronary artery disease, unreconstructable chronic limb ischaemia or a vasospastic condition such as Raynaud's disease in a patient who is cognitively competent, and a technically satisfactory spinal cord stimulator can be inserted, then sustained clinical and physiological improvement will follow in at least 80% of cases. If a patient has suffered damage to the brachial plexus with complete avulsion of nerve roots from the spinal cord, which is something that can be identified radiologically and physiologically, spinal cord stimulation (SCS) will not relieve pain in those dermatomes because the relevant neurones have been destroyed and/or disconnected. Patients with spinal cord damage short of complete transection are all unique and because they differ from each other it should not be surprising that in these cases the effect of SCS varies widely. This is reasonable and understandable but much greater difficulties arise with neuropathic conditions such as peripheral nerve damage, lumbar or brachial plexus damage (but not complete avulsion), lumbar or cervical radiculopathy (including post-surgical), phantom pain, complex regional pain syndromes (CRPS) types 1 and 2 (formerly reflex sympathetic dystrophy and causalgia) and post-herpetic neuralgia (PHN). SCS can be very effective in these

conditions but it is not effective in all cases even though they have the same diagnosis and appear clinically identical or very similar. Indeed, the average success rate in this group of conditions has generally been in the region of 50–70% of cases (North et al., 1993; Simpson, 1994; Stanton-Hicks, 1997; Barolat et al., 1998; Kumar et al., 1998; Simpson, 1999; Van Buyten et al., 2001), with slightly better results in CRPS.

Our failure to understand why a technically satisfactory stimulator does not provide pain relief in one patient with neuropathic pain, but gives excellent relief in the next two patients with the same diagnosis is one of the fundamental problems of this entire field. Of direct relevance to this is the fact that we do not yet completely understand the aetiology and pathophysiology of these neuropathic conditions. Thus we do not know why only a minority of people develop CRPS after an injury; even if there is a genetic predisposition it does not explain why CRPS developed after one injury and not after all the previous injuries sustained by that person. We do not know why phantoms are not experienced by all amputees nor why only a proportion of phantoms are painful. Why do only some people go on to develop PHN after an attack of shingles and why does this condition resolve spontaneously in some cases but not others? The response, or lack of response, to SCS may in turn contribute to our understanding of the pathophysiology of these conditions. Despite considerable efforts to improve it (Merskey, 1986; Merskey and Bogduk, 1994), the diagnostic process may still be flawed with what are actually different conditions appearing superficially identical. In this respect a move towards mechanism-based diagnoses of chronic pain syndromes has been proposed (Meyerson, 1997; Woolf et al., 1998). The effectiveness of motor cortex stimulation (MCS) in central post-stroke pain, for example, has been proposed in one study to correlate with a particular drug response profile (Yamamoto et al., 1997).

As the diagnosis alone is, at present, insufficient, additional methods of selection have been sought. Neuropathic pain typically comprises a continuous background element of varying intensity which is often burning, tight or crushing in nature, and a paroxysmal element which is shooting, stabbing or sometimes 'electrical'. Early in the history of SCS, when case selection was very poor, it was recognised that a burning quality was a positive predictor (Nashold and Friedman, 1972). Beyond confirming the neuropathic nature of the pain, the quality of the pain has not provided further clues to case selection except that the use of descriptors with negative emotional overtones such as 'wretched' and 'terrifying' tends to correlate with subsequent failure (North et al., 1993).

1.2. Test/trial stimulation

Other forms of stimulation such as mechanical stimulation of the stump of an amputee (Miles and Lipton, 1978) have been tried but not generally adopted as predictive tests for SCS. Evidence of responsiveness to any counter-irritation, e.g. hot water bottle burns in the painful area, is encouraging but there is a lack of supporting published data. The use of TENS (transcutaneous electrical nerve stimulation) has been advocated as a screening test for SCS (Mittal et al., 1987; Bel and Bauer, 1991) but this has not been supported (Spiegelmann and Friedman, 1991; Le Doux and Langford, 1993), and it appears that there is no useful correlation with the outcome from SCS.

Trial spinal cord stimulation via temporary external connections has considerable intuitive appeal, has become well established and is generally demanded by the 'payers'. It has the advantage of identifying and excluding patients who dislike the experience of electrical neurostimulation. It may also identify those in whom the essential topographical appropriateness of stimulation cannot be achieved for neuropathological or anatomical reasons (the relevant neurones have been destroyed, disconnected or are inaccessible). As to whether trial cord stimulation is a reliable predictor of success, however, the answer is

unequivocally 'no'. If it were, the subsequent response rates with definitive implants would be 100% or close to it (assuming proper technical function), and not the 60–70% that typically obtains. The assumption and assertion of many practitioners, and certainly of reimbursement agencies, is that trial stimulation *must* be a good predictor; several recent publications do not even quote the original number trialled, so great is the extent to which this 'fact' is taken for granted. Success rates undoubtedly rose after the early years, as both expertise and hardware improved, but then plateaued and the failure rate following selection by trial stimulation remains substantial. In three large mixed series, a total of 655 patients (81%) were given definitive implants out of 809 trialled. Of the 655, 515 were available for assessment; long-term success was experienced by 52% (North et al., 1993), by 59% (Kumar et al., 1998) and by 68% (Van Buyten et al., 2001), respectively. Although North's series extended back to 1972 and Van Buyten's to the late 1980s, the selection rates (78 and 85%, respectively) were similar but the success rate increased markedly. The longer trial period (1 month) employed by Van Buyten's group may have been a significant factor. In a prospective multicentre study, Burchiel and colleagues implanted 'permanent' systems in 83% of 219 patients trialled. The follow-up data were relatively limited but at one year only 56% of those who could be analysed were obtaining the level of pain relief that had been required to pass the original trial (Burchiel et al., 1996). The considerable failure rate following selection by even a lengthy period of trial stimulation cannot be ignored and deserves analysis.

One consideration is that trial SCS must, for obvious reasons, utilise percutaneously implantable electrodes rather than the plate systems that require an open operation. Evidence is accumulating for the superior performance and effectiveness of the latter (North et al., 1999; Villavicencio et al., 2000; North et al., 2002). It is possible therefore that some candidates are excluded who would obtain relief with a plate system. In one series of patients with post-surgical back and leg pain, where plate electrodes were used for the trial, the success rate at 2 years was 74% (Le Doux and Langford, 1993). However, this factor probably does not account for many false negatives.

A potentially more significant factor is that trial stimulation may have a placebo effect in some cases and the early occurrence of many of the failures would support this proposal (De La Porte and Van De Kelft, 1993). In a direct demonstration of a placebo effect, a dummy trial stimulator significantly improved the pain scores of patients with diabetic neuropathy (Tesfaye et al., 1996) although an active stimulator improved pain scores more. Allied with this is the suggestion that patients who see stimulation as their 'last hope' may have an intrinsic bias towards passing the trial: there is a positive incentive to pass the trial. These are desperate humans, not laboratory models. Nelson et al. (1996) suggested that those who respond particularly well to a trial tend to have a personality profile which would lead to a negative attitude towards residual pain and physical functioning. On the other hand, recent evidence suggests that those who proceed to a definitive implant are more open to admitting psychological distress, less somatically preoccupied, possibly more submissive (Ruchinskas and O'Grady, 2000), less depressed and with more energy (Olson et al., 1998) than are those who do not. This highlights the difficulty of interpreting psychological evidence.

The selection criterion '50% or better pain relief/reduction in pain scores' is now applied almost universally but may itself be one of the main reasons for the inability of trial stimulation to predict one failure in every three candidates with neuropathic pain. The notation '50% pain relief' has no intrinsic meaning and was generalised to neuropathic pain from analgesic drug trials in acute pain and chronic nociceptive pain (e.g. arthritis) where it is also an arbitrary, but possibly more valid, measure. The not inconsiderable shortcomings of this notation are discussed more completely in Section 2, but suffice to say at this point that a clinically significant reduction in pain may equate to a reduction in pain scores of around 30% rather than 50% (Farrar et al., 2000, 2001). It also poses the question of whether such a test is paradoxically too stringent when the aim is to help a group of patients who are particularly unresponsive to all other treatments, so that some who would have obtained useful relief may be excluded and others are encouraged to 'cheat'. As in the assessment of long-term outcomes, the importance of *functional* improvements and not just pain scores is now increasingly being recognised in interpreting trial stimulation. In some cases these might even be more important than a simple pain score. This should improve the power and reliability of the test whose discriminatory powers have never, in fact, been properly validated. The relative efficacy of definitive SCS in patients who did not meet the arbitrary standard required to 'pass' a trial, usually a 50% or greater reduction in pain scores on a visual analogue scale (VAS), is simply not known. Without such a comparator the discriminatory power of the test cannot be stated. An early report in which trial 'failures' were implanted suggests that the success rate of SCS in the rejected cohort would certainly not be zero (Nielsen et al., 1975). The validity of trial stimulation could also be evaluated by informing all the candidates that they could have a definitive stimulator if they wanted one, *whatever the trial showed*, and then later correlating the long-term outcome with the trial results.

Finally, the defenders of trial stimulation have to explain the published series in which it was not employed but the success rate was comparable to many where it was used (Racz et al., 1989; Barolat et al., 1998; Simpson et al., 2003). Barolat makes the point that 20% of his patients who never had any pain relief from a definitive stimulator would have been excluded had they been submitted to a trial but this makes the assumption that they would have reported 'less than 50% pain relief' in a trial, which is not necessarily the case. His observation that those with high initial levels of pain relief did not experience a decline over time but those with only moderate initial relief did, does lend support to the use of trial stimulation. Barolat also reminds us that some patients who go on to have long-term pain relief develop their response slowly; the duration of the trial is an important factor. Doleys suggests using repeated cycles of evaluation rather than a single trial and suggests that "*The search for a specific test that will predict outcomes may be an exercise in futility*" (Doleys et al., 1997). It should, however, be possible to improve the position with regard to trial stimulation; it would seem to be the way in which it is applied and interpreted rather than the *principle* of trial stimulation that is at fault and which causes its efficacy as a tool to fall short of expectations. Physiological assessments can be incorporated into trial stimulation in PVD and angina. In neuropathic pain many practitioners are now using trial stimulation in a more sophisticated way rather than relying simply on the draconian application of the '50% rule'. However, the incidence of false negatives, i.e. inappropriate rejections, is not known and remains a worry and the fact that, as a selection procedure, it rarely scores better than two out of three is often not acknowledged.

1.3. Psychological factors

An obvious source of clues to the differentiation of potential responders from those who will not obtain pain relief from a neurostimulator might lie within the realms of psychological factors. In some countries a (positive) psychological assessment is a prerequisite for reimbursement. However, although a considerable literature has built up on this rather broad subject, there is no compelling evidence that such assessments materially influence the subsequent success rate (see, for example, Doleys et al., 1997 for extensive discussion). The difficulty in interpreting psychological evidence has already been mentioned, and as long ago as 1974 it was pointed out that it is not the *existence* of psychological factors that is relevant to the management of these patients but rather their significance that needs to be understood (Sweet

and Wepsic, 1974). More recent studies (North et al., 1996) have shown that little progress has been made. Chronic severe pain that is at best only partially responsive to medication cannot be considered in isolation from its effects on the patient and on those close to him or her. Thus, not only the pain itself but also reduced mobility, loss of independence, social isolation, sleep deprivation, the often not inconsiderable side effects of medication and, in many cases, poverty can all lead to depression, fear and anxiety, frustration and despair which may in turn exacerbate the pain. To dissect out from this background, the psychological factors which may have predictive value is a formidable challenge.

In contrast with psychological testing, Nielsen recognised that a psychiatric opinion could be helpful (Nielsen et al., 1975). A Belgian study has since confirmed the usefulness of psychiatric input, the success rate being substantially higher where a psychiatrist had no reservations (Kupers et al., 1994). Psychoanalytical factors such as guilt feelings and attitude towards authority may also have predictive value (Dumoulin et al., 1996), but these isolated studies lack the support of additional published evidence. It is perhaps self-evident that serious personality disorders and some forms of mental illness will militate against a good outcome (Nelson et al., 1996).

Thorough preoperative counselling of all patients is essential, and the physician or surgeon should be alert to the fact that some patients have, or develop, an emotional aversion to implants; precisely what the definitive treatment entails must be made very clear to the patient. The patient's expectations regarding possible outcomes are of course crucially important and sometimes surprisingly unrealistic. This must also be carefully addressed. Psychological input may contribute more in terms of counselling than through preoperative selection, at least at our present level of knowledge.

The complexity and chronicity of many of the cases, and their expectations, colour the whole issue; there is a strong suggestion that neurostimulation should be used earlier, before secondary factors become too established, and not regarded so much as a last resort (see, for example, Kumar et al., 1998). Nonetheless, it is invasive, particularly when applied to the brain rather than spinal cord or nerve, and although serious complications are rare, the invasiveness, although completely justified in most cases, is an important factor to consider in the selection of patients.

2. Assessment of outcome

Just as outcomes depend heavily upon case selection, so does case selection depend, indirectly, upon the assessment, and therefore knowledge, of the efficacy of the treatment. As with case selection, this is more straightforward for ischaemic pain, where physiological markers, exercise tolerance, glyceryl trinitrate (GTN) intake, etc. can be used, than it is for neuropathic pain. Complete removal of the underlying cause, and therefore of the pain, may be possible in ischaemic pain (the anti-ischaemic effect of stimulation) but in neuropathic pain this option does not exist in such a direct way. From the clinical standpoint a really good outcome in neuropathic pain is not difficult to recognise, at least in the short to medium term; the problems arise clinically when it falls short of this ideal and with the passage of time and, academically, as soon as we try to gain any understanding of the phenomenon. In neuropathic pain, a reduction in (the often considerable) medication intake with SCS may increase general well-being and the ability to cope with any residual pain. Increased exercise tolerance with SCS in peripheral ischaemia may improve perfusion and itself reduce the pain level. In angina pectoris, SCS may break the vicious circle of fear/anxiety and sympathetic overactivity. In these examples, what is the analgesic effect of SCS? Determination of the effect of the treatment can be far more complex than many published reports would imply, as others have pointed out (see, for example, Turk et al., 1993; Williams, 1995; Williams et al., 2000),

and the relatively simplistic approach which has often been adopted disregards a considerable literature (see, for example, Melzack, 1983; Turk and Melzack, 1992a). The effect of neurostimulation also tends to be evaluated in isolation. The combined effects of stimulation and physical therapy, stimulation and pain management programmes, and even drug interaction with stimulation have received relatively little attention.

2.1. Percentage pain relief

The convenient 50% standard has been very widely adopted and will have been encountered throughout this volume as in much published work on neurostimulation. The use of percentage pain relief, particularly 'greater or less than 50% pain relief', has become a well-trodden path but that does not by itself bestow legitimacy. We should remind ourselves that it is only a convention, albeit a very convenient one, which has no intrinsic meaning. It was taken from drug trials in acute pain and chronic nociceptive pain and applied to neuropathic syndromes without validation. Recognition of the distinction between neuropathic and nociceptive pain has not been consistently accompanied by a differential approach to this aspect. The convenience and apparent (but not real) standardization that characterises a percentage change in a metric scale has seduced practitioners, with the complicity of healthcare purchasers (commissioners, insurers) and peer reviewers, with little regard for the relationship between pain scales and clinically meaningful changes in pain (Burchiel et al., 1996; Rowbotham, 2001). 'Fifty percent' is almost more a figure of speech than a matter of mathematical or statistical veracity. Where the relationship has been studied, it has been suggested that a reduction in a rating scale of approximately 30% equates better to a clinically significant level of pain relief (Farrar et al., 2000, 2001). Furthermore, it is unlikely that a 50% reduction in angina, in cancer pain, in phantom pain, in postoperative pain, in CRPS and in arthritis are somehow equivalent phenomena. A reduction on a VAS from 10 to 5 will not mean the same as a reduction from 4 to 2. Patients' approach to rating scales is idiosyncratic, not stereotyped; in one study, 8 out of 10 on a VAS was 'average everyday pain' to one patient and 'barely tolerable' to another (Williams et al., 2000). As Turk and Melzack (1992b) reminded us: "*The appropriateness of norms of tests has rarely been considered in the pain literature. In the absence of normative information, the raw score on any test is meaningless.*" Good and excellent pain relief are often equated to 50% and 75% changes respectively on a VAS, but as Barolat points out (Barolat et al., 1998) this does not do justice to an average of 20% of patients who continue to use their stimulators long term with 'moderate' pain relief. In one prospective study only 26% of patients with leg pain reported 50% or greater pain relief but 70% said SCS helped them and they would recommend it. After 2 years, two-thirds had reduced or discontinued their narcotic intake (Ohnmeiss et al., 1996). Fifty-five percent of De La Porte and Van De Kelft's patients reported at least 50% pain relief but 90% were able to stop or reduce their medication (De La Porte and Van De Kelft, 1993). Patients suffering from long-term pain for whom nothing else has been effective may be very pleased with a relatively small reduction on a pain scale, particularly if it is consistent and is accompanied by functional improvements and decreased medication. Their own estimates of percentage relief may, however, be relatively meaningless and the position is made worse by the vernacular use of percentages, as in "I'm 100% better but the pain's still there" and "He's 100% worse everyday."

2.2. The holistic approach

Pain is a perception and as such it is influenced by many factors including mood, experience, expectation, tiredness, activity level, etc. It is not simple, unitary or directly quantifiable. Even the process of assessing and reporting pain may influence the perception. Pain is multidimensional and although this is still poorly defined, it follows that the assessment of any analgesic therapy is greatly enhanced if functional changes and not just pain scores are taken into account. This is now increasingly recognised and, following the early lead of Long (Long et al., 1981) and of Koeze et al. (1987), a more holistic approach to assessment of the effects of stimulation, including quality of life (QoL) measures is being taken. Mobility, activities of daily living, social interaction, recreation, alertness and sleep are increasingly taken into account (see, for example, De La Porte and Van De Kelft, 1993; North et al., 1993; Burchiel et al., 1996; Vulink et al., 1999; Kemler et al., 2000; Anderson et al., 2001; May et al., 2002). In CRPS, Kemler reported an 11% improvement in the overall score for the health-related QoL. Changes in pain severity over time have been shown to correlate with changes in physical and social functioning, energy and vitality and general health (Elliott et al., 2000). Verbal ratings and the reports of partners and other third parties are probably not given sufficient prominence. The question of changes in medication is complex but in some cases this can provide useful information. Although very long-term trial stimulation is not feasible, the increasing incorporation of functional and QoL measures into the use of trial stimulation for case selection should improve its predictive power and reduce the potentially inappropriate rejection of candidates who might benefit from long-term stimulation.

Return to work is frequently quoted as a marker of success, which indeed it probably is when it occurs. However, for a group of patients many of whom are physically disabled and have been off work for a long time in societies with high unemployment rates and decreasing employer tolerance, it certainly cannot be a *necessary* condition for success.

2.3. The assessor

Assessment by a 'disinterested' third party should remove, or at least reduce, observer bias and there is some evidence for this. Some of North's patients, with definitive stimulators implanted after a trial, told a third party that they had *never had any* pain relief and one in five said they had never actually experienced the '50% or more' pain relief that had been required to pass the trial (North et al., 1993). It does not follow that careful, thorough, repeated face-to-face assessments by an experienced practitioner have no value; in fact Koeze et al. (1987) found that the reports of the patient, of a close friend and of an involved clinician all correlated well. Nevertheless, observer bias must be a potential source of error even in multidisciplinary teams.

2.4. Chronicity and late failure

The chronicity of the conditions being treated generates further potential inaccuracy and misinterpretation concerning the patient's own assessment of the degree of pain relief afforded by an implanted neurostimulator. It is well recognized that many patients report diminishing pain relief over the years but continue to use their technically satisfactory stimulator. In some cases this 'late failure' may be due to true tolerance, about which very little is known. There is at least anecdotal evidence that in many more cases late failure reflects a reporting error on the part of the patient. It is a relatively common experience to find a patient who has reported only moderate or slight pain relief, demands urgent repair or replacement when battery depletion or a technical failure of their device occurs. This is typically accompanied by a comment such as "I had forgotten just how bad the pain used to be." There is evidence that chronic pain is remembered less well than acute pain (Hunter et al., 1979; Erskine et al., 1990; Babul and Darke, 1994) and that patients with chronic pain do not accurately recall the intensity of previous pain (Linton and Melin, 1982; Jamison et al., 1989; Bryant, 1993) particularly if the present pain intensity is low, when previous pain may be remembered as being less severe than it was (Eich et al., 1985). The effect of this flexibility

of memory on the assessment might be considerable but it should be borne in mind that this evidence comes mostly from studies of nociceptive pain. Memory for neuropathic pain and the interaction between present neuropathic pain and memory are very poorly understood. Neuropathic pain has little or no survival value, only deleterious effects, and it would not be surprising if memory for neuropathic pain were inaccurate and unreliable. A thorough psychological study of 'late failures' might be illuminating.

Prompted by this, Monhemius and Simpson (2003) conducted an abstinence study of patients with spinal cord stimulators implanted a median 42 months earlier for neuropathic pain. The stimulator was to be off completely for 2 weeks followed by 1 week of normal usage and then the cycle was repeated. Twice daily VAS scores were recorded along with sleep, activity and medication data. Compliance was poor partly because 2 weeks was probably too long. The biggest *average* 'pain relief' score recorded was 42%; differences as low as 13% were recorded in patients who appeared to derive considerable benefit from SCS, and such differences were statistically significant. Burchiel et al. (1996) similarly reported a reduction in *average pain* VAS score of only 14% after one year of SCS, yet this gave a P value of <0.0005. The relationship between clinical and statistical significance in pain relief indicates yet another facet of the problem of assessment (Turk et al., 1993). Repeated assessments over time may indicate that relatively small reductions in pain scores can be significant both clinically and statistically. In other words, 'single shot' assessments may be misleading and relatively meaningless in a chronic paradigm. When a long-term treatment is applied to a chronic condition which is typically complicated by a penumbra of factors and which may be subject to diurnal and other temporal variations, it should perhaps not be surprising if a snapshot assessment can be misleading and there is some evidence to support this (Jensen and McFarland, 1993). The abstinence model may provide a useful method of assessing efficacy in the context of a chronic therapy for a chronic condition.

In some cases of late failure, the alteration in the patient's circumstances caused by the (initially) effective treatment may have brought about an unrecognised change in the treatment parameters now required to maintain that change. Very little has been reported on dynamic changes in stimulation requirements and on what changes may be required to recapture previous efficacy.

2.5. Cost-effectiveness

The socio-economic dimension is probably as important as the clinical and the technological; cost-effectiveness data should be able to provide a measure of group average efficacy, yet very few studies have been carried out. This is perhaps surprising given the emphasis on cost-containment in many healthcare systems, the high initial cost of neurostimulators and the problems with reimbursement in some countries (Simpson, 1998). Considerable cost-savings have been demonstrated with SCS for angina (Rasmussen et al., 1992). In studies of the so-called failed back surgery syndrome (FBSS), the rather variable factor of return to work has the biggest impact on cost-effectiveness (Bel and Bauer, 1991), but in a recent article, Budd (2002) has highlighted the difficulty in obtaining data relating to social benefit payments, accurate indications of disability, etc. In some circumstances there may be advantages in not having formal employment. Nonetheless, in this condition (FBSS), SCS can attain cost-neutrality after about 5 years or less, possibly as early as 2 years (Bell et al., 1997; Budd, 2002). In the most comprehensive cost-effectiveness study of SCS to date (Kumar et al., 2002), 15% of patients with FBSS treated with SCS returned to work compared with none of the controls. Cost-equivalence was reached after 2.5 years. Over 5 years, SCS saved approximately US $9,000 per patient. Healthcare commissioners and reimbursers do not seem to be as impressed by such evidence of efficacy and cost-saving as one might

expect, perhaps because the holder of one budget may not be concerned about savings made in another.

2.6. Prospective-controlled trials

What these bodies do demand, increasingly, is Level 1 evidence of efficacy, i.e. randomised, fully controlled trials (RCTs). Such evidence is lacking in the field of therapeutic neuromodulation. Studies of SCS cannot be blind because of the necessary evoked paraesthesiae, but MCS and stimulation of some deep brain targets do not induce any sensations and can be studied with observer and subject blinding. Most of the published evidence concerning neurostimulation comprises retrospective case series often comprising a mixture of indications. Two meta analyses of SCS (Turner et al., 1995: 39 case series of chronic low-back pain (CLBP) and FBSS, and Wetzel et al., 2000: 35 case series and one RCT of FBSS) concluded that only limited conclusions could be drawn about efficacy. In their recent systematic review, Taylor and colleagues similarly concluded that although 65 studies of FBSS/CLBP consistently associated SCS with pain relief (50% or greater pain relief achieved in a mean of 62% of patients and in 16 studies an average of 53% discontinued analgesic medication), and there was some evidence of improved functional capacity and QoL; the quality of the evidence was such that "*Until further evidence becomes available it is not possible to recommend SCS as routine treatment for CLBP/FBSS*" (Taylor et al., submitted for publication). The same review was more positive about CRPS, largely because of the results from the well-conducted RCT of Kemler et al. (2000). In 19 case series, a mean of 67% achieved '50% pain relief'. The review was again critical of the quality of the case-series evidence, which was analysed in detail, but concluded "*Evidence from a well-controlled RCT supports the conclusion that SCS, combined with physical therapy, is a clinically effective and cost effective treatment for CRPS Type 1.*" Although some prospective studies of neurostimulation have been published, mainly in ischaemic pain, the number of controlled studies remains extremely small. In FBSS there have been only two (North et al., 1994, 1995; Dario et al., 2001) and only North's study was randomised. North's group has published another RCT but that was primarily a comparison of surgical versus percutaneous electrodes (North et al., 2002). In the Italian cohort study (Dario et al., 2001), the comparator was medical treatment, and in the US study it was back surgery. By 6 months, 67% of the surgical group in the latter had requested crossover to SCS but only 17% of the SCS group requested back surgery.

There is an obvious need for more RCTs of neurostimulation but they should include assessments of QoL and of cost-effectiveness. The way in which relief of chronic neuropathic pain is assessed needs to be addressed and developed, and the limitations of isolated VAS scores recognised. The power of any trial depends not only on the design and size of the trial but also on the method of assessment of the individual cases; if the latter is not meaningful the largest, best-designed and most controlled trial will not generate legitimate results.

3. Conclusions

3.1. Case selection

- The outcome depends heavily upon case selection.
- The indications are, broadly, neuropathic and ischaemic pain.
- The success rate is higher in ischaemic pain and case selection relatively more straightforward, being assisted by radiological and physiological factors and greater diagnostic specificity.
- In neuropathic pain it is not understood why two-third of patients respond to stimulation and one-third do not, with the same clinical diagnosis. The diagnostic process may not yet be sufficiently sophisticated and there is much about the underlying conditions, e.g. CRPS, which is not understood.
- Preliminary trial stimulation, whether for SCS, MCS or deep brain stimulation, does not yield the long-term success rates that would be expected. It is probably the way in which the outcome of the trial is assessed that is at fault, rather than the principle, e.g. the requirement of a 50% reduction on a VAS may be inappropriate. Functional assessment is also needed, where possible. A placebo effect of trial stimulation may be relevant in some cases and others may be influenced by seeing stimulation as their last chance. A trial will exclude some non-responders but the false negative rate is not known and this should be studied, as should the 30–40% of patients with neuropathic pain who 'pass' a trial and then fail later. The discriminative power of trial stimulation has always been assumed but has never been properly tested.
- Psychological factors are integral to chronic pain but psychological testing has not improved case selection, whereas a psychiatric opinion has. Preoperative counselling of patients is essential; expectations are often unrealistic and inappropriate. In some conditions the earlier use of neurostimulation, before secondary factors become established, might facilitate the selection procedure and improve outcomes.

3.2. Outcome assessment

- The lack of a generally agreed and validated measure of success, at least in neuropathic pain, compromises the evaluation of selection procedures.
- Evaluation of the effect in ischaemic pain is generally less complex and less difficult than in neuropathic pain. The option to remove, or at least reduce, the underlying cause of the pain is not available in neuropathic pain in the way that it can be in ischaemic pain (the anti-ischaemic effect of stimulation).

- Assessment of long-term treatment of long-term neuropathic conditions, which are complicated by many secondary factors and by temporal variation, cannot be simplistic. Unidimensional snapshot assessments are likely to be misleading.

- The use of percentage changes in visual analogue or numerical rating scales is widespread and well established but has important limitations which should be recognised. The use of 50% reduction is an almost universal convention but is arbitrary and has no intrinsic meaning. The relationship between pain scales and clinically meaningful changes in pain is poorly understood. Relatively small percentage changes can correlate with considerable patient satisfaction.

- The 'feed-forward' effect of pain relief can fuel itself to some extent: in PVD a greater exercise tolerance may improve peripheral perfusion, in angina the sympathetic vicious circle of fear, etc. may be broken, and in neuropathic pain a reduction in medication reduces malaise and increases the ability to cope with residual pain.

- Pain is a multidimensional perception, influenced by many factors including mood, expectation, activity level and so on. Functional changes and QoL measures should be taken into account and may sometimes be more important than simple pain scores.

- Memory for chronic pain, particularly neuropathic pain, is poorly understood but is known to be plastic and unreliable. This may influence long-term reporting and probably contributes to the phenomenon of 'late failure'.

- Cost-effectiveness data have shown considerable savings with SCS in angina, thereby providing indirect evidence of efficacy. Data are limited and can be difficult to obtain, but for neuropathic pain all studies show cost-neutrality occurring between 2 and 5 years after implantation followed by savings thereafter. The complexity of healthcare finance systems defuses the implications of this but many more studies are needed.

- Many retrospective case series have been published and a small number of systematic reviews but virtually no randomised controlled trials. Studies of SCS cannot be blind because of the essential evoked paraesthesiae but there is a great need for well-designed prospective controlled trials of all applications of neuro-stimulation. These must incorporate evaluations of the individual cases that are as appropriate and meaningful as possible.

References

Anderson, V.C., Carlson, C., and Shatin, D. (2001) Outcomes of spinal cord stimulation: patient validation. Neuromodulation, 4: 11–17.

Babul, N. and Darke, A.C. (1994) Reliability and accuracy of memory for acute pain. Pain, 57: 131–132.

Barolat, G., Ketcik, B., and He, J. (1998) Long-term outcome of spinal cord stimulation for chronic pain management. Neuromodulation, 1: 19–29.

Bel, S. and Bauer, B.L. (1991) Dorsal column stimulation (DCS): cost to benefit analysis. Acta Neurochir., Suppl. 52: 121–123.

Bell, G.K., Kidd, D., and North, R.B. (1997) Cost-effectiveness analysis of spinal cord stimulation in treatment of failed back surgery syndrome. J. Pain Symptom Manage., 13: 286–295.

Bryant, R.A. (1993) Memory for pain and affect in chronic pain patients. Pain, 54: 347–351.

Budd, K. (2002) Spinal cord stimulation: cost-benefit study. Neuromodulation, 5: 75–78.

Burchiel, K.J., Anderson, V.C., Brown, F.D., Fessler, R.G., Friedman, W.A., Pelofsky, S., Weiner, R.L., Oakley, J., and Shatin, D. (1996) Prospective, multicenter study of spinal cord stimulation for relief of chronic back and extremity pain. Spine, 21: 2786–2794.

Dario, A., Fortini, G., Bertollo, D., Bacuzzi, A., Grizzetti, C., and Cuffari, S. (2001) Treatment of failed back surgery syndrome. Neuromodulation, 4: 105–110.

De La Porte, C. and Van De Kelft, E. (1993) Spinal cord stimulation in failed back surgery syndrome. Pain, 52: 55–61.

Doleys, D.M., Klapow, J.C., and Hammer, M. (1997) Psychological evaluation in spinal cord stimulation therapy. Pain Rev., 4: 189–207.

Dumoulin, K., Devulder, J., Castille, F., DeLaht, M., Van Bastelaere, M., and Rolly, G. (1996) A psychoanalytic investigation to improve the success rate of spinal cord stimulation as a treatment for chronic failed back surgery syndrome. Clin. J. Pain, 12: 43–49.

Eich, E., Reeves, J.L., Jaeger, B., and Graff-Radford, S.B. (1985) Memory for pain; relation between past and present pain intensity. Pain, 23: 375–379.

Elliott, A.M., Smith, B.H., Smith, W.C., and Chambers, W.A. (2000) Changes in chronic pain severity over time: the Chronic Pain Grade as a valid measure. Pain, 88: 303–308.

Erskine, A., Morley, S., and Pearce, S. (1990) Memory for pain: a review. Pain, 41: 255–265.

Farrar, J.T., Portenoy, R.K., Berlin, J.A., Kinman, J.L., and Strom, B.L. (2000) Defining the clinically important difference in pain outcome measures. Pain, 88: 287–294.

Farrar, J.T., Young, J.P., LaMoreaux, L., Werth, J.L., and Poole, R.M. (2001) Clinical importance of changes in chronic pain intensity measured on an 11-point numerical pain rating scale. Pain, 94: 149–158.

Hunter, M., Philips, C., and Rachman, S. (1979) Memory for pain. Pain, 6: 35–46.

Jamison, R.N., Sbrocco, T., and Parris, W.C.V. (1989) The influence of physical and psychosocial factors on accuracy of memory for pain in chronic pain patients. Pain, 37: 289–294.

Jensen, M.P. and McFarland, C.A. (1993) Increasing the reliability and validity of pain intensity measurement in chronic pain patients. Pain, 55: 195–203.

Kemler, M.A., Barendse, G.A.M., van Kleef, M., de Vet, H.C.W., Rijks, C.P.M., Furnée, C.A., and van den Wildenberg, F.A.J.M. (2000) Spinal cord stimulation in patients with chronic reflex sympathetic dystrophy. N. Engl. J. Med., 343: 618–624.

Koeze, T.H., Williams, A.C. De C., and Reiman, S. (1987) Spinal cord stimulation and the relief of chronic pain. J. Neurol. Neurosurg. Psychiatry, 50: 1424–1429.

Kumar, K., Toth, C., Nath, R.K., and Laing, P. (1998) Epidural spinal cord stimulation for treatment of chronic pain – some predictors of success. A 15-year experience. Surg. Neurol., 50: 110–121.

Kumar, K., Malik, S., and Demeria, D. (2002) Treatment of chronic pain with spinal cord stimulation versus alternative therapies: cost-effectiveness analysis. Neurosurgery, 51: 106–116.

Kupers, R.C., Van den Oever, R., Van Houdenhove, B., Vanmechelen, W., Hepp, B., Nuttin, B., and Gybels, J.M. (1994) Spinal cord stimulation in Belgium: a nation-wide survey on the incidence, indications and therapeutic efficacy by the health insurer. Pain, 56: 211–216.

Le Doux, M.S. and Langford, K.H. (1993) Spinal cord stimulation for the failed back syndrome. Spine, 18: 191–194.

Linton, S.J. and Melin, L. (1982) The accuracy of remembering chronic pain. Pain, 13: 281–285.

Long, D.M., Erickson, D., Campbell, J., and North, R. (1981) Electrical stimulation of the spinal cord and peripheral nerves for pain control. A 10-year experience. Appl. Neurophysiol., 44: 207–217.

May, M.S., Banks, C., and Thomson, S. (2002) A retrospective long-term, third-party follow-up of patients considered for spinal cord stimulation. Neuromodulation, 5: 137–144.

Melzack, R. (Ed.) (1983) *Pain Measurement and Assessment*, Raven Press, New York.

Merskey, H. (Ed.) (1986) Classification of chronic pain. Descriptions of chronic pain syndromes and definition of pain terms. Pain, Suppl 3: S1–S226.

Merskey, H. and Bogduk, N. (Eds.) (1994) *Classification of Chronic Pain. Descriptions of Chronic Pain Syndromes and Definitions of Pain Terms.* 2nd ed., IASP Press, Seattle, WA.

Meyerson, B.A. (1997) Guest Editorial. Pharmacological tests in pain analysis and in prediction of treatment outcome. Pain, 72: 1–3.

Miles, J. and Lipton, S. (1978) Phantom limb pain treated by electrical stimulation. Pain, 5: 373–382.

Mittal, B., Thomas, D.G.T., Walton, P., and Calder, I. (1987) Dorsal column stimulation (DCS) in chronic pain: report of 31 cases. Ann. R. Coll. Surg., 69: 104–109.

Monhemius, R. and Simpson, B.A. (2003) Efficacy of spinal cord stimulation for neuropathic pain – assessment by abstinence. Eur. J. Pain, in press.

Nashold, B.S. and Friedman, H. (1972) Dorsal column stimulation for control of pain. Preliminary report on 30 patients. J. Neurosurg., 36: 590–597.

Nelson, D.V., Kennington, M., Novy, D.M., and Squitieri, P. (1996) Psychological considerations in implantable technology. Pain Forum, 5: 121–126.

Nielsen, K.D., Adams, J.E., and Hosobuchi, Y. (1975) Experience with dorsal column stimulation for relief of chronic intractable pain: 1968–1973. Surg. Neurol., 4: 148–152.

North, R.B., Kidd, D.H., Zahurak, M., James, C.S., and Long, D.M. (1993) Spinal cord stimulation for chronic, intractable pain: experience over two decades. Neurosurgery, 32: 384–395.

North, R.B., Kidd, D.H., Lee, M.S., and Piantadosi, S. (1994) A prospective, randomized study of spinal cord stimulation versus reoperation for failed back surgery syndrome: initial results. Stereotact. Funct. Neurosurg., 62: 267–272.

North, R.B., Kidd, D.H., and Piantadosi, S. (1995) Spinal cord stimulation versus reoperation for failed back surgery syndrome: a prospective, randomized study design. Acta Neurochir., Suppl. 64: 106–108.

North, R.B., Kidd, D.H., Wimberly, R.L., and Edwin, D. (1996) Prognostic value of psychological testing in patients undergoing spinal cord stimulation: a prospective study. Neurosurgery, 39: 301–311.

North, R.B., Kidd, D., Davis, C., Olin, J., and Sieracki, J.M. (1999) Spinal cord stimulation electrode design: a prospective randomized, controlled trial comparing percutaneous and laminectomy electrodes. Stereotact. Funct. Neurosurg., 73: 134.

North, R.B., Kidd, D.H., Olin, J.C., and Sieracki, J.M. (2002) Spinal cord stimulation electrode design: prospective, randomized, controlled trial comparing percutaneous and laminectomy electrodes – Part 1: Technical outcomes. Neurosurgery, 51: 381–390.

Ohnmeiss, D.D., Rashbaum, R.F., and Bogdanffy, G.M. (1996) Prospective outcome evaluation of spinal cord stimulation in patients with intractable leg pain. Spine, 21: 1344–1351.

Olson, K.A., Bedder, M.D., Anderson, V.C., Burchiel, K.J., and Villanueva, M.R. (1998) Psychological variables associated with outcome of spinal cord stimulation trials. Neuromodulation, 1: 6–13.

Racz, G.B., McCarron, R.F., and Talboys, P. (1989) Percutaenous dorsal column stimulator for chronic pain control. Spine, 14: 1–4.

Rasmussen, M.B., Andersen, C., Andersen, P., and Frandsen, F. (1992) Cost-benefit analysis of electric stimulation of the spinal cord in the treatment of angina pectoris. Ugeskrift For Laeger, 154: 1180–1184.

Rowbotham, M.C. (2001) Editorial: What is a 'clinically meaningful' reduction in pain? Pain, 94: 131–132.

Ruchinskas, R. and O'Grady, T. (2000) Psychological variables predict decisions regarding implantation of a spinal cord stimulator. Neuromodulation, 3: 183–189.

Simpson, B.A. (1994) Spinal cord stimulation. Pain Rev., 1: 199–230.

Simpson, B.A. (1998) Neuromodulation in Europe – regulation, variation and trends. Pain Rev., 5: 124–131.

Simpson, B.A. (1999) Spinal cord and brain stimulation. In: P.D. Wall and R. Melzack (Eds.), *Textbook of Pain*. 4th ed. (pp. 1353–1381). Churchill Livingstone, Edinburgh.

Simpson, B.A., Bassett, G., Davis, K., Herbert, C., and Pierri, M. (2003) Cervical spinal cord stimulation for pain: a report on 41 patients. Neuromodulation, 6: 20–26.

Spiegelmann, R. and Friedman, W.A. (1991) Spinal cord stimulation: a contemporary series. Neurosurgery, 28: 65–71.

Stanton-Hicks, M. (1997) Stimulation of the central and peripheral nervous system for the control of pain. J. Clin. Neurophysiol., 14: 46–62.

Sweet, W.H. and Wepsic, J.G. (1974) Stimulation of the posterior columns of the spinal cord for pain control: indications, technique and results. Clin. Neurosurg., 21: 278–310.

Taylor R., Van Buyten J.-P., and Buchser E. (submitted for publication) Spinal cord stimulation for chronic low back pain/failed back surgery syndrome and complex regional pain syndrome: a systematic review of the clinical effectiveness and cost effectiveness literature.

Tesfaye, S., Watt, J., Benbow, S.J., Pang, K.A., Miles, J., and MacFarlane, I.A. (1996) Electrical spinal cord stimulation for painful diabetic peripheral neuropathy. Lancet, 348: 1698–1701.

Turk, D.C. and Melzack, R. (Eds.) (1992) *Handbook of Pain Assessment*, The Guildford Press, New York and London.

Turk, D.C. and Melzack, R. (1992) Trends and future directions in human pain assessment. In: D.C. Turk and R. Melzack (Eds.), *Handbook of Pain Management* (pp. 473–479). The Guildford Press, New York and London. Chapter 26.

Turk, D.C. and Rudy, T.E. (1992) Classification logic and strategies in chronic pain. In: D.C. Turk and R. Melzack (Eds.), *Handbook of Pain Management* (pp. 409–428). The Guildford Press, New York and London. Chapter 23.

Turk, D.C., Rudy, T.E., and Sorkin, B.A. (1993) Neglected topics in chronic pain treatment outcome studies: determination of success. Pain, 53: 3–16.

Turner, J.A., Loeser, J.D., and Bell, K.G. (1995) Spinal cord stimulation for chronic low back pain: a systematic literature synthesis. Neurosurgery, 37: 1088–1096.

Van Buyten, J.-P., Van Zundert, J., Vueghs, P., and Vanduffel, L. (2001) Efficacy of spinal cord stimulation: 10 years of experience in a pain centre in Belgium. Eur. J. Pain, 5: 299–307.

Villavicencio, A.T., Leveque, J.-C., Rubin, L., Bulsara, K., and Gorecki, J.P. (2000) Laminectomy versus percutaneous electrode placement for spinal cord stimulation. Neurosurgery, 46: 399–406.

Vulink, N.C.C., Overgaauw, D.M., Jessurun, G.A.J., Ten Vaarwerk, I.A.M., Kropmans, T.J.B., van der Schans, C.P., Middel, B., Staal, M.J., and De Jongste, M.J.L. (1999) The effects of spinal cord stimulation on quality of life in patients with therapeutically chronic refractory angina pectoris. Neuromodulation, 2: 33–40.

Wetzel, F.T., Hassenbusch, S., Oakley, J.C., Willis, K.D., Simpson, R.K., and Ross, E.L. (2000) Treatment of chronic pain in failed back surgery patients with spinal cord stimulation: a review of current literature and proposal for future investigation. Neuromodulation, 3: 59–74.

Williams, A.C. De C. (1995) Pain measurement in chronic pain management. Pain Rev., 2: 39–63.

Williams, A.C. De C., Davies, H.T.O., and Chadury, Y. (2000) Simple pain rating scales hide complex idiosyncratic meanings. Pain, 85: 457–463.

Woolf, C.J., Bennett, G.J., Doherty, M., Dubner, R., Kidd, B., Koltzenburg, M., Lipton, R., Loeser, J.D., Payne, R., Torebjork, E. (1998) Editorial. Towards a mechanism-based classification of pain? Pain, 77: 227–229.

Yamamoto, T., Katayama, Y., Hirayama, T., and Tsubokawa, T. (1997) Pharmacological classification of central post stroke pain: comparison with the results of chronic motor cortex stimulation therapy. Pain, 72: 5–12.

Electrical Stimulation and the Relief of Pain
Pain Research and Clinical Management, Vol. 15
Edited by Brian A. Simpson

The future of spinal cord stimulation and related 'neuroaugmentative' procedures

Eric Buchser[a],* and Simon Thomson[b]

[a]*Anaesthesia and Pain Management Services, Hôpital de Morges, 1110 Morges, Switzerland*
[b]*Basildon and Thurrock University Hospitals NHS Trust, Pain Management Services, Orsett Hospital, Rowley Road, Orsett, Essex RM16 3EU, UK*

Abstract

Over the last 40 years, we have seen how electrical stimulation for the relief of pain has progressed from an experimental treatment based upon clinical theory to being on the threshold of a standard of medical practice.

Severe persistent pain is a complex clinical problem which has not been solved by Cartesian-inspired medical techniques. Electrical stimulation of the nervous system is efficacious in the relief of some neuropathic and ischaemic pain states. The uses of these treatments have in themselves contributed to the understanding of these clinical entities and have broadened our range of treatable conditions.

To truly come of age as a standard medical practice, neuromodulation has not only to demonstrate its efficacy in well-conducted prospective-randomised comparison trials but also its cost-utility.

Partnership between medical practitioner, technology and industry has brought us up to the present point. The future of these treatments may well depend upon health technology assessments, health economics and patient power.

Keywords: Spinal cord stimulation; Cost-utilisation; Neuromodulation; Failed back surgery syndrome; Chronic back and leg pain; Complex regional pain syndrome; Angina pectoris; Peripheral vascular disease; Health economics

1. Introduction

"Predictions are difficult, particularly when regarding the future," said the French humorist Sacha Guitry. More seriously, the future of a therapy in general, and spinal cord stimulation (SCS) in particular, is an exercise that is unavoidably tainted by personal bias, whether optimistic or pessimistic. Looking at the broad picture, it appears that the development of SCS will be influenced by a variety of factors. While aspects related to the equipment and its improvement are important, their impact on the wider application of spinal neuromodulation may be outweighed by the scientific, social and economic factors that eventually determine the framework in which medicine is practised. For the purposes of this chapter, we are discussing the future of both spinal cord stimulation and peripheral nerve stimulation (PNS) as the two modalities are conceptually linked, use similar equipment or are even actually combined. We have not tried to examine the future of other electrical neuroaugmentative techniques separately.

---

*Correspondence to: Phone: +41 (21) 804-2211; Fax: +41 (21) 804-2787; E-mail: eric.buchser@hospvd.ch

2. Present status of SCS and PNS

The first human application of SCS was published more than 30 years ago (Shealy et al., 1967) but its acceptance by the medical community is still limited to a relatively small number of physicians, predominantly those who are dealing with chronic pain problems. It is now generally recognised that SCS can be effective in the treatment of pain, particularly when of neuropathic or vascular origin. Hence, the use of this treatment has increased, mostly in the last 10 years. This is largely due to technological improvements of the equipment and the development of other applications of neurostimulation in the area of pain management as well as in the treatment of functional disorders such as faecal and urinary incontinence or retention.

It is difficult to obtain precise information of the current level of SCS implantation. In the late 1990s it was estimated that about 15,000 SCS systems were implanted worldwide each year, of which approximately 5000 were in Europe (Linderoth and Meyerson, 2002). In 2002, extrapolated figures suggest that around 26,000 SCS systems will be implanted worldwide, with about two-thirds in the US. Although the numbers of SCS devices implanted globally appears small, the high unit price results in an overall budget that has substantial impact – approximately one-third of the total active neuroimplant (stimulators and intrathecal drug pumps) budget of some one billion US dollars (Linderoth and Meyerson, 2002), and the market is expected to grow at least 15% per year.

While the application of SCS is expanding (Barolat and Sharan, 2000), its mechanism of action, though partially elucidated, is still unclear. The controlled randomised studies that support the clinical impression of efficacy have started to appear only in the last 5 years. It should be recognised that the performance of a controlled randomised study is very difficult with any treatment requiring a surgical procedure however minor, and the production of Level 1 evidence is

further impaired by the virtual impossibility to blind the treatment because of the need for evoked paraesthesiae. Nevertheless, the recognition of SCS as an effective treatment is dependent upon credible evidence regarding its efficacy and a convincing explanation of its mechanism of action. Furthermore, its widespread use is further impeded by incomplete prospective cost-utilisation data whereby downstream patient costs, often expressed as cost per quality-adjusted life-years (QALY), can be demonstrated to be less than that of existing management strategies. Kemler's study for complex regional pain syndrome (CRPS) does include this information (Kemler et al., 2001; Kemler and Furnee, 2002) but the data remain incomplete for failed back surgery syndrome/chronic low back pain (FBSS/CBLP) and angina.

2.1. Current practice

In the early days, the use of SCS was within the realm of academic centres. As the equipment became more reliable and its use easier, the technique was increasingly used in private hospitals and non-academic institutions. Today SCS is carried out equally in university hospitals and in other institutions, where those countries have insurance systems that reimburse these treatments.

Two nationwide surveys of SCS practice have been published to date. The first study, funded by the Belgian health authorities, was conducted between 1983 and 1992 (Kupers et al., 1994). Over that period, 697 SCS devices were implanted in 28 hospitals. In 14 hospitals (50%), not more than two implants were registered over the 3-year sampling period and in only seven hospitals (28%) there were more than 10 implantations over the 3 years. Of the patients, 53.6% were implanted in teaching and 46.4% in general hospitals.

A second study, from the US (Fanciullo et al., 1999), is a questionnaire survey of 95 institutions with anaesthesiology pain fellowship programmes (i.e. academic teaching centres) across the US. Of the 76 (80%) programmes that replied, 66 reported implanting SCS systems. On average 12.4 SCS devices per institution were implanted in the previous year, representing some 4.6 SCS systems per implanting physician. The survey indicated a range of implantation practice and procedures across centres. It appears that the average number of implants per physician is low, and may not guarantee the high level of experience and clinical skill that is required for success with this technique.

There is no comparable study regarding PNS. PNS has not undergone the same development as that of SCS, essentially because of technical problems with the equipment (electrode breakage) and surgical implant techniques, resulting in variable success (Stanton-Hicks and Salamon, 1997). Hence, PNS remains limited to a small number of centres and patients. However, easier procedures using modified spinal approaches (Alo et al., 1999) or subcutaneous electrode placement (Weiner and Reed, 1999; Stinson et al., 2001) may stimulate a revival of PNS.

2.2. Current indications

The controversies mentioned earlier may explain, at least in part, the uneven use of SCS across developed western countries. Estimations of indications for SCS based on figures given by the industry indicate that, worldwide, around two-thirds of all SCS systems are implanted for FBSS/CLBP. The second most important indication in Europe is peripheral vascular disease (PVD; around 20%) in contrast to the US where it is barely used for this. Similarly, SCS for the treatment of refractory angina pectoris, although still very limited, seems to be more accepted in Europe (7%) than in the US (1%). CRPS accounts for 5% of all implants in Europe contrasting with the US at around 15%.

The variation of SCS implantation rates across Europe appears to be influenced more by the differences in funding systems than by the incidence or prevalence of disease. Belgium is the only European Union (EU) country with a full official reimbursement system (until recently restricted to neuropathic causes). Belgium has the highest rate of implanted SCS systems at more than 30 per million per annum, followed by Switzerland where reimbursement is also approved for neuropathic and vascular pain. In the UK, where access to SCS is restricted by budget rather than indication, the relative number of SCS devices implanted is about one-quarter of those of Belgium (Simpson, 1998).

2.3. Current clinical and technical difficulties

2.3.1. Patient selection

The proper selection of patients for neuroaugmentative treatment modalities has been, and in certain conditions still is, a difficult clinical problem. This is largely due to incomplete understanding of the mechanism of both the pain and the action of SCS and is further complicated by the broadening of the indications that result from accumulated clinical experience.

Trial stimulation is widely advocated although there is no consensus on how and under what conditions it should be carried out and for how long. The performance of a test stimulation before the 'permanent' implantation of an expensive device makes intuitive sense, and in some countries is a prerequisite for reimbursement. However, there is little evidence that, as such, trial stimulation provides any predictive information on long-term outcome. Of concern is that the outcome of patients who fail the trial has never been evaluated prospectively (Simpson, 1999). A retrospective, third party follow-up of patients who were 'screened out' and not implanted suggested that their pain worsened compared to those who passed the trial test and were subsequently implanted (May et al., 2002). Despite these shortcomings, trial stimulation has the merit of allowing patients to test SCS both for efficacy and for paraesthesia perception, which sometimes cannot be tolerated despite achieving good pain relief.

Psychiatric and personality disorders have long been identified as unfavourable factors in the long-term success of SCS. Hence, psychological screening has become a standard requirement in the evaluation of patients considered for SCS therapy. However, the usefulness of psychological evaluation remains unclear. Even though there are suggestions that psychiatric clinical evaluation has predictive value (Kupers et al., 1994), other studies found no correlation between systematic psychological testing and medium- or long-term success rate of SCS therapy (Burchiel et al., 1995; North et al., 1996).

2.3.2. Paraesthesia coverage

Another persisting major challenge is to achieve the ideal placement of the lead, so as to elicit paraesthesiae over the entire painful area, and this is regardless of the type of lead used. Over the years, knowledge regarding the best probable location for the lead has accumulated (Barolat et al., 1993). Most implanters prefer to position their electrodes in an awake and cooperative patient to allow precise localisation of electrodes for maximal topographical coverage. The technique that has become known as 'trawling' has been developed with this in mind. In experienced hands, this technique reduces the time spent trying to achieve optimal paraesthesia coverage.

Techniques have been developed to maximise charge density over those areas of the dorsal columns that serve sensation over the low back whilst at the same time providing stimulation in the neuropathic limb. This has involved using multiple leads, electrodes and configurations, although the rationale for this has been challenged (Holsheimer, 2000). Other techniques combine PNS with dorsal column stimulation in an attempt to maximise paraesthesia topography. Yet, eliciting optimal paraesthesiae remains a problem, not only at the time of the implantation of the electrode, but also at later stages, when the paraesthesia coverage becomes inadequate either because of the migration of the leads or the progression of the underlying disease. It has been recognised that in many patients frequent reprogramming is required to ensure appropriate paraesthesia coverage in the long term (Sharan et al., 2002). Unpublished data from a systematic registry carried out by one of the present authors (E.B.) shows that, on average, combined nursing and physician time devoted to reprogramme a four-contact, single-lead, single-channel system is in the order of 30 min. When reprogramming is needed in a patient carrying a two-electrode (eight contacts) dual-channel system, this time nearly doubles (50 min).

2.3.3. Lead-related technical problems

The technological advances that have been achieved in SCS equipment have been spectacular. The leads have become more flexible and yet more resilient, resulting in fewer electrode breakages. However, this improvement is difficult to quantify since the stress imposed upon the lead varies with the location of the implant, the spontaneous mobility of the patient and the length of time the device has been implanted. Earlier series have quoted fracture rates of up to 6% (Davis and Gray, 1981) while recent series reported 3% or less (Spincemaille et al., 2001).

More important is the problem of lead migration, particularly with wire electrodes that tend to dislocate far more frequently than the surgically implanted leads. Here again, both the location of the implant and the functional status of the patient play an important role. Yet, most series report a dislodgement rate between 8% (May et al., 2002) and 27% for percutaneous leads (De Jongste et al., 1994), the majority occurring within the first year after implant (Andersen, 1997). In contrast, surgically implanted plate electrodes are more stable and migration rates as low as 2% or less have been reported (Barolat, 1993). However, these advantages are outweighed by an implant procedure that is significantly more invasive, requiring at least a small laminotomy and often general anaesthesia.

When patients cannot cooperate with the optimal placement of the electrode, as in general anaesthesia or profound sedation, the ideal location cannot be searched for (by 'trawling' or any other way). In addition, when dislodgement occurs, the repositioning of a plate electrode is often difficult because of local fibrosis. Finally, it is a fact that the vast majority of 'implanters' are anaesthesiologists and it would further reduce patient access to SCS therapy if over-stretched neurosurgeons with other neurosurgical priorities were to take on the implantation of all electrodes.

2.3.4. Pulse generator-related problems

The most recent pulse generators, whether totally implantable or passive radiofrequency (RF) coupled systems driven from an external trans-mitter, have multichannel capabilities, sometimes providing for multiple programmes, each of which activate a specific set of contacts to produce paraesthesiae in a variety of locations. Although largely regarded as a significant improvement by most authors (North et al., 1992; Barolat and Sharan, 2000), the clinical difficulties of maintaining adequate topography of evoked paraesthesiae remain. The main difficulty resulting from the use of an increased number of active contacts is that the number of possibilities increases exponentially from 50 combinations with four contacts to tens of millions when 16 or more contacts are available. In an effort to solve the dilemma, a patient-interactive computerised system was developed by the group at Johns Hopkins (North et al., 1992). The software was designed to facilitate direct patient interaction with the device and reduce the considerable amount of time that staff was to invest in programming the pulse generators. Despite encouraging initial results, it appears that this system has not gained wide popularity but further development of this approach is ongoing (see Chapter 12).

The industry has tended to evolve its pulse generators into fully implantable, multiple channel devices. Apart from the commercial advantage of having to replace an exhausted intracorporeal pulse generator (IPG), there are other factors supporting this strategy. For example, a post-marketing surveillance study by Medtronic Inc. has suggested that, in patients who have had experience with both the RF coupled and fully implantable IPG, the latter is preferred. The pros and cons of both systems need to be carefully balanced in order to ensure that both patient and health payer are getting best benefit at best value.

Multiple channels do allow a patient to switch between pre-set electrode arrays and thereby change the emphasis of stimulation topography. This, however, often requires the activation of a large number of contacts, which tends to exhaust implanted batteries prematurely, hence the use of extracorporeal RF-coupled pulse generators. In some patients this feature is important but in many well-selected patients it is not.

3. Future perspective of SCS

While aspects related to the equipment and its improvement are important, the viability and the future development of neuromodulation in general and SCS in particular will be largely influenced by other aspects including scientific, social and economic factors that eventually determine the framework in which medicine is practised.

3.1. Technical developments

An innovative concept for SCS was proposed in 1996 by Holsheimer and colleagues (Struijk and Holsheimer, 1996). Based on a previously described three-dimensional computer model representing the geometry and electrical character-istics of the spinal cord, the nerve fibres and the surrounding tissues (Holsheimer et al., 1991; Holsheimer, 1998), a transversely orientated tripolar plate electrode was evaluated with a new dual-channel stimulator. The new stimulator allows for a balanced stimulation by moving the electrical field from one side to the other, electronically. Similar to the balance of stereo-phonic audio equipment, the electrical field can be shifted from left to right through the manipulation of a 'joystick', resulting in an easy steering of the evoked paraesthesiae over a large surface of the body.

The predicted performance of this new approach was verified in a clinical setting. In a first study (Holsheimer et al., 1998), a transverse tripolar electrode, with a central cathode, was implanted in the lower thoracic region in four patients with chronic neurogenic pain. The steering of the electrical field resulted in para-esthesia coverage ranging from 70 to 100% of the body up to the level of the lead in all but one patient. Similar results were obtained in two patients with cervical (C4–C5) transverse tripolar lead implants (Struijk et al., 1998). Building on these preliminary results, a new generation of devices and electrodes might significantly improve the ease of use of SCS and contribute to an improvement in clinical results. The energy cost of this new stimulation modality is, however, high, rising to more than twice the current consumption of a comparable conventional mono- or bipolar longitudinal configuration (Struijk et al., 1998).

Although high current consumption is pre-dominantly a feature of percutaneous wire electrodes (Greco et al., 1999; Spincemaille et al., 2001), it is also encountered in patients carrying plate leads, particularly in those who have undergone previous spinal surgery. Given the current trend towards a totally implanted pulse generator, an increased current requirement would lead to the shortening of the lifespan of the battery and result in increased costs. Improved battery lifespan can be achieved with optimal program-ming and cycling of stimulation. Improved efficiency in current delivery can be achieved by design modifications such as insulated arrays of electrodes (North et al., 2002) and low-impedance electrodes and extensions. The trend towards the use of fully implanted pulse generators appears to be driven predominantly by factors related to convenience and comfort rather than by consid-erations of efficacy or cost-effectiveness. The use of implanted but rechargeable stimulators would

seem to be a compromise that might offer the most versatile options.

Miniaturised pulse generators and connecting equipment will increase patient tolerance and reduce the incidence of local tenderness or pain due to protrusion of parts of the system, whether connectors or pulse generators. Other modifica-tions may include patient data registration and more sophisticated physician (and patient)/gen-erator interfaces. Improvement in the telemetry technology and device isolation could decrease the risk of interference with cardiac pacemakers and environmental RF energy. The development of remote-programming capabilities, using either the internet or conventional telephone lines may facilitate doctor/patient/therapy interaction and hence patient access to neuromodulation thera-pies. Although valuable for patients who live far away, it should be remembered that the manage-ment of chronic pain is primarily based on proper doctoring that is unlikely to be achieved purely electronically, whatever the sophistication of the system.

In summary, it appears that technological improvement of the equipment used for SCS is likely to facilitate the use and the follow-up of neuromodulation treatment modalities. Improved electrodes might be less likely to break and to migrate; better implant technique and anchoring may also reduce migration. The use of new stimulation principles with adjustable electrical fields should greatly reduce the difficulties in finding and maintaining adequate paraesthesia coverage. However, the need for higher energy requirements will necessitate innovative strategies that might allow fully implanted pulse generators to be recharged non-invasively or the recourse to being powered by RF-coupled devices.

Despite all this progress, however, it seems improbable that technical modifications alone will substantially augment the practice of neuromodu-lation. Health commissioners inform their deci-sion-making by using the data made available to them from health technology assessments (HTAs). An HTA provides not only evidence of efficacy of the treatment but also its cost-effectiveness. From prospective cost-utilisation data and quality of life indices, it is possible to calculate a cost per QALY (Quality Adjusted Life-Year) for a given treatment of a given condition. The maximum cost per QALY to be considered good value currently stands at about 50,000 euros (Raftery, 2001; O'Brien et al., 2002). In essence, treatments costing more than this per QALY are unlikely to be commissioned. It should be recognised that the cost of new devices, including the refinements of existing apparatus, has considerably increased in recent years due to modern requirements in quality control and to the medico-legal environment. Increasing complexity and unit cost of the devices may merely serve to price the therapy out-of-reach of most healthcare budgets.

3.2. Research

The development of SCS has been – and still is – largely driven by the device industry. Unlike the pharmaceutical industry, which has fuelled and participated in the development of scientific fields such as pharmacology and physiology, SCS has not been as closely integrated, nor has it benefited from any major basic science discipline. As a result of this relative isolation, the investments that have been made have been predominantly devoted to the development and the refinement of the equipment. Unfortunately, there has been inadequate support of basic science research into the mechanism of action and insufficient support for high-quality clinical trials to demonstrate efficacy and cost-effectiveness.

3.2.1. Basic research

Most of our understanding regarding the electrical stimulation of dorsal column nerve fibres with epidural electrodes derives from the work of Holsheimer and colleagues at the Department of Electrical Engineering, University of Twente, Enschede, The Netherlands. Since the late seventies, this group has been developing a series of three-dimensional volume-conductor computer models representing the anatomical structures in the spinal canal, as well as cable models representing the electrical behaviour of nerve fibres (Holsheimer, 1998). A high degree of correlation was found between empirical data and the models' predictions for most of the characteristics of SCS. This resulted in a number of publications, which have contributed to our understanding of various aspects of SCS including the best combination of active contacts in relation to the thickness of the CSF layer (Holsheimer et al., 1991) and the effects of both anatomic and electrode geometry factors on the recruitment of dorsal column (Holsheimer and Struijk, 1991; Struijk et al., 1992; Holsheimer et al., 1995; Rijkhoff et al., 1995; Holsheimer and Wesselink, 1997) and dorsal root (Struijk et al., 1993) fibres. Recently, the same group suggested a novel approach to both the geometry of the lead (transverse tripolar) and the mode of stimulation (balanced) that might lead to a significant improvement and greater ease of use of SCS (Holsheimer et al., 1998; see Section 3.1).

The mechanisms of action of SCS are reviewed extensively in another chapter of this book and will not be specifically addressed here. It is expected that further research into the mechanism of both the pain and the action of SCS is likely to be an important factor in helping to improve patient selection for SCS. In addition, this knowledge is one of the key factors to understanding and possibly preventing late failures of the treatment.

It should be pointed out that SCS produces a number of different effects, both electrophysiological and biochemical, and that these effects can differ depending upon the integrity, or lack of integrity, of the nervous system. It has also been recognised that SCS-related changes differ according to the condition that is being treated (Linderoth and Foreman, 1999).

Until recently, conventional approaches to neuromodulation as a whole have focused either on stimulation or on drug delivery. An attempt to combine these two techniques has been proposed. Experimental evidence suggests that the relief of neuropathic pain is mediated by GABAergic (gamma-amino butyric acid) mechanisms (Cui et al., 1996, 1997). A clinical study involving SCS and simultaneous spinal administration of baclofen (a GABA-B agonist) has been started (Meyerson et al., 1997). Similar studies have been carried out in rats with the anticonvulsant drugs gabapentin and pregabalin. Using photochemically induced allodynia in a rat model, Wallin and colleagues could demonstrate that in SCS non-responding animals, the combination of SCS and subeffective intrathecal doses of either drug could markedly decrease allodynia (Wallin et al., 2002). Devices of a future generation could therefore include both stimulation and drug-delivery capabilities incorporated in a single catheter/electrode allowing a suitable combination of electrical and chemical modulation of the central and/or the peripheral nervous system.

3.2.2. Clinical studies

The literature regarding SCS, although abundant, comprises predominantly retrospective, uncontrolled case series, the quality of which is in general relatively poor, scoring a median quality score of one out of a potential maximum score of seven (Taylor et al., submitted for publication). In particular, very few publications have used a case-series design that prospectively studied consecutive patients using independently assessed and validated outcome measures. This unfortunate situation is explained, at least in part, by the nature of the therapy which includes the need for evoked paraesthesiae. This factor prevents adequate blinding, and the requirement of a surgical procedure restricts or complicates the use of randomisation. In addition, with certain indications such as chronic low back and leg pain, the patient populations are lacking homogeneity and are therefore difficult to define. Indeed, a comprehensive systematic literature review which examined FBSS/CLBP suggested that no conclusions could be drawn concerning the effectiveness of SCS relative to other treatments, placebo or no treatment (Turner et al., 1995).

Randomised-controlled studies on the efficacy of SCS have, however, started to appear in the last few years. This much needed work has provided convincing evidence in a number of SCS applications, including FBSS/CBLP (North et al., 1994, 1995), CRPS (Kemler et al., 2001), PVD (Suy et al., 1994; Jivegard et al., 1995; Claeys and Horsch, 1996; Klomp et al., 1999; Ubbink et al., 1999a,b) and angina pectoris (De Jongste and Staal, 1993; Mannheimer et al., 1998; Jessurun et al., 1999).

3.2.3. Recommendations for the design of future studies

In the era of evidence-based medicine, it has become increasingly clear that clinical research of inadequate quality is unproductive in promoting a therapy, and in some instances might even have deleterious effects. However, given the drive for publication, particularly in academic institutions, it is likely that the number of uncontrolled studies will continue to rise. Decisions about the nature of further research would best be made through involvement of clinicians, patients, researchers, policy makers and the device industry. The quality could be improved by following some basic rules.

3.2.3.1. Case series. Case series undertaken in the future should be conducted prospectively, in consecutive patients and use validated outcome measures and independent assessors. Detailed description of the methods used and a complete reporting of the results of all outcomes, particularly adverse events and complications, should be provided. In case series that include more than one clinical indication, results should be reported disaggregated according to each indication. In addition, all studies concerning SCS should report the extent of paraesthesia coverage, and include a detailed description of the implanted system (single or multiple lead) and the number and configuration of active poles that were used.

3.2.3.2. Registries. Other procedures, in particular hip prostheses and cardiac pacing (Crick, 1991; Moller and Arnsbo, 1996), have benefited from the centralised collection of good quality, comprehensive, independent and validated outcome data in the form of a registry (Herberts and Malchau, 2000). The development of a nationwide registry, that included independent assessment of patient outcomes, supported a central decision to reimburse SCS in Belgium (Kupers et al., 1994).

3.2.3.3. Controlled studies. There is a paucity of prospective randomised-controlled or comparison trials for any of the main indications for SCS. Many commentators have described the difficulties in undertaking the 'classic' randomised-controlled trial design in this area (Kemler and De Vet, 2000; Wetzel et al., 2000): firstly, the inability to 'blind' patients to SCS; secondly, the difficulty in selecting an appropriate comparative therapy (medical, rehabilitative or surgical) and thirdly, the ethical reluctance of individual clinicians to participate in such a trial.

A recently proposed solution is to undertake a cluster randomised-controlled trial of SCS. In this design, patients are randomised to a centre that provides SCS or to a centre that provides comparative therapy (Wetzel et al., 2000). The principal advantage of such a design is that centres can participate in a trial yet continue with their preferred approach to the treatment. For 'non-SCS' centres this could include surgical or optimal non-surgical care. The implementation of a cluster trial would depend on the ability to recruit a sufficient number of centres.

Another improvement to the case-series evidence would be to undertake well-conducted observational-controlled studies (such as a prospective cohort design) of SCS. An observational design could also incorporate a cluster design so that the comparison is of patients treated by different centres, some with SCS and some without. A detailed description of both patient characteristics (e.g. demographic information, duration and severity of pain) and characteristics of the centres (e.g. package of care delivered) are fundamental to the interpretation and analysis of a well-conducted observational study.

3.3. The changing views regarding symptomatic treatment

Unlike traditional Chinese medicine, modern western medicine is based on the paradigm of Cartesian science. Empirical- and logical-thought processes have used measurable variables to build a rational science in which objective (i.e. measurable) signs prevailed over subjective, essentially non-quantifiable symptoms, which were mostly regarded as disease indicators. Hence, some disorders such as neurogenic pain with its allodynic component have been neglected and regarded as a psychiatric behavioural malady rather than as an organic disease. As a result of advances in medical knowledge and understanding concerning the pathophysiology and psychosocial dimensions of pain, these outdated concepts have been profoundly modified in recent years.

An initiative stemming from the European Federation of IASP (International Association for the Study of Pain) Chapters (EFIC) is aiming to alter the status of chronic pain from being considered as a symptom towards one of a '...major healthcare problem, a disease in its own right.' The 'Declaration on Chronic Pain' was part of a campaign that was launched in 2001 at the European Parliament in Brussels. The aim is to raise awareness of chronic pain amongst European political authorities as well as with the general public and medical community. It tries to prevent attitudes that prevailed in the past, whereby patient care would be denied if a pain problem could not find an explanation that would fit the current concepts and theories. Although the scientific community has come a long way towards a more caring and open attitude to patients suffering from unexplained symptoms, the controversies surrounding unclear disorders such as fibromyalgia serve as a useful reminder for those who have forgotten the early days of what we now call CRPS.

One of the merits of SCS is that it has significantly contributed to this change of perspective. By offering a totally novel, largely mysterious but remarkably effective pain-relieving treatment in patients who had failed any other treatment, it stimulated interest in pragmatic symptom control.

3.3.1. SCS at the crossroads of modern requirements and attitude

Another interesting by-product of the application of SCS and related neuroaugmentative techniques is their contribution to redefining our understanding of medical conditions and the management of chronic-disabling conditions. SCS started out as an experiment to try to utilise in practice the existing basic concept of the Gate Control theory. The treatment failed as the pain was nociceptive in nature, and as we know now SCS does not block C-fibre transmission by enhancing large fibre-mediated inhibition as predicted by the simple theory. Presumably through trial and error, SCS has been attempted in more and more clinical situations where established treatment ideas have been exhausted. In some there have been treatment successes which when reported have led to further investigation. In many areas this endeavour has helped redefine our understanding of disease and chronic disability such as in spinal pain, angina pectoris and critical limb ischaemia. Other potential areas of interest are in pelvic, perineal and visceral pain syndromes and migraine (see Section 4).

In a similar way, neuroaugmentative therapies have stimulated research into the evaluation of treatment benefits. Neuromodulation therapies, whatever the indication, are symptomatic treatments and their benefits are therefore measured in terms of quality of life rather than disease cure. Questionnaires and other semi-quantitative tools that are currently used to measure the quality of life, although validated, are time consuming and cumbersome to use. One of the main features of the quality of life measures is the ability to perform unlimited physical activity. Any condition that results in a decrease of physical activity is associated with a decrease in the quality of life, and vice versa. The developments of sophisticated

activity monitors have allowed the detailed quantification of the usual physical activities of daily life (Aminian et al., 1999). They allow a detailed analysis of the actual physical activity under normal life conditions, providing information on the walking distance, the stride length, the time-spent lying or sitting, etc. The objective information that is provided by these sensors is validated (Bussmann et al., 1998; Aminian et al., 1999), is opening new avenues in the evaluation of the quality of life and is likely to be used in other areas such as the management of heart failure and neurodegenerative diseases. It is plausible that future generations of these tools will be incorporated into the assessment of neuromodulation devices.

3.3.2. Future trends in the practice of SCS

In an editorial comment, Palmer stressed the need for training and development of clinical skills that are required in 'the art and science of implantation' (Palmer, 1999). Looking at today's trend one can assume that SCS and other forms of neurostimulation will become more popular, that the number of indications will increase and that the complication rate will be more closely monitored. From other areas of technical medical care, it appears that the quality of care is related to volume (Birkmeyer et al., 2002; Prystowsky et al., 2002). This implies that in the future there will be a shift from large numbers of low-volume neurostimulator implanting centres to fewer but larger-volume centres of excellence, a trend that is already apparent today. However, this centralising trend must be accompanied by an appropriate organisation of the healthcare network that should include trained physicians, nurses and other medical personnel capable of providing suitable patient monitoring and follow-up. This is an essential step, if two conflicting goals such as a wider access to neuroaugmentative treatment modalities and a smaller number of implanting centres are to be achieved. Moreover, it is an inescapable development if neuromodulation techniques become more frequently employed.

The treatment of chronic pain and disability is complex, and draws on our understanding of the bio-psycho-social model of disease and disability in order to manage it. Neurostimulation, including SCS, is just one aspect of a package of treatment that addresses the needs of the patient. As such it is widely agreed that neuromodulation treatments should be positioned within a multidisciplinary team.

With the evolution of knowledge concerning chronic disabling conditions and neuromodulation has also come better medical interdisciplinary team working. New medical relationships have been built such as between pain anaesthetist and cardiologist, orthopaedic surgeon, urologist or colorectal surgeon. It is likely that with the many therapeutic applications of neuromodulation, the implanting pain anaesthetist or neurosurgeon will start to see himself more as a 'neuromodulator' who offers his case selection, implantation and management skills to a wider number of patients and disciplines. In these circumstances, a more critical appraisal of therapeutic options for the patients suffering from a particular condition is likely to evolve. Services of excellence are more likely to advocate a patient-centred approach to care drawing from a sensible and increasingly evidence-based therapeutic armamentarium.

4. Future indications

As the numerous biochemical and neurophysiological changes that result from either SCS or PNS are increasingly elucidated, new applications of neuromodulation are likely to emerge, both for the treatment of pain conditions and for the improvement of functional disorders. In a number of cases, however, the recognition of new treatment modalities will also require a reappraisal of the pathophysiology of the disease process. As an example, interstitial cystitis may undergo a re-evaluation with an ensuing redefinition of some visceral pain states as neuropathic disorders. A case series published recently (Feler et al., 1999) is consistent with the unpublished experience of one of the present authors (S.T.), which indicates

that long-term pain relief can be achieved in interstitial cystitis with nerve root stimulation (see also Chapter 5). The electrodes are placed within the sacral canal using a retrograde technique via the lumbar epidural route (Alo et al., 1999). Similarly, diffuse chronic abdominal or pelvic, pain occurring either spontaneously or after multiple surgical operations might, in the future, be understood as a neuropathic process and treated accordingly.

The re-evaluation of pathophysiological concepts could also lead to a different positioning of currently accepted indications for SCS. In angina pectoris, for example, the present understanding is largely restricted to the imbalance between oxygen demand and supply to the myocardium. While this concept does not account for silent ischaemia, it does not provide a satisfactory explanation for the pain occurring in syndrome X either (see Chapter 10). In addition, it neglects all the autonomically mediated interactions between the brain and the heart which are crucial, at least in the development of malignant dysrhythmias such as ventricular fibrillation in the ischaemic heart (Ebert et al., 1970; Davis and Natelson, 1993). It is therefore quite conceivable that a broader approach to the pathophysiology could lead to a repositioning of SCS earlier in the treatment algorithm for angina pectoris.

Other areas of exciting potential development include cerebral–vascular disorders. It is well established that cervical SCS increases cerebral blood flow both in animal (Isono et al., 1995) and in man (Meglio et al., 1991a,b). The use of SCS in the treatment of stroke has been suggested by earlier pre-clinical studies (Matsui and Hosobuchi, 1989) and its potential benefit further supported by subsequent human clinical trials in cerebral ischaemia (Hosobuchi, 1991; Shinonaga and Takanashi, 2001; Visocchi et al., 2001a,b). Similarly, it is conceivable that cervical SCS could be used, alone or in combination with unilateral or bilateral occipital nerve stimulation, to prevent and even treat migraine attacks. Other blood flow-related disorders such as intestinal ischaemia may respond to SCS in some instances (Ceballos et al., 2000) and this potential indication merits further evaluation.

In addition to the management of pain, there are a number of indications and potential developments for SCS and PNS in the treatment of functional disorders. Currently, the use of neurostimulation in the management of refractory urge incontinence of urine, urgency-frequency and voiding difficulty is becoming established (Bemelmans et al., 1999). In the same way, the ability to manage faecal incontinence by sacral nerve stimulation is increasingly recognised (Kenefick et al., 2002) and the number of patients receiving the treatment is growing.

It is well established that SCS can modulate the autonomic nervous system, particularly its sympathetic component. It follows that body functions that are under significant autonomic control could potentially be subject to modulation through SCS, PNS or both. It has been suggested that, in certain circumstances, oesophageal motility disorders are due to neurophysiological abnormalities (Rate et al., 1999), and the effects of SCS on specific disturbances of gastrointestinal motility are currently being evaluated.

By analogy, SCS-induced autonomic modulation might affect airway resistance in some instances. In an intriguing unpublished observation, one of the authors (E.B.) noted a substantial decrease in bronchospasm episodes in a patient treated with SCS for intractable angina. Although no pulmonary function tests were performed to document this effect, the clinical context suggested that the decreased airway resistance was not due to improved cardiac function. It is suggested that bronchospastic, gastrointestinal and possibly metabolic disorders could become a focus for neuromodulation in the future.

5. Social and economic aspects

Healthcare cost are taking an increasing share of total public expenditure in all WHO member states (Musgrove et al., 2002), and the latest spending projections in the US suggest that health expenditure will account for 16.8% of gross domestic product (GDP) by 2010 (Heffler et al., 2002). As a result, cost-containment in healthcare has become an obsession with nearly all governments around the world. Politicians seldom publicise, though privately recognise, that increased health expenditure is inescapable, at least for several years to come. The challenge is to reconcile the diverging trends of the economic requirement (to spend as little as possible) with the social demand (to treat everybody) and the consequent need for the political acceptance of the unavoidable choices that will have to be imposed. Empirical research has suggested that there is a causal and statistically significant relationship between growth in health spending and growth in GDP. However, when used to predict health-policy development, the validity of this relationship has been challenged (Kanavos and Mossialos, 1999). It follows that, regardless of the increase in wealth, the resources devoted to healthcare will not increase indefinitely and restriction of some kind is likely to be implemented one way or another.

In western countries, the state is supporting an ever-growing share of healthcare expenditure, mostly because of social and political enticement. As a result, governments, including that of the US, are increasingly committed to broaden the entitlement to public care (Badham, 1998; Belien, 2000). At the same time considerable effort and resources are devoted to a variety of schemes designed to restrain healthcare expenditure. In Europe, new policies aimed at reducing costs while maintaining the quality and equity of healthcare have been introduced in a number of ways suited to each country's social, political and cultural reality. Contradictory measures such as market-orientated incentives and increased government control have been taken simultaneously. Rather than empowering patients, the intent was to limit the growth of the healthcare sector by restricting consumption (Belien, 2000).

Neuromodulatory treatment modalities can be cost-effective but they are expensive and cannot be supported by the vast majority of potential patients. Hence, the growth and long-term development of neuroaugmentative treatment modalities are subject to their reimbursement by some kind of health insurance. It may be of importance to keep in mind that private insurance, by freeing patients from the concern for cost, undermines cost-effectiveness whilst state-provided healthcare systems may make cost-effectiveness easier to achieve (Musgrove, 1995).

As the competition for healthcare resources increases, evidence-based criteria such as cost-effectiveness and efficacy will be necessary but may not be sufficient (Stolk et al., 2002) and other factors are likely to play an important role as well. Whatever the means, it seems clear that painful choices will have to be made but there are no simple solutions to the setting of healthcare priorities (Holm, 1998). Priority lists do not necessarily result in rankings that are correlated with cost-effectiveness (Tengs et al., 1996). On the other hand, in the eyes of the general public, not all QALYs are equal and the value of a treatment depends on the patient's state of health before the development of a life-threatening illness (Ubel et al., 1999). This means that consumers' willingness to accept monetary compensation to reject a treatment is greater than their willingness to pay for the benefit, so that the selling price of a QALY is higher than the buying price (O'Brien et al., 2002).

Other factors that are not directly related to health economics may play an increasingly important role in a context of limited resources. For instance, the preponderance of societal over moral values in healthcare allocation may become more significant (Walker and Siegel, 2002). This may challenge the current popularity of symptomatic treatments, which are valued in modern and wealthy societies that are preoccupied with the quality of life. It seems clear that any system of healthcare prioritisation such as the Oregon approach (Tengs et al., 1996), QALYs or some

other system such as that based upon a definition of necessary care as in the Netherlands, or on the severity of disease as in Norway, does not necessarily result in legitimate and rational decisions. More complex priority-setting processes are likely to be used in the future, using a variety of criteria (Singer et al., 2000).

Any of the considerations above might have an impact on future decisions regarding the acceptance and the funding of SCS and related therapies.

6. Conclusion

The future of SCS and related techniques is dependent on a variety of scientific, technical, social and economic factors, each of which is essential but will probably have relatively little impact if considered separately. Research in the mechanisms of pain, of diseases and of the action of SCS is likely to result in a broadening of the indications for therapeutic neuromodulation, not only for pain management but also for the control of functional disorders.

Technological improvements of the equipment will improve treatment reliability and ease of application. This should eventually decrease the total cost by reducing the need for revision and device replacement as well as the recourse to expensive and time-consuming procedures.

The provision of neuromodulation therapies on a large scale requires an appropriate organisation of the healthcare system. To ensure both treatment access and high standard of care, a small number of centres that provide optimal conditions for the evaluation of patients as well as the performance of the implant will have to be assisted by an infrastructure in the community that can offer appropriate follow-up and specific patient care with regards to implanted devices.

Cost-effectiveness and efficacy are key issues in the acceptance of the therapy and proper studies as well as adequate information for the public, the physicians and the healthcare decision makers are crucial. However, other factors such as complex priority-setting processes and moral and societal issues may play a significant role.

Basic notions regarding neuromodulation have to be incorporated in under-graduate curricula in order for the young physician to be familiarised with these techniques. This is of particular importance since healthcare decision-making processes are becoming more complex and multi-factorial, and awareness of the treatment is playing an important role. For neuromodulation to expand, it must be shown to be effective but also be perceived that way if physicians are to recommend the treatments and patients are to be willing to accept them.

References

Alo, K.M., Yland, M.J., Redko, V., Feler, C.A., and Naumann, C. (1999) Lumbar and sacral nerve root stimulation (NRS) in the treatment of chronic pain: a novel anatomic approach and neurostimulation technique. Neuromodulation, 2: 23–31.

Aminian, K., Robert, P., Buchser, E., Rutschmann, B., Hayoz, D., and Depairon, M. (1999) Physical activity monitoring based on accelerometry: validation and comparison with video observation. Med. Biol. Eng. Comput., 37: 304–308.

Andersen, C. (1997) Complications in spinal cord stimulation for treatment of angina pectoris. Differences in unipolar and multipolar percutaneous inserted electrodes. Acta Cardiol., 52: 325–333.

Badham, J. (1998) Future financial impact of the current health financing system. Aust. Health Rev., 21: 96–110.

Barolat, G. (1993) Experience with 509 plate electrodes implanted epidurally from C1 to L1. Stereotact. Funct. Neurosurg., 61: 60–79.

Barolat, G. and Sharan, A.D. (2000) Future trends in spinal cord stimulation. Neurol. Res., 22: 279–284.

Barolat, G., Massaro, F., He, J., Zeme, S., and Ketcik, B. (1993) Mapping of sensory responses to epidural stimulation of the intraspinal neural structures in man. J. Neurosurg., 78: 233–239.

Belien, P. (2000) Healthcare systems. A new European model? Pharmacoeconomics, 18 Suppl. 1: 85–93.

Bemelmans, B.L., Mundy, A.R., and Craggs, M.D. (1999) Neuromodulation by implant for treating lower urinary tract symptoms and dysfunction. Eur. Urol., 36: 81–91.

Birkmeyer, J.D., Siewers, A.E., Finlayson, E.V., Stukel, T.A., Lucas, F.L., Batista, I., Welch, H.G., and Wennberg, D.E. (2002) Hospital volume and surgical mortality in the United States. N. Engl. J. Med., 346: 1128–1137.

Burchiel, K.J., Anderson, V.C., Wilson, B.J., Denison, D.B., Olson, K.A., and Shatin, D. (1995) Prognostic factors of spinal cord stimulation for chronic back and leg pain. Neurosurgery, 36: 1101–1110. discuss.

Bussmann, J.B., Van De Laar, Y.M., Neeleman, M.P., and Stam, H.J. (1998) Ambulatory accelerometry to quantify motor behaviour in patients after failed back surgery: a validation study. Pain, 74: 153–161.

Ceballos, A., Cabezudo, L., Bovaira, M., Fenollosa, P., and Moro, B. (2000) Spinal cord stimulation: a possible therapeutic alternative for chronic mesenteric ischaemia. Pain, 87: 99–101.

Claeys, L.G. and Horsch, S. (1996) Transcutaneous oxygen pressure as predictive parameter for ulcer healing in endstage vascular patients treated with spinal cord stimulation. Int. Angiol., 15: 344–349.

Crick, J.C. (1991) European multicenter prospective follow-up study of 1,002 implants of a single lead VDD pacing system. The European Multicenter Study Group. Pacing Clin. Electrophysiol., 14: 1742–1744.

Cui, J.G., Linderoth, B., and Meyerson, B.A. (1996) Effects of spinal cord stimulation on touch-evoked allodynia involve GABAergic mechanisms. An experimental study in the mononeuropathic rat. Pain, 66: 287–295.

Cui, J.G., O'Connor, W.T., Ungerstedt, U., Linderoth, B., and Meyerson, B.A. (1997) Spinal cord stimulation attenuates augmented dorsal horn release of excitatory amino acids in mononeuropathy via a GABAergic mechanism. Pain, 73: 87–95.

Davis, A.M. and Natelson, B.H. (1993) Brain-heart interactions. The neurocardiology of arrhythmia and sudden cardiac death. Tex. Heart Inst. J., 20: 158–169.

Davis, R. and Gray, E. (1981) Technical factors important to dorsal column stimulation. Appl. Neurophysiol., 44: 160–170.

De Jongste, M.J. and Staal, M.J. (1993) Preliminary results of a randomized study on the clinical efficacy of spinal cord stimulation for refractory severe angina pectoris. Acta Neurochir. Suppl. (Wien), 58: 161–164.

De Jongste, M.J., Nagelkerke, D., Hooyschuur, C.M., Journee, H.L., Meyler, P.W., Staal, M.J., De Jonge, P., and Lie, K.I. (1994) Stimulation characteristics, complications, and efficacy of spinal cord stimulation systems in patients with refractory angina: a prospective feasibility study. Pacing Clin. Electrophysiol., 17: 1751–1760.

Ebert, P.A., Vanderbeek, R.B., Allgood, R.J., and Sabiston, D.C., Jr. (1970) Effect of chronic cardiac denervation on arrhythmias after coronary artery ligation. Cardiovasc. Res., 4: 141–147.

Fanciullo, G.J., Rose, R.J., Lunt, P.G., Whalen, P.K., and Ross, E. (1999) The state of implantable pain therapies in the United States: a nationwide survey of academic teaching programs. Anesth. Analg., 88: 1311–1316.

Feler, C.A., Whitworth, L.A., Brookoff, D., and Powell, R. (1999) Recent advances: sacral nerve root stimulation using a retrograde method of lead insertion for the treatment of pelvic pain due to interstitial cystitis. Neuromodulation, 2: 211–216.

Greco, S., Auriti, A., Fiume, D., Gazzeri, G., Gentilucci, G., Antonini, L., and Santini, M. (1999) Spinal cord stimulation for the treatment of refractory angina pectoris: a two-year follow-up. Pacing Clin. Electrophysiol., 22: 26–32.

Heffler, S., Smith, S., Won, G., Clemens, M.K., Keehan, S., and Zezza, M. (2002) Health spending projections for 2001–2011: the latest outlook. Faster health spending growth and a slowing economy drive the health spending projection for 2001 up sharply. Health Aff. (Millwood), 21: 207–218.

Herberts, P. and Malchau, H. (2000) Long-term registration has improved the quality of hip replacement: a review of the Swedish THR Register comparing 160,000 cases. Acta Orthop. Scand., 71: 111–121.

Holm, S. (1998) The second phase of priority setting. Goodbye to the simple solutions: the second phase of priority setting in health care. Br. Med. J., 317: 1000–1002.

Holsheimer, J. (1998) Computer modelling of spinal cord stimulation and its contribution to therapeutic efficacy. Spinal Cord, 36: 531–540.

Holsheimer, J. (2000) Does dual lead stimulation favor stimulation of the axial lower back?. Neuromodulation, 3: 55–57.

Holsheimer, J. and Struijk, J.J. (1991) How do geometric factors influence epidural spinal cord stimulation? A quantitative analysis by computer modeling. Stereotact. Funct. Neurosurg., 56: 234–249.

Holsheimer, J. and Wesselink, W.A. (1997) Optimum electrode geometry for spinal cord stimulation: the narrow bipole and tripole. Med. Biol. Eng. Comput., 35: 493–497.

Holsheimer, J., Nuttin, B., King, G.W., Wesselink, W.A., Gybels, J.M., and De Sutter, P. (1998) Clinical evaluation of paresthesia steering with a new system for spinal cord stimulation. Neurosurgery, 42: 541–547.

Holsheimer, J., Struijk, J.J., and Rijkhoff, N.J. (1991) Contact combinations in epidural spinal cord stimulation. A comparison by computer modeling. Stereotact. Funct. Neurosurg., 56: 220–233.

Holsheimer, J., Struijk, J.J., and Tas, N.R. (1995) Effects of electrode geometry and combination on nerve fibre selectivity in spinal cord stimulation. Med. Biol. Eng. Comput., 33: 676–682.

Hosobuchi, Y. (1991) Treatment of cerebral ischemia with electrical stimulation of the cervical spinal cord. Pacing Clin. Electrophysiol., 14: 122–126.

Isono, M., Kaga, A., Fujiki, M., Mori, T., and Hori, S. (1995) Effect of spinal cord stimulation on cerebral blood flow in cats. Stereotact. Funct. Neurosurg., 64: 40–46.

Jessurun, G.A., DeJongste, M.J., Hautvast, R.W., Tio, R.A., Brouwer, J., Van Lelieveld, S., and Crijns, H.J. (1999) Clinical follow-up after cessation of chronic electrical neuromodulation in patients with severe coronary artery disease: a prospective randomized controlled study on putative involvement of sympathetic activity. Pacing Clin. Electrophysiol., 22: 1432–1439.

Jivegard, L.E., Augustinsson, L.E., Holm, J., Risberg, B., and Ortenwall, P. (1995) Effects of spinal cord stimulation (SCS) in patients with inoperable severe lower limb ischaemia: a prospective randomised controlled study. Eur. J. Vasc. Endovasc. Surg., 9: 421–425.

Kanavos, P. and Mossialos, E. (1999) International comparisons of health care expenditures: what we know and what we do not know. J. Health Serv. Res. Policy, 4: 122–126.

Kemler, M.A. and De Vet, C.W. (2000) Does randomisation introduce a bias?. Epidemiology, 11: 228.

Kemler, M.A. and Furnee, C.A. (2002) Economic evaluation of spinal cord stimulation for chronic reflex sympathetic dystrophy. Neurology, 59: 1203–1209.

Kemler, M.A., Barendse, G.A., Van Kleef, M., De Vet, H.C., Rijks, C.P., Furnee, C.A., and Van Den Wildenberg, F.A. (2001) Spinal cord stimulation in patients with chronic reflex sympathetic dystrophy. N. Engl. J. Med., 343: 618–624.

Kenefick, N.J., Vaizey, C.J., Cohen, R.C., Nicholls, R.J., and Kamm, M.A. (2002) Medium-term results of permanent sacral nerve stimulation for faecal incontinence. Br. J. Surg., 89: 896–901.

Klomp, H.M., Spincemaille, G.H., Steyerberg, E.W., Habbema, J.D., and Van Urk, H. (1999) Spinal-cord stimulation in critical limb ischaemia: a randomised trial. ESES Study Group. Lancet, 353: 1040–1044.

Kupers, R.C., Van den Oever, R., Van Houdenhove, B., Vanmechelen, W., Hepp, B., Nuttin, B., and Gybels, J.M. (1994) Spinal cord stimulation in Belgium: a nation-wide survey on the incidence, indications and therapeutic efficacy by the health insurer. Pain, 56: 211–216.

Linderoth, B. and Foreman, R.D. (1999) Physiology of spinal cord stimulation: review and update. Neuromodulation, 2: 150–164.

Linderoth, B. and Meyerson, B. (2002) Spinal cord stimulation: mechanisms of action. In: K. Burchiel (Ed.), *Surgical Management of Pain* (pp. 505–526). Thieme Medical Publisher Inc, New York.

Mannheimer, C., Eliasson, T., Augustinsson, L.E., Blomstrand, C., Emanuelsson, H., Larsson, S., Norrsell, H., and Hjalmarsson, A. (1998) Electrical stimulation versus coronary artery bypass surgery in severe angina pectoris: the ESBY study. Circulation, 97: 1157–1163.

Matsui, T. and Hosobuchi, Y. (1989) The effects of cervical spinal cord stimulation (cSCS) on experimental stroke. Pacing Clin. Electrophysiol., 12: 726–732.

May, M.S., Banks, C., and Thomson, S.J. (2002) A retrospective, long-term, third-party follow-up of patients considered for spinal cord stimulation. Neuromodulation, 5: 137–144.

Meglio, M., Cioni, B., and Visocchi, M. (1991a) Cerebral hemodynamics during spinal cord stimulation. Pacing Clin. Electrophysiol., 14: 127–130.

Meglio, M., Cioni, B., Visocchi, M., Nobili, F., Rodriguez, G., Rosadini, G., Chiappini, F., and Sandric, S. (1991b) Spinal cord stimulation and cerebral haemodynamics. Acta Neurochir. (Wien), 111: 43–48.

Meyerson, B.A., Cui, J.G., Yakhnitsa, V., Sollevi, A., Segerdahl, M., Stiller, C.O., O'Connor, W.T., and Linderoth, B. (1997) Modulation of spinal pain mechanisms by spinal cord stimulation and the potential role of adjuvant pharmacotherapy. Stereotact. Funct. Neurosurg., 68: 129–140.

Moller, M. and Arnsbo, P. (1996) Appraisal of pacing lead performance from the Danish Pacemaker Register. Pacing Clin. Electrophysiol., 19: 1327–1336.

Musgrove, P. (1995) Cost-effectiveness and the socialization of health care. Health Policy, 32: 111–123.

Musgrove, P., Zeramdini, R., and Carrin, G. (2002) Basic patterns in national health expenditure. Bull. World Health Organ., 80: 134–142.

North, R.B., Fowler, K., Nigrin, D.J., and Szymanski, R. (1992) Patient-interactive, computer-controlled neurological stimulation system: clinical efficacy in spinal cord stimulator adjustment. J. Neurosurg., 76: 967–972.

North, R.B., Kidd, D.H., Lee, M.S., and Piantodosi, S. (1994) A prospective, randomized study of spinal cord stimulation versus reoperation for failed back surgery syndrome: initial results. Stereotact. Funct. Neurosurg., 62: 267–272.

North, R.B., Kidd, D.H., and Piantadosi, S. (1995) Spinal cord stimulation versus reoperation for failed back surgery syndrome: a prospective, randomised study design. Acta Neurochir. Suppl. (Wien), 64: 106–108.

North, R.B., Kidd, D.H., Wimberly, R.L., and Edwin, D. (1996) Prognostic value of psychological testing in patients undergoing spinal cord stimulation: a prospective study. Neurosurgery, 39: 301–310.

North, R.B., Kidd, D.H., Olin, J.C., and Sieracki, J.M. (2002) Spinal cord stimulation electrode design: prospective, randomised, controlled trial comparing percutaneous and laminectomy electrodes – part I: technical outcomes. Neurosurgery, 51: 381–389. discussion 389–390.

O'Brien, B.J., Gertsen, K., Willan, A.R., and Faulkner, L.A. (2002) Is there a kink in consumers' threshold value for cost-effectiveness in health care?. Health Econ., 11: 175–180.

Palmer, P.P. (1999) Implantable pain therapies – what training is required? [editorial; comment]. Anesth. Analg., 88: 1203–1204.

Prystowsky, J.B., Bordage, G., and Feinglass, J.M. (2002) Patient outcomes for segmental colon resection according to surgeon's training, certification, and experience. Surgery, 132: 663–670. discussion 670–672.

Raftery, J. (2001) NICE: faster access to modern treatments? Analysis of guidance on health technologies. Br. Med. J., 323: 1300–1303.

Rate, A.J., Hobson, A.R., Barlow, J., and Bancewicz, J. (1999) Abnormal neurophysiology in patients with oesophageal motility disorders. Br. J. Surg., 86: 1202–1206.

Rijkhoff, N.J., Holsheimer, J., Debruyne, F.M., and Wijkstra, H. (1995) Modelling selective activation of small myelinated nerve fibres using a monopolar point electrode. Med. Biol. Eng. Comput., 33: 762–768.

Sharan, A.D., Cameron, T., and Barolat, G. (2002) Evolving patterns of spinal cord stimulation in patients implanted for intractable low back and leg pain. Neuromodulation, 5: 167–179.

Shealy, C.N., Mortimer, J.T., and Reswick, J.B. (1967) Electrical inhibition of pain by stimulation of the dorsal columns: preliminary clinical report. Anesth. Analg., 46: 489–491.

Shinonaga, M. and Takanashi, Y. (2001) Vasodilating effect of spinal cord stimulation for cerebral vasospasm. Acta Neurochir., Suppl. 77: 229–230.

Simpson, B.A. (1998) Neuromodulation in Europe: regulation, variation and trends. Pain Rev., 5: 124–131.

Simpson, B.A. (1999) Spinal cord and brain stimulation. In: P.D. Wall and R. Melzack, (Eds.), *Textbook of Pain* (pp. 1353–1381). Churchill Livingstone, Edinburgh, London, New York, Philadelphia, St. Louis, Sidney, Toronto.

Singer, P.A., Martin, D.K., Giacomini, M., and Purdy, L. (2000) Priority setting for new technologies in medicine: qualitative case study. Br. Med. J., 321: 1316–1318.

Spincemaille, G.H., Klomp, H.M., Steyerberg, E.W., Van Urk, H., and Habbema, J.D. (2001) Technical data and complications of spinal cord stimulation: data from a randomized trial on critical limb ischemia. Stereotact. Funct. Neurosurg. 2000, 74(2): 63–72.

Stanton-Hicks, M. and Salamon, J. (1997) Stimulation of the central and peripheral nervous system for the control of pain. J. Clin. Neurophysiol., 14: 46–62.

Stinson, L.W., Jr., Roderer, G.T., Cross, N.E., and Bennet, E.D. (2001) Peripheral subcutaneous electrostimulation for control of intractable post-operative inguinal pain: a case report series. Neuromodulation, 4: 99–104.

Stolk, E.A., Brouwer, W.B., and Busschbach, J.J. (2002) Rationalising rationing: economic and other considerations in the debate about funding of Viagra. Health Policy, 59: 53–63.

Struijk, J.J. and Holsheimer, J. (1996) Transverse tripolar spinal cord stimulation: theoretical performance of a dual channel system. Med. Biol. Eng. Comput., 34: 273–279.

Struijk, J.J., Holsheimer, J., Van Der Heide, G.G., and Boom, H.B. (1992) Recruitment of dorsal column fibers in spinal cord stimulation: influence of collateral branching. IEEE Trans. Biomed. Eng., 39: 903–912.

Struijk, J.J., Holsheimer, J., and Boom, H.B. (1993) Excitation of dorsal root fibers in spinal cord stimulation: a theoretical study. IEEE Trans. Biomed. Eng., 40: 632–639.

Struijk, J.J., Holsheimer, J., Spincemaille, G.H., Gielen, F.L., and Hoekema, R. (1998) Theoretical performance and clinical evaluation of transverse tripolar spinal cord stimulation. IEEE Trans. Rehabil. Eng., 6: 277–285.

Suy, R., Gybels, J., Van Damme, H., Martin, D., Van Maele, R., and Delaporte, C. (1994) Spinal cord stimulation for ischaemic rest pain. The Belgian randomised study. In: S. Horsch and L. Claeys, (Eds.), *Spinal Cord Stimulation. An Innovative Method in the Treatment of PVD* (pp. 197–202). Steinkopff, Darmstadt.

Taylor, R., Van Buyten, J.P., and Buchser, E. (submitted for publication) Spinal cord stimulation for chronic low back pain/failed back surgery syndrome and complex regional pain syndrome: a systematic review of clinical effectiveness and cost effectiveness literature.

Tengs, T.O., Meyer, G., Siegel, J.E., Pliskin, J.S., Graham, J.D., and Weinstein, M.C. (1996) Oregon's Medicaid ranking and cost-effectiveness: is there any relationship?. Med. Decis. Making, 16: 99–107.

Turner, J.A., Loeser, J.D., and Bell, K.G. (1995) Spinal cord stimulation for chronic low back pain: a systematic literature synthesis. Neurosurgery, 37: 1088–1095.

Ubbink, D.T., Spincemaille, G.H., Prins, M.H., Reneman, R.S., and Jacobs, M.J. (1999a) Microcirculatory investigations to determine the effect of spinal cord stimulation for critical leg ischemia: the Dutch multicenter randomized controlled trial. J. Vasc. Surg., 30: 236–244.

Ubbink, D.T., Spincemaille, G.H., Reneman, R.S., and Jacobs, M.J. (1999b) Prediction of imminent amputation in patients with non-reconstructible leg ischemia by means of microcirculatory investigations. J. Vasc. Surg., 30: 114–121.

Ubel, P.A., Richardson, J., and Prades, J.L. (1999) Life-saving treatments and disabilities. Are all QALYs created equal?. Int. J. Technol. Assess. Health Care, 15: 738–748.

Visocchi, M., Di Rocco, F., and Meglio, M. (2001a) Protective effect of spinal cord stimulation on experimental early cerebral vasospasm. Conclusive results. Stereotact. Funct. Neurosurg., 76: 269–275.

Visocchi, M., Giordano, A., Calcagni, M., Cioni, B., Di Rocco, F., and Meglio, M. (2001b) Spinal cord stimulation and cerebral blood flow in stroke: personal experience. Stereotact. Funct. Neurosurg., 76: 262–268.

Walker, R.L. and Siegel, A.W. (2002) Morality and the limits of societal values in health care allocation. Health Econ., 11: 265–273.

Wallin, J., Cui, J.G., Yakhnitsa, V., Schechtmann, G., Meyerson, B.A., and Linderoth, B. (2002) Gabapentin and pregabalin suppress tactile allodynia and potentiate spinal cord stimulation in a model of neuropathy. Eur. J. Pain, 6: 261–272.

Weiner, R.L. and Reed, K.L. (1999) Peripheral neurostimulation for control of intractable occipital neuralgia. Neuromodulation, 3: 217–221.

Wetzel, F.T., Hassenbusch, S.J., Oakley, J., Willis, K.D., Simpson, R.K., Jr., and Ross, E. (2000) Treatment of chronic pain in failed back surgery patients with spinal cord stimulation: a review of current literature and proposal for future investigation. Neuromodulation, 3: 59–74.